PAIN

Howard L. Fields, M.D., Ph.D.

Professor of Neurology and Physiology
Department of Neurology
University of California, San Francisco
San Francisco, California

Foreword by Patrick D. Wall

McGraw-Hill Information Services Company
HEALTH PROFESSIONS DIVISION

New York   St. Louis   San Francisco   Colorado Springs   Auckland   Bogotá   Hamburg
Lisbon   London   Madrid   Mexico   Milan   Montreal   New Delhi   Panama   Paris
San Juan   São Paulo   Singapore   Sydney   Tokyo   Toronto

PAIN

Copyright © 1987 by McGraw-Hill, Inc. All rights reserved. Printed in the United States of America. Except as permitted under the United States Copyright Act of 1976, no part of this publication may be reproduced or distributed in any form or by any means, or stored in a data base or retrieval system, without the prior written permission of the publisher.

45678910 KPKP 99876543

ISBN 0-07-020701-1

This book was set in Times New Roman by Compset, Inc.; the editor was William Day; the production supervisors were Avé McCracken and Elaine Gardenier; the cover was designed by Edward R. Schultheis. Project supervision was done by Bermedica Production.
Arcata Graphics/Halliday was printer and binder.

Library of Congress Cataloging-in-Publication Data

Pain.

Includes bibliographies and index.
1. Fields, Howard L. [DNLM: 1. Pain.   WL 704 P1443]
RB127.P3319   1987   616'.0472   87-2969
ISBN 0-07-020701-1

For my father, Charles Fields, and for my other teachers—Donald Kennedy, Patrick D. Wall, and Norman Geschwind

Contents

Foreword

Howard Fields is particularly suited to write this book for three reasons. First, he has been an eyewitness to a series of coincident revolutions which have changed the scene and he has participated in them. Second, he is deep into the neurosciences and into clinical medicine, both of which had to cooperate to produce one of the revolutions. Third, he thinks and writes clearly.

The 1950s witnessed the beginning of a new attitude toward pain. By then the awful pains of emergencies and of surgery had been largely brought under control. This had a number of consequences. One was that it brought back some minimal respectability to symptom control. Previously, doctors and their patients had focused on diagnosis and cure. Signs and symptoms such as fever or pain were regarded as mere signposts along the road which medicine must travel. However, by the time Fields started his career, many patients and some doctors were beginning to request a proper study of symptom control until such time as the fundamentalists provided adequate diagnosis and cure. Chronic and intractable pains became recognized as an urgent and special problem demanding attention both for understanding and for help. Ninety percent of patients with persistent pain still fall into four categories: those with (1) deep tissue damage such as arthritis and cancer, (2) peripheral nerve damage such as amputation, (3) root damage such as arachnoiditis, and (4) pains with no objective pathology and no adequate explanation, for example, most low back pains and headaches.

The success of the anesthesiologists in controlling acute pain brought along with it some unfortunate impedimenta. They had worked on the assumption that the brain contained a special fire alarm system and that all you had to do to stop pain was to cut the lines chemically or surgically. Using this simplistic explanation of chronic pain as a guide to therapy has clearly failed, since many pains remain untreatable. There are then two alternatives—abandon the theory or declare the troublesome patients mad. The latter solution is still accepted by all too many but some, including Howard Fields, decided to reexamine the theory.

One aspect of rethinking had to consider psychology and philosophy. Our society usually accepts a dualistic explanation of sensation. Dualism proposes that a reliable reporting system collects information in the periphery and generates a sensory process within the brain. Then an entirely separate entity, the mind, examines the sensory process and, according to quite different rules, perceives a sensation and dresses it in the clothes of affect. The discovery that descending controls from the highest reaches of the brain affect the messages transmitted to the brain had a revolutionary impact. It was no longer possible to propose a separate system continuously delivering an accurate account of events in the periphery and generating innocent sensation without value judgment. Howard Fields is one of those who have helped to unravel the anatomy, physiology, and chemistry of descending control systems in modern precise terms.

These discoveries changed not only ways of thinking and of experimenting but also the attitude to patients. Phenomena such as the placebo response and the variable relation between pain and injury could be faced rather than dismissed as irrational perversities. Once the variability of pain could be explained in neural terms, psychology and psychiatry became respectable parts of an integrated approach to understanding and treating pain patients, rather than being considered a last resort when medicine had failed. It is curious that just at the time when medicine was moving from a philistine, mechanistic stimulus-response pain system to a sophisticated interacting sensation-perception system, large numbers of the lay population came to reject the entire medical establishment in favour of anti-intellectual mystical ways of thinking and alternative medical practices (e.g., acupuncture, herbal medicine, homeopathy). A future historian who enjoys social paradoxes may like to study the present book, generated in a precise, powerful scientific intellectual atmosphere during the years when so many, especially Californians, were passionately turning to non-medical solutions to pain, based on unproven theories.

This book should be considered a preliminary first edition, it cannot be the definitive text. Every chapter offers exciting prospects for the future, because all work is still in progress. Puzzles remain but the old questions are asked in much more answerable ways. It looks possible that pain and its mechanism will be integrated into sensation and perception in general rather than considered as a separate special system bolted onto the outside of the real brain. Furthermore, pain and its mechanism are not single but multiple and change in time during the course of disease. This book is a concise description of where we stand now and an exciting invitation to anticipate the future.

Patrick D. Wall
Department of Anatomy and Embryology
University College London
London, England

Preface

This book is written primarily for the medically trained reader who encounters patients with difficult pain problems and who seeks to know more about basic mechanisms of pain. It is also for neurobiologists who wish to know more about this clinically relevant sensory system. My impetus for writing it was the significant expansion of knowledge about pain mechanisms that has occurred recently. Among the advances have been greater knowledge of pain-transmitting pathways, the discovery of a network in the brain that selectively inhibits pain, and the isolation of substances from the brain that have the same pharmacologic properties as opiate painkillers like morphine.

The challenge before us is to translate these and other scientific advances into improvements in patient care. This task is made easier by the fact that, over the years, clinicians have had a major interest in pain research. Clinical observations and human experiments have repeatedly served as an impetus and guide for experimental studies in animals. For example, the earliest evidence that the spinothalamic tract is the major pain pathway came from clinical observations. Furthermore, it is unlikely that a phenomenon like referred pain would even have been suspected without patient descriptions. The continued interplay between laboratory and clinic is clearly essential for greater understanding of pain and for improved pain treatment. To foster this interplay, I have attempted to show how clinical observations have contributed to our knowledge of the anatomy and physiology of pain. Wherever possible, I have discussed the neural models that have been used to explain these clinical phenomena.

In addition to progress in understanding the neural mechanisms of pain, there has also been progress in the evaluation and treatment of pain patients. For example, a combination of clinical observations and animal studies has brought us closer to understanding the pathophysiology of painful nerve injuries. Another advance, of special relevance for patients with chronic pain, is the shift to psychosocial evaluation and treatment based on operant control of behaviors related to pain such as inactivity and drug taking. For many, this approach has provided an important alternative to disability and a repetitive cycle of drug-taking and surgical procedures.

This broadened knowledge of physiology and psychology and the improvements in patient evaluation and treatment have drawn clinicians of various specialties to the care of pain patients. There are many physicians who now spend most of their time caring for these patients, and it has even been suggested that because such an extensive body of knowledge needs to be mastered, there should be a separate specialty for pain treatment. Although there is some merit to this position, the field of pain treatment encompasses almost all of medicine. It is not reasonable, therefore, to expect that any individual can be an expert in the treatment of pain in such varied areas as arthritis, cancer, labor, and headache. Ideally, many different specialists and all primary care providers should be able to manage appropriately the common pain problems they most frequently encounter.

The organization of this book reflects the experimental and descriptive biases of modern medicine. Since knowledge of pain is most extensive for the sensory transmission system, the pain modulation system, and standard analgesic treatment modalities, these subjects will be covered in most detail. In addition, since psychological reactions become very prominent in patients with persistent pain, I will outline some of the major psychological factors that are thought to either perpetuate or exacerbate suffering and functional impairment. My goal is not so much to provide the reader with an exhaustive review of these subjects as to provide a foundation for deeper understanding.

The physician who cares for a patient in pain is often in the dark about how to proceed. The cause of the pain, or of its persistence, may be obscure. The patient wants an explanation and demands relief. Often, in such circumstances, the best the physician can do is to give an opinion about the cause and to try a therapy. These opinions and treatments are often based more on an educated guess than definitive information. This book is intended to help the physician give better explanations and make better therapeutic guesses when the available information is incomplete.

Acknowledgments

I would like to thank those who have helped me by reading and suggesting changes in early drafts, especially Mary Heinricher and John Day. Illustrators included Walter Denn of Biomed Arts, Ann Burke, Annette Lowe, and Gwen Watson. Peter J. Dyck, Allan I. Basbaum, and John Adams provided photographs. Barry Fogel, Nick Barbaro, Mike Rowbotham, and Jon Levine provided important information, discussion, and suggestions on key references. Christine Haws and Pat Littlefield made significant contributions through editorial work. Wendy Ng, Kathy Weimelt, and Susan Elliott assisted in manuscript preparation, correspondence, and administrative matters related to publication. I would also like to thank Eliot Licht, Allen Gruber, Stu Eisendrath, John Walker, Jon Levine, John Adams, and Bob Lutz for major contributions to the development of the UCSF Pain Questionnaire. Others have had an impact through informal discussions on various issues related to the material in the book; they include George Engel, Dennis Turk, and Fernette Fang.

The research and training support received from the National Institute of Neurological, Communicative Disorders and Stroke, the National Institute of Drug Abuse, and the National Migraine Foundation have played a critical role in the development of an environment for pain research and treatment at the University of California, San Francisco. This environment has been a tremendous educational resource for me and has provided much of the motivation for writing this book.

Finally, I would like to thank my family for their patience and unwavering support.

Chapter 1

Introduction

Physicians are familiar with pain as a common symptom in people who seek medical help. They use the description of its location, quality, and time course to determine its cause and they use the reported intensity to judge the efficacy of treatment. The person who is experiencing pain is obviously less objective about it. From his or her point of view, the pain complaint is a cry for help. The subjective experience includes an urge to escape from the cause or, if that is not possible, to obtain relief. It is this overwhelming desire to make it stop that gives pain its power. It can produce fear and, if it persists, depression. Ultimately, the pain sufferer may lose the will to live. People have understood this power for millenia, using painful punishment (or the fear of it) to control the behavior of others. Parents, for example, will punish their children physically when they have done something wrong. Children learn to associate pain with actions that are disapproved of by others. Because much of our behavior, especially in early life, is shaped by the desire to avoid pain, the psychological reaction to it can be as complex as the individual who experiences it. This complexity has been a major stumbling block for physicians trying to understand and treat pain patients, particularly those with chronic pain.

Because it is a common experience with diverse psychological conse-quences, there have been many definitions of pain. *Webster's New Collegiate Dictionary* (2nd ed.) defines it as "a distressing feeling due to disease, bodily injury, or organic disorders." For clinical purposes, I would define pain in the following way: an unpleasant sensation that is perceived as arising from a specific region of the body and is commonly produced by processes which damage or are capable of damaging bodily tissue. It is necessary to emphasize that pain is perceived as arising from a *specific place* in the body in order to distinguish it from moods (e.g., sadness) or body feelings such as hunger or warmth, which may be felt as arising from the body but not necessarily a particular body region. Another reason for this refinement is that the word "pain" is commonly used to denote emotional rather than bodily suffering ("a painful loss") and it is used metaphorically to describe irritation ("a pain in the neck"; "that person is a pain").

The Physiological Function of the Pain Sensory System

In most cases the sensation of pain is produced either by injury or by stimuli that are intense enough to be potentially injurious (noxious). Along with the subjective experience of pain, noxious stimuli elicit a variety of behaviors that all serve to protect uninjured tissues. Under different circumstances, tissues can be protected either by withdrawal reflexes, escape, immobilization of the injured part, or avoiding future encounters with similar damaging stimuli.

The protective function of the pain sensory system is vividly illustrated by the rare condition of congenital insensitivity to pain. Individuals with this condition lack the neural apparatus for detection of noxious stimuli. They repeatedly injure themselves by failing to avoid high temperatures, intense pressure, extreme twisting, or corrosive substances. They may be totally unaware of internal diseases that would be very painful in a normal person. On examination, they are usually found to have pressure sores, missing digits, and damaged weight-bearing joints. The following case, excerpted from a report by Dyck and his colleagues (1), is an example of congenital insensitivity to pain:

> At five months of age the patient was noted to be "floppy" and had no response when her blood was drawn. She lost her teeth prematurely, possibly due to trauma sustained by chewing hard objects. She said her first words at 13 months, though she was unable to walk unsupported until she was 23 months. Her parents were concerned that she did not cry when her hands were spanked. At 15 months she sustained a severe burn on one foot and, three weeks later she severely burned her hand (Figure 1.1). In neither instance was there any overt sign of pain. She frequently bit her tongue and cheek severely enough to draw blood but without crying. On one occasion she ran a pencil through her cheek without crying.
>
> On exam (at age 26 months), noxious stimuli delivered to the extremities elicited no sign of discomfort. Histological examination of this girl's peripheral

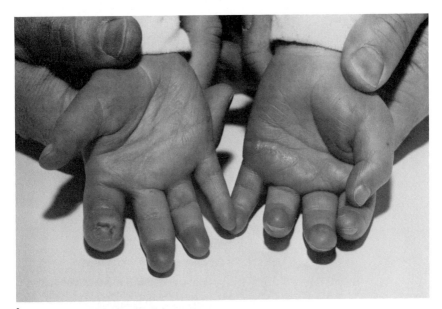

A

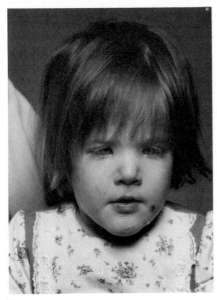

B

Figure 1.1 A: Hands of patient with congenital insensitivity to pain. Note especially the right index finger. **B:** Face of same patient showing scar on left cheek from running pencil through it. Photographs courtesy of P. J. Dyck.

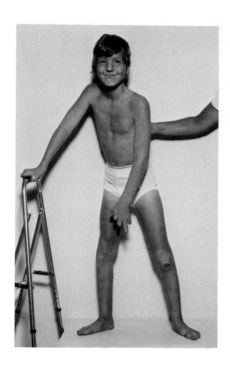

Figure 1.2 Twelve-year-old boy with insensitivity to pain (see text). Note missing digits on his hands and sore on left knee. Photograph courtesy of P. J. Dyck.

nerve revealed a significant reduction of the small diameter axons that are usually associated with pain transmission. (see Chapter 2)

This case illustrates the consequences of not having the normal neural apparatus for detecting intense stimuli. The child repeatedly injured herself when exposed to intense stimuli because the stimuli did not elicit the normal protective behaviors such as withdrawal or immobilization.

Figure 1.2 illustrates a 12-year-old boy with a similar condition. Note the missing distal digits and the open sore over the knee, presumably due to repeated and prolonged pressure from kneeling.

Loss of pain sensation can also lead to traumatic injury in adults. Figure 1.3 illustrates a case in which the sensory nerves of the leg were damaged by syphilis infection. The loss of sensory input from the hip has led to its virtual destruction, presumably as a result of repeated trauma.

These cases clearly illustrate that a major function of the pain sensory system is to prevent injury. Individuals who lack the system do not react to or avoid noxious stimuli, nor do they appear to be particularly disturbed by them. Because of its close linkage with injury-avoiding behaviors, it is useful to think of pain as a perceptual correlate of the protective responses elicited by noxious stimuli.

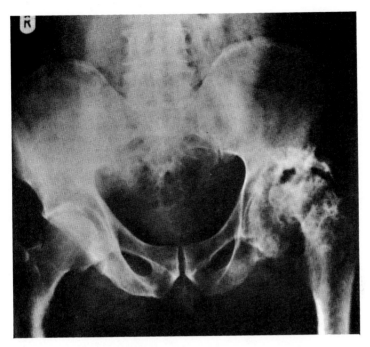

Figure 1.3 Hip damaged due to loss of afferent input. This radiograph is from an adult patient with neurosyphilis, which destroys primary afferent fibers. (From Spillane, J. D.: *An Atlas of Clinical Neurology.* Oxford University Press, London, 1968.)

The Neural Pathways That Transmit and Modulate Pain

Between the stimulus of tissue injury and the subjective experience of pain is a series of complex electrical and chemical events. There are four distinct processes involved: transduction, transmission, modulation, and perception.

Figure 1.4 is a greatly simplified diagram of the pain system. Embedded in the various tissues are nerve endings that respond best to noxious stimuli. *Transduction* is the process by which noxious stimuli lead to electrical activity in the appropriate sensory nerve endings. The second process, *transmission*, refers to the neural events subsequent to transduction. Once the noxious stimulus has been coded by the impulses in the peripheral nerve, the sensations that result are determined by the neurons of the pain transmission system. There are three major neural components of the pain transmission system: the peripheral sensory nerves, which transmit impulses from the site of transduction to their terminals

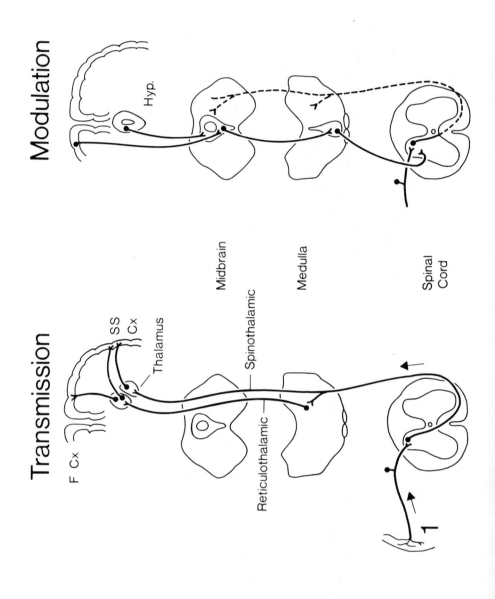

in the spinal cord; a network of relay neurons that ascend from the spinal cord to brainstem and thalamus; and reciprocal connections between thalamus and cortex.

Modulation, the third process, refers to the neural activity leading to control of the pain transmission neurons. A distinct pathway has been discovered in the central nervous system that selectively inhibits pain transmission cells at the level of the spinal cord. This pathway can be activated by stress or by certain analgesic drugs like morphine. When the pain modulation system is active, noxious stimuli produce less activity in the pain transmission pathway. The activity of this modulatory system is one reason why people with apparently severe injuries may deny significant levels of pain.

The final "process" is *perception.* Somehow, the neural activity of the pain transmission neurons produces a subjective correlate. How this comes about is totally obscure, and it is not even clear in which brain structures the activity occurs that produces the perceptual event. Even if this problem were solvable, many questions would remain, the most immediate being whether it is possible to explain how objectively observable neural events produce subjective experience. Unfortunately, since pain is fundamentally a subjective experience, there are inherent limitations to understanding it.

The Variability of Pain

It is common experience that the pain responses to a given stimulus cannot be predicted with certainty. In some individuals innocuous stimuli produce excruciating pain. In other situations, patients with severe injuries deny any significant pain. Over the years, this variability has bedevilled physicians and patients alike. There are several reasons for this variability (Table 1.1). One, mentioned above, is the activity of the pain modulation system. Presumably, under certain contingencies, its activity will reduce the perceived intensity of the sensation produced by a noxious stimulus. Pain modulation will be described in detail in Chapter 5. Another reason for variability in response is abnormal functioning of the nervous system. As discussed above, damage to the transmission system can block pain

---

◀ **Figure 1.4** **Left:** Transmission system for nociceptive messages. Noxious stimuli activate the sensitive peripheral ending of the primary afferent nociceptor by the process of transduction (*1*). The message is then transmitted over the peripheral nerve to the spinal cord, where it synapses with cells of origin of the two major ascending pain pathways, the spinothalamic and spinoreticulothalamic. The message is relayed in the thalamus to both the frontal (*F Cx*) and the somatosensory cortex (*SS Cx*). **Right:** Pain modulation network. Inputs from frontal cortex and hypothalamus (*Hyp.*) activate cells in the midbrain, which control spinal pain transmission cells via cells in the medulla.

Table 1.1   Sources of Variability in Responses to Noxious Stimuli

Process	Result
Injury to pain transmission system	Lower pain intensity
Activity of the modulatory system	Lower pain intensity
Abnormal neural activity	Increased pain intensity Pain without stimulus
Individual psychological differences	Normal pain intensity; unpredictable response

perception. Paradoxically, lesions of the nervous system can also produce a situation in which there is an *overreaction* to noxious stimuli. Furthermore, ongoing pain and hypersensitivity can result from self-sustaining processes that are set in motion by injury but that persist beyond the time it takes for the original injury to heal (see Chapter 6). In these conditions there is pain without an active tissue-damaging process. The pain has acquired, so to speak, a life of its own, sustained by abnormal function of the nervous system. An example of this is causalgia, a burning pain that is occasionally observed following trauma to a peripheral nerve. In causalgia, pain is sustained by activity in the sympathetic nervous system and can be immediately and completely terminated when the sympathetic supply to the painful region is blocked. Such neuropathic pains will be discussed in detail in Chapter 6.

Sensory and Affective Aspects of Pain

The neural mechanisms discussed above can cause significant differences in reported pain due to apparently similar injuries. If pain were simply a sensation, these mechanisms would probably be sufficient to explain most of the clinically observed variability. However, pain is more than a sensation. The close association of the pain sensory system with the function of protection of the body from damage is unique among the sensory systems. It is essential for understanding pain patients that the desire to escape from or terminate the sensation be considered. To this end it is useful to think of pain as consisting of two distinct components: the sensory and the affective or motivational. In its purely sensory aspect, pain has much in common with other somatic sensations; there are specific receptors for pain, and the stimulus that activates them can be identified, located to a particular region of the body, and graded with respect to intensity. The affective or unpleasantness component of pain correlates with the urge to escape. It is related to but distinct from intensity. It is the unpleasantness aspect that makes pain an important clinical issue: if it isn't unpleasant it isn't pain. Conversely, even if the patient does not call it pain, an unpleasant or uncomfortable somatic sensation should be considered as painful.

Table 1.2 lists some of the important differences between the sensory and affective aspects of pain. Clinically, the most important distinction to make is between pain detection threshold and pain tolerance. Detection threshold is a property of the sensory system that depends on the type of stimulus used. *Pain detection threshold* is highly reproducible in different individuals and in the same individual at different times. In contrast to this reproducibility of pain threshold, *pain tolerance* is highly variable. No two individuals react to pain in quite the same way. For example, some people are not bothered by having their teeth drilled, whereas others want to be well anesthetized.

Keeping this difference between pain threshold and pain tolerance in mind is a major key to understanding the variability of pain. Pain tolerance is a manifestation of a person's reaction to pain and it is highly dependent on psychological variables. Not only does it vary between different individuals in the same situation, but the same individual may react differently in different situations. For example, one can imagine how the response of an individual to a moderately severe headache would be changed if a close relative had recently died of a brain tumor.

The importance of individual differences in determining pain threshold is clearly illustrated in studies described by Turk and Kerns (2). Pain tolerance was measured by asking individuals to place one hand in ice water and to leave it submerged for as long as they could bear it, to a maximum of 5 minutes. Pain threshold was also assessed using subjective reports of pain intensity. All subjects reported a definite feeling of pain within 30 seconds of immersing the hand. The subjects fell into two very distinct groups, those who kept their hand submerged for the full 5 minutes (60 percent) and a second group (40 percent) who removed their hand from the water after 1 minute or less. Written reports of subjective feelings revealed that individuals in the low-tolerance group were more worried about possible irreversible damage to the submerged limb.

This study illustrates the point that, although the sensory aspect (i.e., detection threshold) of pain is quite uniform in different people, the affective as-

Table 1.2 The Two Aspects of Pain

Sensory	Affective
Intensity	Unpleasantness
Pain threshold/detection	Escape threshold/tolerance
Identification/location	Reaction
Reproducible	Variable

pect, as manifested by pain tolerance, is highly variable and depends on both personality traits and situational factors.

One can conclude from this that there is a wide range of possible responses to any level of pain intensity. It appears that the meaning of the pain to the individual is one important factor in determining his or her pain tolerance. Different individuals have learned different ways of coping with pain; some minimize its importance and others overreact. Thus for many patients it may be as important to know what they think their pain means as to know what its cause is. For example, back pain in an otherwise healthy person who spent the previous day moving furniture may not be a serious concern. However, in a patient with cancer, back pain of the same intensity may be a reminder of impending death and therefore intolerable. Because of the importance of the patient's interpretation, it is imperative, especially for persistent or recurrent pain, to make some inquiry about this issue. Often this can be very helpful in treatment. In fact, there are a variety of apparently successful treatment approaches that use cognitive methods to help patients develop strategies for coping with their pain (3). Sometimes this type of approach can obviate the need for more powerful painkillers or for surgical intervention. The important point is that differences in the meaning of the pain and in coping strategies produce tremendous variation in patients' responses to similar pain-producing stimuli.

Summary

I have defined and described pain, briefly outlined its underlying neural pathways, and discussed the major sources of variability in the subjective experience of it. In the following chapters I will go into each of these topics in more detail. In reading this material keep in mind that the individual's report of his or her subjective experience is still the best available method of assessing pain, and that this experience has both sensory and affective aspects. Since it is natural to concentrate on what we best understand, I have tended to dwell on the sensory aspect. As this book will document, research in this area has been very productive and has provided extensive knowledge in the areas of anatomy, physiology, and pharmacology. In contrast, progress in understanding the affective aspect of pain and the psychological variables that influence it has been slow, and our knowledge remains primitive. Unfortunately, it is the affective aspect, in all its complexity, that makes pain an important and vexing clinical problem. Until we know more about it, we will have to apply what little information is available and hope for better understanding in the future.

References

1 Dyck, P. J., Mellinger, J. F., Reagan, T. J., Horowitz, S. J., McDonald, J. W., Litchy, W. J., Daube, J. R., Fealey, R. D., Go, V. L., Kao, P. C., Brimijoin, W. S., and Lambert, E. H.: Not 'indifference to pain' but varieties of hereditary sensory and autonomic neuropathy. *Brain* **106:**373–390, 1983.

2 Turk, D. C., and Kerns, R. D.: Conceptual issues in the assessment of clinical pain. *Int. J. Psychiatry Med.* **13:**57–68, 1983–84.

3 Weisenberg, M.: Cognitive aspects of pain. In P. D. Wall and R. Melzack, (eds.): *Textbook of Pain,* Chpt. 13. Churchill Livingstone, Edinburgh, 1984.

Chapter 2

The Peripheral Pain Sensory System

When a stimulus of sufficient intensity to be tissue damaging (i.e., noxious) is applied to a sensitive part of the body such as the skin, a chain of events is set in motion that eventually results in a sensation identifiable as painful. The capacity of tissues to elicit pain when noxious stimuli are applied to them depends on their innervation by nociceptors. Nociceptors are primary afferent nerves with peripheral terminals that can respond differentially to noxious stimuli. These primary afferent nociceptors have two major functions: transduction and transmission. In the process of *transduction,* or receptor activation, one form of energy (either chemical, mechanical, or thermal) is converted to another form, in this case, the electrochemical nerve impulse in the primary afferent. By this process the information about the stimulus is converted to a form that is accessible to the brain. The information is coded by the frequency of impulses in the population of primary afferents activated by the stimulus. *Transmission* refers to the process by which this coded information is relayed to those structures of the central nervous system whose activity produces the sensation of pain. The first stage of transmission is the conduction of impulses in primary afferents to the spinal cord. At the spinal cord, activity in the primary afferents activates spinal neurons that relay the pain message to the brain. This message elicits a variety of responses ranging from withdrawal reflexes to the subjective perceptual event ("It hurts!") that is familiar to all of us. This chapter will describe the properties of the different primary afferent nociceptors and discuss the contribution of each

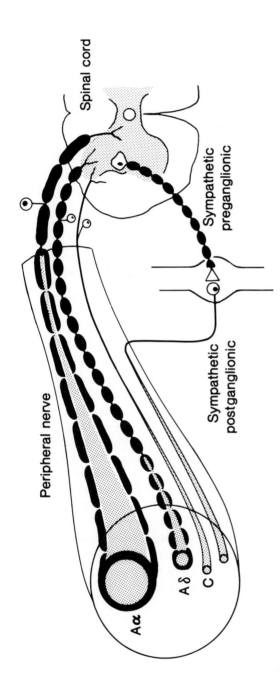

Figure 2.1 Components of a typical cutaneous nerve. **A:** Illustrates that there are two distinct functional categories of axon: primary afferents with cell bodies in the dorsal root ganglion and sympathetic postganglionic fibers with cell bodies in the sympathetic ganglion. Primary afferents include those with large-diameter myelinated (Aα), small-diameter myelinated (Aδ), and unmyelinated (C) axons. All sympathetic postganglionic fibers are unmyelinated. **B:** Electron micrograph of cross-section of a cutaneous nerve illustrating the relative sizes and degree of myelination of its complement of axons. The myelin appears as black rings of varying thickness. The unmyelinated axons (C) occur singly or in clusters. (From Ochoa, J. L.: In P. J. Dyck et al. (eds.): *Peripheral Neuropathy* (1st ed.). Saunders, Philadelphia, 1975.)

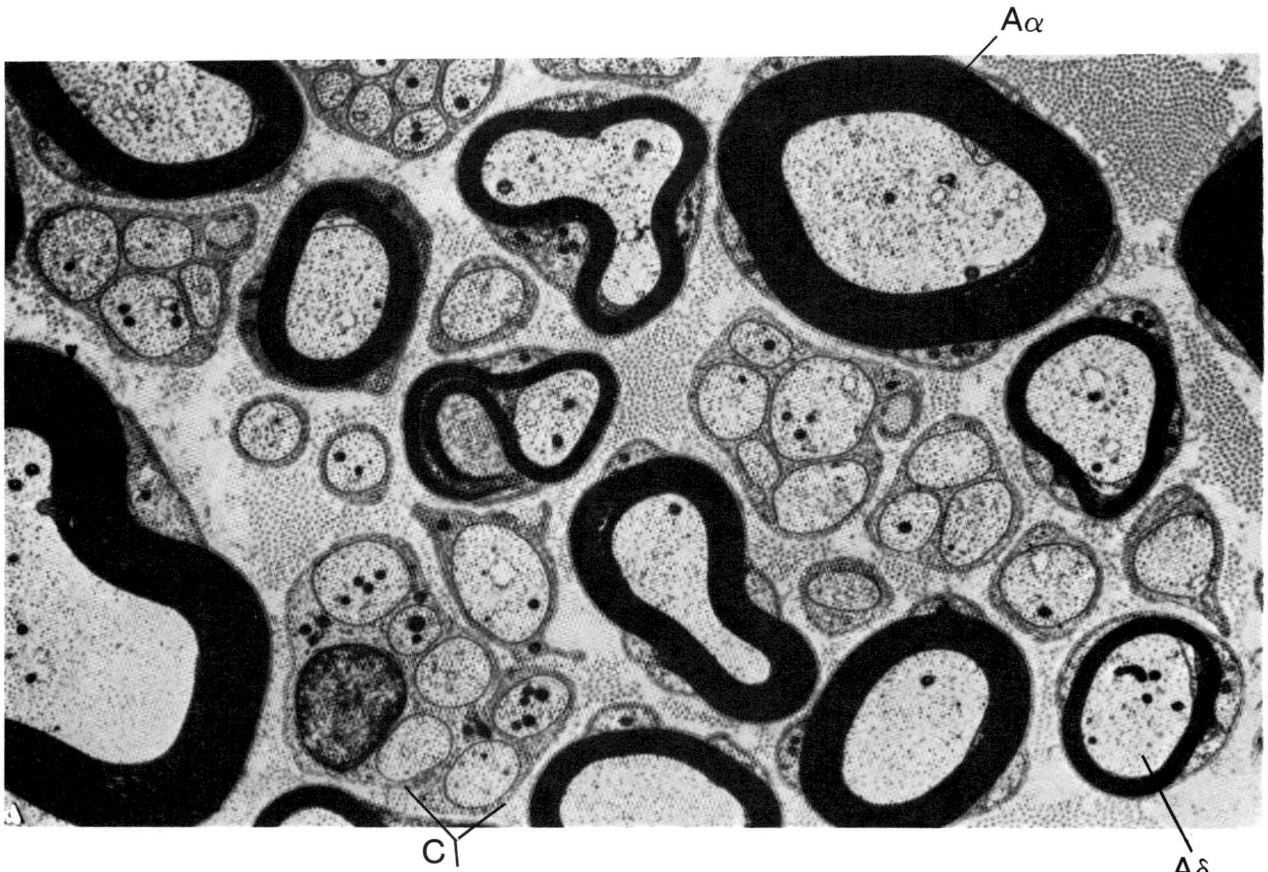

B

Figure 2.1 (*Continued*).

to human pain perception. It will also cover the chemical factors that produce or enhance activity in primary afferent nociceptors.

The Primary Afferent Nociceptor

Our most detailed knowledge of the pain transmission system is derived from studies of primary afferent axons in peripheral nerve. Peripheral nerves are complex transmission lines that subserve a variety of functions, including motor and autonomic control as well as sensory transmission. This diversity of function of a peripheral nerve is reflected in the heterogeneity of its constituent axons (5, 6). Examination of a peripheral nerve in cross-section reveals axons that vary widely in diameter and the presence or absence of a myelin sheath (Figure 2.1). When the numbers of axons of each diameter are counted, it is clear that they can be grouped into distinct populations (Figure 2.2). The major groups are Aα (6–22 μM), Aδ (2–5 μM), and C (0.3–3.0 μM). This grouping of axons by their diameter is reflected in the compound action potential, which is the electrical potential generated by simultaneous activity in the entire population of axons in a peripheral nerve. As illustrated in Figure 2.2, the compound action potential consists of several components corresponding to axon groups conducting at different velocities. These conduction velocity groups correspond to the diameter groupings mentioned above (Figure 2.2).

Different functional classes of primary afferents tend to cluster within a restricted diameter and conduction velocity range. The slowly conducting C axons have the smallest diameter and are unmyelinated. They conduct at velocities of less than 2 m/sec. Although most unmyelinated axons are primary afferents with cell bodies in the dorsal root ganglion; approximately 20 percent are sympathetic postganglionic efferents with cell bodies located in the paraspinal ganglia of the sympathetic chain (Figure 2.1A).

The myelinated axons have conduction velocities ranging from 5 to over

---

Figure 2.2   A: Axon diameter histogram of human cutaneous nerve, in this case the sural nerve. Unmyelinated axons (*thin bars*) comprise about 80 percent of the total number of axons in a cutaneous nerve. Approximately 25 percent of these are sympathetic postganglionics. (From Ochoa, J. and Mair, W. G. P.: The normal sural nerve in man. I. Ultrastructure and numbers of fibers and cells. *Acta Neuropathol.* **13:**197–216, 1969.) **B:** Compound action potential. This is an electrical recording from the whole nerve. It represents the summated action potentials of all the component axons in the nerve. Note that even though there are many more unmyelinated axons, the major voltage deflections are produced by the relatively small number of myelinated axons. This is because action potentials in the population of more slowly conducting axons are dispersed in time and each generates a smaller extracellular current than the myelinated axons.

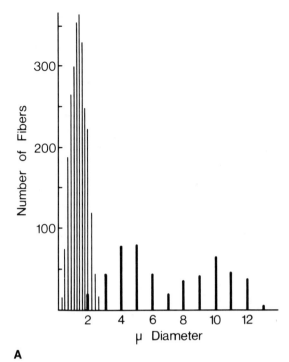

A

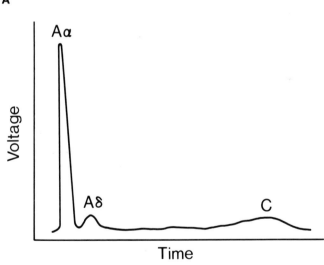

B

100 m/sec. Among the myelinated group are the axons of motoneurons and primary afferents. There are several classes of myelinated primary afferents. The afferents having the largest diameter (Aα) include the muscle proprioceptors (muscle spindles and Golgi tendon organs). In a cutaneous nerve there are two groups of myelinated afferents, the larger diameter Aα fibers which respond to light mechanical stimuli and the smaller diameter Aδ fibers.

NEUROPHYSIOLOGICAL CHARACTERIZATION
OF PRIMARY AFFERENT NOCICEPTORS

The weight of evidence indicates that the great majority of nociceptive primary afferents conduct either in the Aδ or C velocity range. The most direct evidence for this comes from studies of the axons of single primary afferent nociceptors in cutaneous nerves. Cutaneous nerves have been studied most extensively for several reasons. The skin is one of the most densely innervated structures and it is simple to apply controlled noxious stimuli to it. Cutaneous nerves are readily identified, and easily isolated for electrophysiological study, and each supplies a well-defined region of the skin. Figure 2.3 illustrates a typical experiment. Recordings are usually made from axons in the nerve at a distance from the site of application of stimuli. Stimuli are applied to the general area of skin supplied by the nerve until the region is found that excites the axon being recorded. The receptive field of the sensory neuron is defined as that region (or structure) which upon stimulation, causes a change in its discharge frequency.

With these methods, primary afferents can be characterized physiologically by their conduction velocity and the stimuli that cause them to discharge. In order for a neuron to transmit nociceptive information it must respond differentially to noxious and innocuous stimuli. The majority of the larger myelinated primary afferents (Aα) are not capable of transmitting such information (6). Most are excited by mild mechanical stimuli, including light touch and the bending of hairs. Since these afferents do not increase their discharge when more intense stimuli are applied they cannot signal the application of noxious stimuli. Furthermore, when these large-diameter primary afferent axons are electrically stimulated in normal awake humans, the subjects report a variety of feelings but not pain (5, 11). Thus, not only do large-diameter primary afferents not respond to noxious stimuli but, in normal subjects, their activity does not produce pain. In contrast, a significant number of both small-diameter myelinated fibers (Aδ) and unmyelinated (C) primary afferents can be classified as nociceptors because they respond maximally only when noxious stimuli are applied to their receptive fields (e.g., Figure 2.3B).

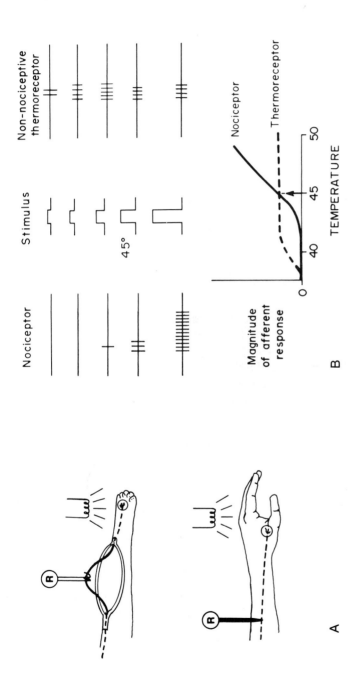

Figure 2.3 Comparison of response properties of thermal nociceptor and non-nociceptive thermoreceptor. Recordings are made from the trunk of a peripheral nerve at a distance from the stimulus. **A:** In animals, the nerve can be dissected free. In humans, small metal microelectrodes can be passed through the skin directly into the nerve bundle. **B:** At non-noxious temperatures, both types of receptors may fire. Then, as the temperature is raised into the noxious range, only the nociceptor continues to increase in discharge frequency. Both receptors can signal warming, but only the nociceptor can transmit the message that the temperature is in the noxious range.

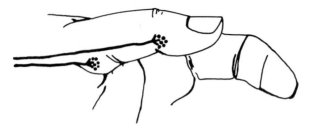

Figure 2.4   The multipunctate receptive field of an Aδ nociceptor.

Myelinated Nociceptors

Although a few nociceptors have been found that conduct in the Aα range, the overwhelming majority of myelinated nociceptors are Aδ fibers. In human limb nerve their mean conduction velocity is about 20 m/sec (1). Aδ nociceptors respond to noxious mechanical stimuli. Some may respond to stimuli that are innocuous, although none of the Aδ afferents are as sensitive to mechanical stimuli as Aα mechanoreceptors. By definition, Aδ nociceptors increase their discharge as the stimulus intensity is increased into the range that produces tissue damage, as evidenced by erythema or visible edema and pain when applied to the skin of a human subject. Aδ nociceptors are particularly sensitive to stimulation with sharp-pointed instruments such as pins or toothed forceps. Their receptive fields consist of a cluster of sensitive spots about 1 mm in diameter (Figure 2.4). In primate hairy skin, the average total area of the receptive field is about 5 mm² (17).

A significant percentage (20–50 percent) of Aδ nociceptors respond to heat as well as mechanical stimuli (1, 17). Some of these heat-sensitive Aδ nociceptors respond to skin temperatures below pain threshold, but all respond more as temperatures are raised into the noxious range (45–47°C). Some of these nociceptors also respond to cooling in their receptive field.

The Aδ nociceptors that respond readily to heat are called mechanothermal nociceptors; the others are called high-threshold mechanoreceptors (HTMs). Both have a property called *sensitization*. Sensitization refers to the increased sensitivity of a receptor following repeated application of a noxious stimulus. Sensitization has been studied quantitatively using thermal stimuli (7, 15). The process is most striking in the high threshold mechanoreceptor because, by definition, it does not respond at all to the *first* application of a thermal stimulus. With repeated noxious thermal stimuli the Aδ HTMs begin to respond and then give progressively larger responses (Figure 2.5A). Furthermore, the threshold temperature drops so that lower and lower temperatures are required to activate it. In fact, a sensitized HTM behaves very much like the mechanothermal nociceptor. It is of interest that the threshold of HTMs to *mechanical* stimuli is unaffected by stimuli that produce thermal sensitization (7).

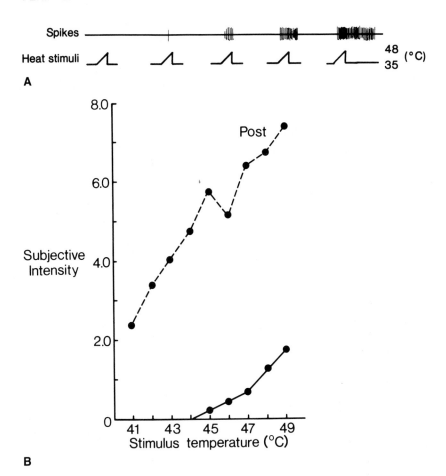

Figure 2.5 Sensitization of primary afferent nociceptors and human hyperalgesia. **A:** Sensitization of an Aδ HTM using thermal stimuli. By definition, this receptor is initially insensitive to noxious thermal stimuli, but with repeated stimulation it begins to respond. **B:** Psychophysiological study of hyperalgesia in humans. The *solid line* indicates measurements made prior to sensitization of skin; the *dashed line* (Post) indicates subjective responses to the same stimuli following a small cutaneous burn. The ordinate is subjective pain intensity, on a relative scale (pain threshold between 0 and 1). (From Meyer, R. A., and Campbell, J. N.: Myelinated nociceptor afferents account for the hyperalgesia that follows a burn to the hand. *Science* **213:**1527–1529, 1981.)

Both high-threshold mechanical and mechanothermal myelinated nociceptors are present in human cutaneous nerve (1). Furthermore, in awake human subjects it has been possible to show a positive correlation between the activity in myelinated mechanothermal nociceptors and the reported intensity of pain. This supports the concept that these myelinated nociceptors contribute to pain sensation in man.

In summary, there are at least two types of myelinated nociceptors; mechanical and mechanothermal. Both types have an average conduction velocity in the Aδ range, receptive fields about 5 mm² consisting of a cluster of sensitive spots, and show sensitization with repeated noxious thermal stimuli. The sensitivity of myelinated nociceptors to irritant chemicals has not been systematically studied, although preliminary studies indicate that a significant number have such sensitivity (1).

Unmyelinated Nociceptors

The majority of axons in a peripheral nerve are primary afferents and, of these, three-fourths are unmyelinated (C fibers). In primate cutaneous limb nerves, over 90 percent of the C fiber afferents are nociceptive. Furthermore, in studies of human nerves, all C fiber afferents found have been nociceptive (37). Thus, C fiber afferents are the most common element in most peripheral nerves and, at least in primates, the overwhelming majority of C-fibers are nociceptors.

The major class of C fiber nociceptor is the C-polymodal nociceptor (C-PMN) so named because it responds to noxious thermal, mechanical, and chemical stimuli applied to the skin. The receptive field of the C-PMN is smaller than that of the myelinated nociceptors and usually consists of a single area rather than a cluster of spots. As with the myelinated nociceptors, C-PMNs sensitize with repeated noxious stimuli and frequently develop an ongoing background discharge after sensitization. Paradoxically, C-PMNs may be *less* sensitive immediately (within 2 minutes) after a noxious stimulus is delivered to their receptive field and may be completely inactivated at very high temperatures (>55°C).

C-PMNs are the only type of C fiber afferent so far encountered in human cutaneous nerve. When recordings of C-PMNs are made in awake human subjects, chemical, thermal, or mechanical stimuli sufficient to produce reports of pain concomitantly elicit vigorous discharge in the C-PMNs innervating the area stimulated (18, 37–39). Furthermore, using thermal stimuli, there is a good correlation between subjective pain intensity and the simultaneously recorded activity of C-PMNs (18) (Figure 2.6).

In summary, there are three major classes of primary afferents in peripheral nerve that have been found in significant numbers and are capable of signaling the presence of noxious stimuli applied to the skin. They are the Aδ mechanosensitive nociceptor, the Aδ mechanothermal nociceptor, and the C-PMN.

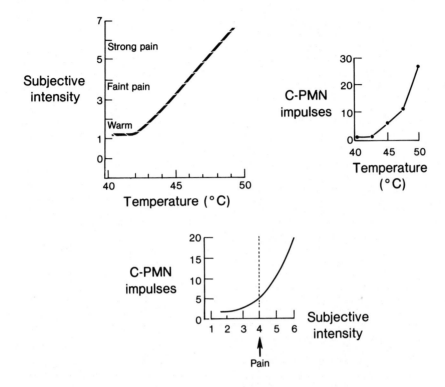

Figure 2.6 Comparison of reported pain intensity in human subjects with responses in either primate or human C-PMNs. **Top left:** Reported pain intensity in human subjects to thermal stimuli of increasing intensity. **Top right:** Responses of primate C-PMNs using identical stimuli. Discharge increases in the noxious range. (Adapted from LaMotte, R. H., and Campbell, J. N.: Comparison of responses of warm and nociceptive C-fiber afferents in monkey with human judgments of thermal pain. *J. Neurophysiol.* **41**:509–528, 1978.) **Bottom:** C-PMN discharge and concomitant subjective pain intensity in human subjects. There is a positively accelerating relationship consistent with a contribution by human C-PMNs to pain. (From Gybels, J., Handwerker, H. O., and Van Hees, J.: A comparison between the discharges of human nociceptive nerve fibers and the subject's ratings of his sensations. *J. Physiol. (Lond.)* **292**:193–206, 1979.)

PERIPHERAL NOCICEPTORS AND PAIN SENSATION (5, 35)

What do each of the nociceptor types contribute to pain sensation? Some answers to this challenging question have been provided by detailed correlations of reported pain sensations in human subjects with activity in defined classes of sensory fiber.

One early approach to this problem was to use electrical stimulation of peripheral nerve in awake human subjects (5, 11). Because the large-diameter axons have the lowest electrical threshold they could be activated selectively. As mentioned previously, these studies indicated that selective activation of Aα fibers does not elicit pain. In contrast, when the stimulus intensity was raised to Aδ threshold, single stimuli evoked a sharp, intense tingling. With repetitive stimulation, a definitely painful sensation was produced. When the stimulus intensity was increased to the C fiber threshold, a single stimulus produced an intense and prolonged painful sensation. These findings implicated both Aδ and C fibers in pain sensation but were inconclusive because, with electrical stimulation of peripheral nerve, the higher intensities required to activate C fibers would also activate all the other sensory fibers.

Corollary evidence was obtained by selectively blocking activity in different fiber groups (5). Unmyelinated fibers are relatively susceptible to the action of local anesthetics, and pain is the first sensation to disappear when local anesthetics are applied to a peripheral nerve. Conversely, unmyelinated fibers are relatively resistant to the blocking effect of pressure on peripheral nerves, and pain sensation survives compression sufficient to block most myelinated fibers. These studies were carried a step further by Torebjork and Hallin (37, 38). They used electrical stimulation of the skin and recorded both the sensations that were reported by the subjects and the activity recorded at the same time from C fibers in the nerve supplying the region stimulated. They were able to show that C fiber activity is associated with a prolonged burning sensation. Both the sensation and the C fiber activity survived compression of the nerve sufficient to block myelinated fibers and were abolished concomitantly by local anesthetic application that only blocked C fibers. Furthermore, discharge in the C fibers showed fatigue with repetitive (5-Hz) stimulation, and the subjects reported a concomitant diminution of the prolonged burning sensation.

Pain Threshold and Intensity

An important approach to evaluating the contribution of nociceptors to sensation has been to compare human pain reports with the responses of primate nociceptors using identical stimuli. Most quantitative studies of pain sensation have used a radiant heat method. Since there is no mechanical contact with the skin, activation of mechanoreceptors is avoided, although some non-nociceptive thermoreceptors are stimulated. The human thermal pain threshold is remarkably reproducible. For example, a temperature pulse lasting 3 seconds at 45°C will evoke a report of pain in about 50 percent of subjects. As the temperature is increased subjects experience an increasingly intense sensation.

Using a CO_2 laser to deliver precisely controlled heat pulses, LaMotte and Campbell (25) applied identical stimuli to the forearm skin of human subjects and, in parallel studies, to the receptive fields of primate C-PMNs. They found that subjective pain ratings and the discharge in primate C-PMNs were similar functions of temperature over the range of 40–50°C (Figure 2.6). In an important extension of these findings, Gybels and his colleagues (18) recorded C-PMN activity and subjective pain reports simultaneously in the same human subjects. Using controlled thermal stimuli they found a direct relationship between C-PMN discharge and the reported intensity of pain (Figure 2.6). Thus, C-PMNs signal the occurrence of thermal stimuli near pain threshold and probably contribute to the perceived intensity of noxious heat. It is likely that Aδ mechanothermal nociceptors also contribute to these functions, but their contribution probably differs in different skin regions (24).

Evidence implicating both Aδ and C fibers in human pain perception comes from the observation that brief, intense stimuli delivered to the distal limb give rise to two distinct sensations: an early sharp and relatively brief pricking sensation (first pain) and a later dull, somewhat prolonged sensation (second pain) (8, 30, 36). When brief thermal stimuli are used the second sensation often has a burning quality. First pain disappears when myelinated fibers are selectively blocked by pressure (36) (Figure 2.7). The second duller, burning pain is abolished when unmyelinated fibers are selectively blocked using low concentrations of local anesthetic. Lewis proposed that the sharp, pricking early pain was elicited by activity in Aδ fibers, a concept supported by recent studies establishing a minimum conduction velocity in the Aδ range (6 m/sec) for the peripheral axons that mediate first pain (8). First pain is detectable using thermal stimuli to skin areas that have not been previously stimulated. Because HTMs do not respond to thermal stimuli unless sensitized, the mechanothermal rather than the high-thresold mechanical nociceptor must be the primary afferent class whose activity underlies first pain elicited by thermal stimuli.

These observations demonstrate that both Aδ and C nociceptors contribute to pain sensation. Furthermore, they suggest that the activity of each contributes in a distinct way to the quality of the pain sensation. Despite this it is an oversimplification to identify a given quality of pain sensation with activity in a single primary afferent or even a single class of primary afferents. It is clear that any naturally occurring stimulus to the skin will activate a broad range of receptors. This is most obviously true for mechanical stimuli, which will activate many Aα mechanoreceptors in addition to nociceptors. Noxious heat will activate thermoreceptors, and irritant chemicals cannot be applied without some accompanying mechanical or thermal stimulus.

The size of the area stimulated, the frequency with which a stimulus is applied, and the duration and location of the stimulus will all affect the quality of sensation (41). Although pain is a specific and singular experience that depends on activity in specific receptors, there is not a simple one-to-one relationship between activity in the primary afferent nociceptor and the perceptual experience. The sensation produced by activity in a single nociceptor will depend

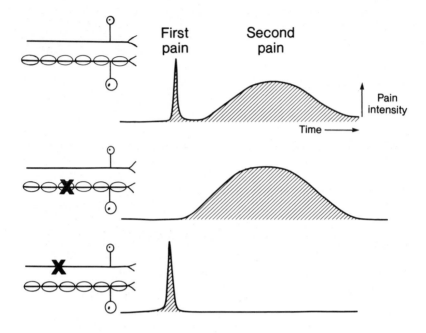

Figure 2.7   Top: First and second pain are carried by two different primary afferent axons. First pain is abolished by selective blockade of myelinated axons (**middle**) and second pain by blocking C fibers (**bottom**).

on which other afferents are active at the same time. Just as a visual experience
is compounded of location, shape, and color and depends on the activity of
multiple photoreceptors, so is the pain experience compounded from the concurrent inputs of multiple somatic receptors.

Peripheral Activation of Nociceptors:
Transduction

The function of a sensory receptor is to respond to a particular type of stimulus
energy while remaining relatively insensitive to all other types. For example, C-
PMNs are sensitive to intense mechanical and thermal stimuli and to irritant
chemicals (Figure 2.8). Somehow, the presence of these stimuli depolarizes the
nociceptor, leading to the generation of nerve impulses. The process by which
noxious stimuli depolarize the nociceptor is called *transduction*. It has not yet
been possible to study directly the nociceptive transduction process at the receptor level. It is not known whether noxious stimuli act directly on the primary
afferent terminal. Another possibility is that noxious stimuli act directly on some

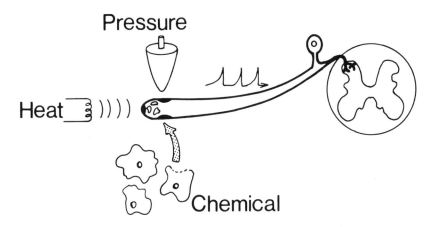

Figure 2.8 Sensitivity range of the C-polymodal nociceptor. Available evidence suggests that the terminals are sensitive to direct heat or mechanical distortion. Thus transduction can occur at the terminal. The terminals are also sensitive to chemicals released from damaged cells. In this manner, any tissue cell can serve as an intermediate in the transduction process. In a sense, all tissue cells are "receptors" for injury.

other cell that secondarily activates the primary afferent terminal. In some sensory systems (visual, auditory) such intermediate cells (called receptor cells) have been identified as the site of transduction. In other cases, the two functions are combined in the peripheral processes of the sensory neuron (e.g., the pacinian corpuscle, a sensitive mechanoreceptor).

The peripheral terminals of one class of nociceptor (the Aδ mechanical nociceptor) have been studied at the ultrastructural level (22). The terminals are wrapped in a Schwann cell sheath, but there is no specialized cell apposed to the nerve terminal. Since there is no evidence for a separate receptor cell, it is most likely that the peripheral terminal of the primary afferent nociceptor is itself mechanosensitive. There are no comparable data available for the other nociceptor types, so it is not known whether any are associated with a separate receptor cell.

There may be more than one nociceptive transduction mechanism. For example, Aδ mechanical nociceptors are relatively insensitive to heat and chemical stimuli and, when sensitized to heat, show no change in sensitivity to mechanical stimuli. In a survey of a large number of C-PMNs, no correlation was found between mechanical and thermal thresholds (17). These observations indicate that separate mechanisms underlie transduction of the two types of stimulus.

In addition to the sensory transduction processes that underlie the immediate responses to noxious stimuli such as heat or pinch, nociceptor terminals are (or can become) sensitive to a variety of chemical factors released into the extracellular space. Release of these substances may occur following tissue damage or activity in the nociceptors themselves. Such factors may produce pain that outlasts the stimulus. Furthermore, there is evidence that the parallel phenomena of nociceptor sensitization and sensory hyperalgesia are produced by such factors.

Persistent Activity in Nociceptors following Noxious Stimuli: Sensitization and Hyperalgesia

Up to this point we have focused on the activity induced in primary afferent nociceptors by brief, controlled stimuli that can be terminated before irreversible damage is produced in the stimulated tissues. Although such brief, mildly painful insults do occur outside the pain research laboratory, painful experiences that provoke an individual's concern accompany more destructive processes that result in pain and hypersensitivity lasting from minutes to days. This persistent pain may reflect ongoing tissue damage or lingering chemical irritants released by the original insult. Other possibilities are that such persistent pain could result from a lasting change in the receptor itself or even in the central nervous system. In fact, there is evidence that all of these factors contribute.

Stimuli that are only slightly above pain threshold (e.g., temperatures of 45.5°C) will result in visible signs of tissue damage such as vasodilatation (erythema) and swelling that may last for hours or days. It is common experience that more extensive injuries such as bruises, burns, and abrasions are accompanied by a local increase in sensitivity to mild stimuli (hyperesthesia). In injured tissues, stimuli that would be innocuous in undamaged tissues are painful (e.g., tenderness) and stimuli above normal pain threshold are perceived as more intense than in uninjured areas (hyperalgesia) (Figure 2.5B).

Hyperalgesia is paralleled by changes in the sensitivity of primary afferent nociceptors. As discussed above, all classes of primary afferent nociceptor become sensitized with repeated application of noxious heat in their receptive fields, and it is likely that sensitization underlies the phenomena of hyperalgesia and tenderness. Recent studies in human subjects correlating subjective pain reports with activity in single primary afferent nociceptors are consistent with the view that sensitization of C-PMNs contributes to hyperalgesia (24).

In addition to sensitizing nociceptors by directly activating them, tissue-damaging stimuli produce effects that spread beyond the site where they are applied. Lewis (29) observed that following a superficial injury to the skin there appears a regular sequence of events. The earliest event is an intense vasodilatation at the site of injury. This is rapidly followed by the development of edema at the same site (wheal) and a secondary vasodilatation that produces a reddening

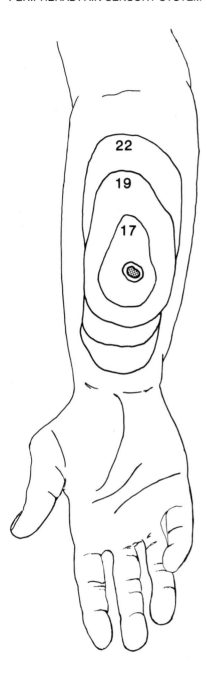

Figure 2.9 Spread of secondary hyperalgesia. A small injury was made with dry ice (*stippled region*). Cutaneous hypersensitivity spread progressively outward over a period of minutes (numbers in the circles). (Data from Lewis, T.: *Pain*. Macmillan, New York, 1942.)

(flare) that spreads for several centimeters into the adjacent, unstimulated skin. After a few minutes, the site of damage develops an increased sensitivity to noxious stimuli (primary hyperalgesia). In addition, hyperalgesia also develops in the unstimulated, undamaged region surrounding the zone of primary hyperalgesia. This region of hypersensitivity, which was not directly stimulated, progressively enlarges with time (Figure 2.9). This phenomenon, called secondary hyperalgesia, seems to depend on activity in the unmyelinated primary afferents. Following injury just outside their receptive fields, C-PMNs are sensitized and may develop spontaneous firing (14, 34). Both the flare (vasodilation) and the remote sensitization of C-PMNs are blocked by local anesthetics injected at the site of injury. The flare is unaffected by sympathectomy but is abolished by destroying the sensory innervation of the skin. If the distal process of the cut peripheral nerve is stimulated so that impulses are propagated antidromically (outward toward the skin) a spreading vasodilatation and edema is produced (Figure 2.10). This manipulation also sensitizes C-PMNs.

Thus activity in C-PMNs, in the absence of tissue damage, causes vasodilatation and activates (and/or sensitizes) other C-PMNs with adjacent receptive fields (Figure 2.10; see Figure 2.12). These observations demonstrate that activation of primary afferent nociceptors is critically dependent on processes outside their receptive fields. Furthermore, nociceptor activity itself produces local tissue changes, including vasodilatation and edema, that outlast the initial stimulus and spread beyond its site of application. These long-lasting changes may play a major role in determining the intensity and quality of clinically significant pains.

Pain-Producing Substances

Among the possible mechanisms of transduction, an attractive proposal is that nociceptor terminals are chemosensitive and that they are activated by pain-producing chemicals released from cells damaged by the noxious stimulus. In fact, a variety of compounds accumulate near nociceptor terminals following tissue injury (Table 2.1). There are at least three sources of these compounds. They may simply leak out from cells damaged by the stimulus. They may be synthesized locally by enzymes from substrates released by damage or that enter the damaged area secondary to plasma extravasation or lymphocyte migration. Finally, they may be released by activity in the nociceptor itself.

Damage to tissue cells produces leakage of intracellular contents. Among the substances released by tissue damage are potassium and histamine, both of which excite polymodal nociceptors and produce pain when injected into human skin (2, 20). Other compounds that may be released by tissue damage and are known to either activate or sensitize nociceptors include acetylcholine, serotonin, and adenosine triphosphate. In fact, there is evidence that several of these

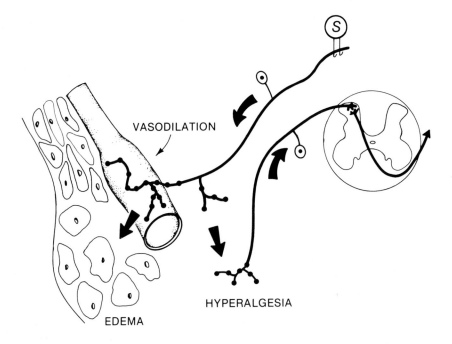

Figure 2.10   Effect of antidromic impulses in primary afferents. Stimulating (*S*) the peripheral cut end of a primary afferent results in impulses being conducted in an antidromic direction (opposite of normal; in this case outward toward the peripheral terminals). The antidromic impulses cause vasodilatation (flare) and edema (wheal), and sensitize nociceptor terminals (hyperalgesia).

compounds can act in combination to sensitize nociceptors (34). It is also possible that different mediators act upon different nociceptors or in different tissues.

One of the most potent pain-producing substances that appears in injured tissue is bradykinin, a 9-amino acid peptide produced at sites of injury by enzymatic cleavage from large plasma proteins. High levels of bradykinin (>8 μM) appear in damaged tissues, especially when there is a visible inflammatory exudate. Bradykinin produces pain in a variety of human and animal tests at concentrations as low as 10nM (2). Polymodal nociceptors can be transiently activated by bradykinin (3, 6) and they then become sensitized to thermal stimuli. Thus bradykinin could contribute to both pain and hyperalgesia.

Another major class of substances that are synthesized in regions of tissue damage are the metabolic products of arachidonic acid. These compounds are among the most potent and ubiquitous of the inflammatory mediators. This class of compounds includes the prostaglandins and leukotrienes. They appear when-

Table 2.1 Chemical Intermediaries in Nociceptive Transduction

Substance	Source	Enzyme	Produces pain in man*	Effect on primary afferent†
Potassium	Damaged cells		++	Activate
Serotonin	Platelets		++	Activate
Bradykinin	Plasma kininogen	Kallikrein	+++	Activate
Histamine	Mast cells		+	Activate
Prostaglandins	Arachidonic acid–damaged cells	Cyclooxygenase	±	Sensitize
Leukotrienes	Arachidonic acid–damaged cells	Lipoxygenase	±	Sensitize
Substance P	Primary afferent		±	Sensitize

*References 3, 4, 6, 19, 20, 21, 31.
†References 3, 4, 6, 27, 28.

ever animal cells are damaged and are present in increased concentration in inflammatory exudates.

The first of these compounds to be identified were the prostaglandins, which are formed from arachidonic acid by the action of the enzyme fatty acid cyclooxygenase. Several of the prostaglandins produce hyperalgesia and sensitize primary afferent nociceptors (20). Prostaglandin E_2 is one of the most potent of this class of compounds. That these metabolic intermediaries in the cyclooxygenase pathway of arachidonic acid metabolism play an important role in nociception is supported by the fact that aspirin and other nonsteroidal anti-inflammatory drugs that are cyclooxygenase inhibitors have significant analgesic potency (40). Some of the arachidonic acid metabolites may contribute to activation of nociceptors by modifying the action of other chemical mediators. For example, low doses of prostaglandin E_1 only produce pain when injected concomitantly with bradykinin or histamine (13).

Another important metabolic pathway of arachidonic acid is the lipoxygenase pathway, which produces the leukotrienes. Leukotrienes produce hyperalgesia in animal models and in humans (4). The hyperalgesia produced by leukotriene B_4 is not blocked by cyclooxygenase inhibitors but is blocked by depletion of polymorphonuclear leukocytes (28). This raises the interesting possibility that leukocytes contribute to nociceptor activation. Because there are no selective lipoxygenase inhibitors it remains uncertain how leukotrienes actually contribute to nociception.

In addition to the chemical mediators that are released from damaged cells or synthesized in the region of damage, the nociceptors themselves release a substance or substances that enhance nociception. Diffusible material is released into the extracellular space by electrical stimulation of unmyelinated afferents. This material has been shown to activate C fibers and to produce pain when injected into human skin (9, 10). It has not yet been determined what the material is, or even if it is only one substance. One likely constituent is substance P, an 11-amino acid polypeptide that is present in a subset of unmyelinated primary afferent fibers and is released when they are active (33). Nerve fibers containing substance P are found in a variety of pain-sensitive tissues. Of particular interest is the plexus of substance P–containing afferent nerves in the walls of blood vessels (16, 32) (Figure 2.11B). Substance P is a very potent vasodilator and also produces edema. The vascular plexus of substance P fibers may underlie these actions.

In addition to its direct action on blood vessels, substance P causes the release of histamine from mast cells (26). Histamine activates nociceptors and can itself produce vasodilatation and edema. It has been proposed that the neurogenically mediated spread of vasodilatation and hyperalgesia following injury to the skin is due to activation of nociceptors, with consequent release of substance P and then histamine from mast cells (Figures 2.11A and 2.12) (27). This hypothesis is supported by the anatomic finding that substance P–containing,

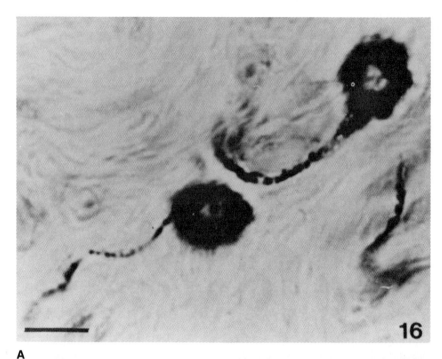

A

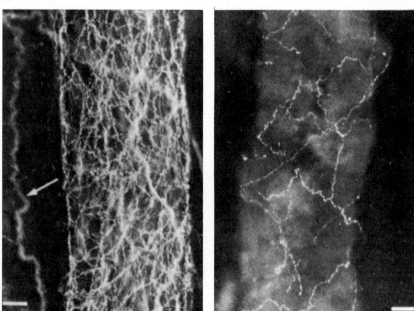

B

presumably sensory, axons are often found in proximity to the histamine-rich mast cells (23) (Figure 2.11A).

Figure 2.12 diagrammatically summarizes these observations and the close interrrelationship between pain and inflammation. Vasodilatation (heat, redness), swelling (edema), and pain are the principal signs of inflammation, all of which can be produced by activity in unmyelinated primary afferents. In a sense, then, nociceptor activity is not merely a passive signal indicating that tissue damage has occurred, but may play an active role in body defenses by participating in the inflammatory process. In fact, destruction of the small-diameter primary afferents of a limb can markedly slow experimental inflammatory arthritis (12). Although the clinical significance of this neurogenic component of inflammation has yet to be determined, there is no doubt that it exists.

Figure 2.11 **A:** Peripheral terminal of a presumed unmyelinated sensory axon (labeled with an antibody to substance P). It is shown terminating near a histamine-containing mast cell (calibration bar 10 μ). (From Kruger, L., Sampogna, S. L., Rodin, B. E., Clague, J., Brecha, N., and Yeh, Y.: Thin-fiber cutaneous innervation and its intraepidermal contribution studied by labeling methods and neurotoxin treatments in rats. *Somatosensory Res.* **2:**335–356, 1985.) **B:** Rich plexus of sensory axons in the wall of a mesenteric (left; calibration bar 100 μ) and cerebral (right; calibration bar 50 μ) artery. The axons are stained using an antibody to substance P. (From Furness, J. B., Papka, R. E., Della, N. G., Costa, M., and Eskay, R. L.: Substance P-like immunoreactivity in nerves associated with the vascular system of guinea-pigs. *Neuroscience* **7:**447–459, 1982.)

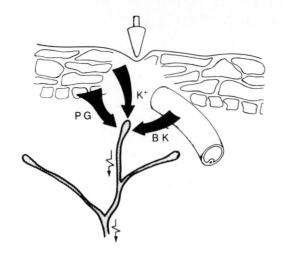

A

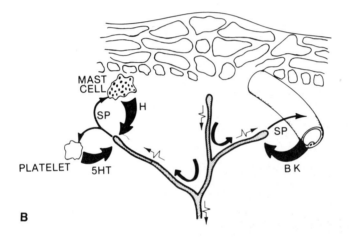

B

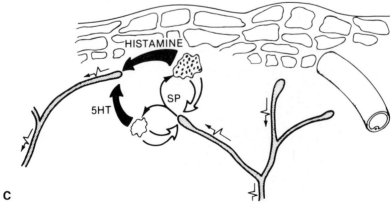

C

36

Conclusions

Nociceptors are primary afferents in peripheral nerve that respond specifically to stimuli that produce pain in humans. There are at least three types of nociceptor and there is evidence that each contributes uniquely to the quality and intensity of pain.

Nociceptor activity is part of a complex combination of processes initiated by noxious stimuli. The peripheral terminals of the nociceptive afferents are directly sensitive to brief intense thermal and mechanical stimuli. In addition to the transient responses to these brief stimuli, nociceptors show relatively long-lasting increases in sensitivity when noxious stimuli are repeatedly applied. Long-lasting enhancement of nociceptor activity can also be produced by a variety of diffusible substances, either released from damaged cells or locally synthesized. Activity in the nociceptors releases neuropeptides, including substance P, which cause vasodilatation, edema, and the release of histamine from mast cells (Figure 2.12). By this complex cascade of events nociceptor activity produces several results. On the perceptual side there is a prolongation of pain long beyond the termination of the stimulus and the development of hyperalgesia. In the peripheral tissues, the activity in nociceptors acts synergistically with the other processes initiated by tissue damage to produce increased blood flow and edema. The primary afferent nociceptor thus not only signals the presence of tissue damage but plays a direct role in local mechanisms of defense and repair.

References

1   Adriaensen, H., Gybels, J., Handwerker, H. O., and Van Hees, J.: Response properties of thin myelinated (A-δ) fibers in human skin nerves. *J. Neurophysiol.* **49**:111–122, 1983.

Figure 2.12 Events leading to activation, sensitization, and spread of sensitization of primary afferent nociceptor terminals. **A:** Direct activation by intense pressure and consequent cell damage. Cell damage leads to release of potassium (K^+) and to synthesis of prostaglandins (*PG*) and bradykinin (*BK*). Prostaglandins increase the sensitivity of the terminal to bradykinin and other pain-producing substances. **B:** Secondary activation. Impulses generated in the stimulated terminal propagate not only to the spinal cord but into other terminal branches, where they induce the release of peptides including substance P (*SP*). Substance P causes vasodilation and neurogenic edema with further accumulation of bradykinin. Substance P also causes the release of histamine (*H*) from mast cells and serotonin (*5HT*) from platelets. **C:** Histamine and serotonin levels rise in the extracellular space, secondarily sensitizing nearby nociceptors. This leads to a gradual spread of hyperalgesia and/or tenderness.

2   Armstrong, D.: Bradykinin, kallidin and kallikrein. In E. G. Erdos (ed.): *Handbook of Experimental Pharmacology*, vol. 25. Springer-Verlag, Berlin, 1970, pp. 434–481.

3   Beck, P. W., and Handwerker, H. O.: Bradykinin and serotonin effects on various types of cutaneous nerve fibres. *Pflugers Arch.* **347**:209–222, 1974.

4   Bisgaard, H., and Kristensen, J. K.: Leukotriene B₄ produces hyperalgesia in humans. *Prostaglandins* **30**:791–797, 1985.

5   Bishop, G. H.: Neural mechanisms of cutaneous sense. *Physiol. Rev.* **26**:77–102, 1946.

6   Burgess, P. R., and Perl, E. R.: Cutaneous mechanoreceptors and nociceptors. In A. Iggo (ed.): *Handbook of Sensory Physiology, Volume II: Somatosensory System.* Springer-Verlag, Berlin, 1973, pp. 29–78.

7   Campbell, J. N., Meyer, R. A., and LaMotte, R. H.: Sensitization of myelinated nociceptive afferents that innervate monkey hand. *J. Neurophysiol.* **42**:1669–1679, 1979.

8   Campbell, J. N., and LaMotte, R. H.: Latency to detection of first pain. *Brain Res.* **266**:203–208, 1983.

9   Chahl, L. A., and Ladd, R. J.: Local oedema and general excitation of cutaneous sensory receptors produced by electrical stimulation of the saphenous nerve in the rat. *Pain* **2**:25–34, 1976.

10 Chapman, L. F., Ramos, A. O., Goodell, H., and Wolff, H. G.: Neurohumoral features of afferent fibers in man. *Arch. Neurol.* **4**:617–650, 1961.

11 Collins, W. F., Jr., Nulsen, F. E., and Randt, C. T.: Relation of peripheral nerve fiber size and sensation in man. *Arch. Neurol.* **3**:381–385, 1960.

12 Colpaert, F. C., Donnerer, J., and Lembeck, F.: Effects of Capsaicin on inflammation and on the substance P content of nervous tissues in rats with adjuvant arthritis. *Life Sci.* **32**:1827–1834, 1983.

13 Ferreira, S. H.: Prostaglandins, aspirin-like drugs and analgesia. *Nature* **240**:200–203, 1972.

14 Fitzgerald, M.: The spread of sensitization of polymodal nociceptors in the rabbit from nearby injury and by antidromic nerve stimulation. *J. Physiol.* **297**:207–216, 1979.

15 Fitzgerald, M., and Lynn, B.: The sensitization of high threshold mechanoreceptors with myelinated axons by repeated heating. *J. Physiol.* **365**:549–563, 1977.

16 Furness, J. B., Papka, R. E., Della, N. G., Costa, M., and Eskay, R. L.: Substance P-like immunoreactivity in nerves associated with the vascular system of guinea-pigs. *Neuroscience* **7**:447–459, 1982.

17 Georgopoulos, A. P.: Functional properties of primary afferent units probably related to pain mechanisms in primate glabrous skin. *J. Neurophysiol.* **39**:71–83, 1974.

18 Gybels, J., Handwerker, H. O., and Van Hees, J.: A comparison between the discharges of human nociceptive nerve fibres and the subject's ratings of his sensations. *J. Physiol. (Lond.)* **292**:193–206, 1979.

19 Hagermark, O., Hokfelt, T., and Pernow, B.: Flare and itch induced by substance P in human skin. *J. Invest. Dermatol.* **71**:233–235, 1978.

20 Juan, H., and Lembeck, F.: Action of peptides and other algesic agents on paravascular pain receptors of the isolated perfused rabbit ear. *Naunyn-Schmiedeberg's Arch. Pharmacol.* **283**:151–164, 1974.

21 Keele, C. A.: Measurement of responses to chemically induced pain. In A. V. S. De Reuck and J. Knight (eds.): *Touch, Heat and Pain.* Little Brown & Co., Boston, 1966.

22 Kruger, L., Perl, E. R., and Sedivec, M. J.: Fine structure of myelinated mechanical nociceptor endings in cat hairy skin. *J. Comp. Neurol.* **198**:137–154, 1981.

23 Kruger, L., Sampogna, S. L., Rodin, B. E., Clague, J., Brecha, N., and Yeh, Y.: Thin-fiber cutaneous innervation and its intraepidermal contribution studied by labeling methods and neurotoxin treatment in rats. *Somatosensory Res.* **2**:335–356, 1985.

24 LaMotte, R. H.: Can the sensitization of nociceptors account for hyperalgesia after skin injury? *Human Neurobiol.* **3**:47–52, 1984.

25 LaMotte, R. H., and Campbell, J. N.: Comparison of responses of warm and nociceptive C-fiber afferents in monkey with human judgments of thermal pain. *J. Neurophysiol.* **41**:509–528, 1978.

26 LaMotte, R. H., Thalhammer, J. G., and Robinson, C. J.: Peripheral neural correlates of magnitude of cutaneous pain and hyperalgesia: A comparison of neural events in monkey with sensory judgments in human. *J. Neurophysiol.* **50**:1–26, 1983.

27 Lembeck, F.: Sir Thoma Lewis's nocifensor system, histamine and substance-P-containing primary afferent nerves. *TINS* **6**:106–108, 1983.

28 Levine, J. D., Lau, W., Kwiat, G., and Goetzl, E. J.: Leukotriene B_4 produces hyperalgesia that is dependent on polymorphonuclear leukocytes. *Science* **225**:743–745, 1984.

29 Lewis, T.: *Pain*. Macmillan, New York, 1942.

30 Lewis, T., and Pochin, E. E.: The double pain response of the human skin to a single stimulus. *Clin. Sci.* **3**:67–76, 1937.

31 Moncada, S., Flower, R. J., and Vane, J. R.: Prostaglandins, prostacyclin, thromboxane A_2 and leukotrienes. In A. G. Gilman et al (eds.): *The Pharmacological Basis of Therapeutics* (7th ed.) Chpt. 28. Macmillan, New York, 1985.

32 Norregaard, T. V., and Moskowitz, M. A.: Substance P and the sensory innervation of intracranial and extracranial feline cephalic arteries. *Brain* **108**:517–533, 1985.

33 Otsuka, M., Konishi, S., Yanagisawa, M., Tsunoo, A., and Takagi, H.: Role of substance P as a sensory transmitter in spinal cord and sympathetic ganglia. *Ciba Found. Symp.* **91**:13–34, 1982.

34 Perl, E. R.: Sensitization of nociceptors and its relation to sensation. In J. J. Bonica and D. Albe-Fessard (eds.): *Advances in Pain Research & Therapy, Vol. 1.* Raven Press, New York, 1976, pp. 17–28.

35 Price, D. D., & Dubner, R.: Neurons that subserve the sensory-discriminative aspects of pain. *Pain* **3**:307–338, 1977.

36 Price, D. D., Hu, J. W., Dubner, R., and Gracely, R. H.: Peripheral suppression of first pain and central summation of second pain evoked by noxious heat pulses. *Pain* **3**:57–68, 1977.

37 Torebjork, H. E.: Afferent C units responding to mechanical, thermal and chemical stimuli in human non-glabrous skin. *Acta Physiol. Scand.* **92**:374–390, 1974.

38 Torebjork, H. E., and Hallin, R. G.: Perceptual changes accompanying controlled preferential blocking of A and C fibre responses in intact human skin nerves. *Exp. Brain Res.* **16**:321–332, 1973.

39 Torebjork, H. E., and Hallin, R. G.: Identification of afferent C units in intact human skin nerves. *Brain Res.* **67**:387–403, 1974.

40 Vane, J. R.: Inhibition of prostaglandin synthesis as a mechanism of action for aspirin-like drugs. *Nature New Biol.* **231**:232–235, 1971.

41 Wall, P. D., and McMahon, S. B.: Microneuronography and its relation to perceived sensation. A critical review. *Pain* **21**:209–229, 1985.

Chapter 3

Pain Pathways in the Central Nervous System

In Chapter 2 the types of stimuli that activate the different primary afferent nociceptors and the relationship of their activity to pain perception in humans was described. In this chapter, the nociceptive message will be traced through the spinal cord, where the primary afferents terminate, to more rostral brain structures such as the brainstem reticular formation, thalamus, and cortex, where the processes underlying pain perception occur.

The study of central nervous system (CNS) pathways for pain is much more complex than that of the peripheral nervous system, and consequently our knowledge of these pathways is less certain. Primary afferents reliably respond to a narrow range of specific stimuli applied to a very small area of the body. In contrast, CNS neurons receive convergent input from numerous primary afferents, often of different types, including both nociceptive and non-nociceptive afferents. CNS neurons have spatially extensive receptive fields that in some cases include the entire body surface. In addition, the responses of CNS neurons to noxious stimuli are variable because they are subject to inhibitory influences either elicited by peripheral stimulation or originating within the brain itself. The ensemble of neurons activated by noxious stimuli and their pattern of activity is thus a complex function of the primary afferent barrage that arrives at the spinal cord and the inhibitory influences that are active at the time.

Despite this complexity, tremendous progress has been achieved over the years as a result of careful clinical observation and extensive studies of the anat-

omy and physiology of pain transmission pathways in the CNS. To briefly outline the pathway (see Figure 1.4); the primary afferent nociceptors terminate in
the dorsal horn of the spinal cord. The axons of spinal neurons activated by these
afferent nociceptors cross to the anterolateral quadrant on the side opposite to
the activated nociceptors. The message then ascends on that side to the brainstem
and via the thalamus to the cortex. Clinical studies have shown that lesions of
this pathway, anywhere from the spinal cord to the cortex, will impair pain sensation. Electrical stimulation at several points along this pathway will produce
pain in humans. This pathway from spinal cord to thalamus and cortex is both
necessary and sufficient for the normal perception of pain.

Primary Afferent Projections
to the Spinal Cord

Primary afferents are unique neurons. Their cell bodies are located in the dorsal
root ganglion. As with all neurons, the cell body is essential for the viability of
all its processes. Unlike other neurons, the cell body of the primary afferent
receives no synaptic connections and probably plays no direct role in the mo-
ment-to-moment processing of nociceptive signals.

The majority of primary afferent axons project from the dorsal root ganglion
to the spinal cord through the dorsal root. A significant number of primary afferents may also project to the spinal cord through the ventral roots. These ventral root afferents may be relevant for pain transmission and will be described in
more detail below.

DORSAL ROOTS AND LISSAUER'S TRACT

The axonal composition of the dorsal roots is a reflection of that of the sensory
component of the peripheral nerve. At least two-thirds of the axons are unmyelinated. It is of interest that there are more dorsal root axons than there are
dorsal root ganglion cells, indicating that there is significant branching of primary afferent axons near the ganglion. As in peripheral nerve, afferent axons of
different sizes are interspersed in the dorsal root through most of its length.
However, as the dorsal root approaches the spinal cord the small-diameter myelinated and unmyelinated axons become segregated in the ventrolateral part of
the root. By the time the root actually penetrates the surface of the cord, the
segregation is virtually complete (Figure 3.1). The larger diameter fibers continue medially, then bifurcate into ascending and descending branches in the
dorsal columns. Collaterals from these main branches penetrate the dorsal horn.
The small-diameter fibers also branch into ascending and descending branches
that extend for one or two segments beyond the level at which the parent axon

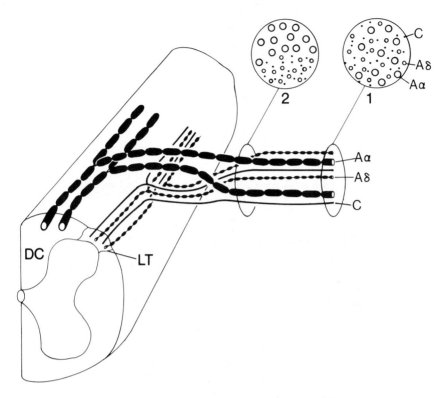

Figure 3.1 Primary afferent entry into the spinal cord. As the dorsal root axons approach the spinal cord, they segregate into two groups: one consists of the large diameter myelinated afferents (Aα), the other is the smaller diameter Aδ and C fibers. The large myelinated axons come to lie dorsal and medial and enter the dorsal columns (*DC*) dorsomedial to the dorsal horn. The small-diameter afferents, which include all nociceptors, assume a ventrolateral position and enter Lissauer's tract (*LT*) at the dorsolateral edge of the dorsal horn.

The insets show cross sections of the dorsal root. **1:** At a distance from the cord, the axons of different diameters are intermingled. **2:** Near the dorsal root entry zone, the Aα axons are gathered into the dorsomedial zone of the dorsal root.

enters. Most of the ascending and descending branches of the small-diameter primary afferents become part of Lissauer's tract, which is located at the dorsolateral edge of the spinal gray matter (Figure 3.1, *LT*). In the primate, about 80 percent of the axons in Lissauer's tract are primary afferents (11). The other axons arise from cells within the adjacent spinal gray matter.

After coursing in Lissauer's tract for a variable distance, the small-diameter primary afferents either enter or send a collateral branch into the adjacent spinal gray matter. There they give rise to an extensive, highly branched terminal field (Figure 3.2). Before further description of the terminal fields, it would be useful to briefly review the anatomy of the spinal gray matter.

The Laminar Organization of the Spinal Cord

The spinal cord gray matter is organized into sheets that are elongated in the rostrocaudal axis. This laminar organization was first described completely by Rexed (50), whose scheme is now generally accepted. He divided the gray matter of the spinal cord into 10 laminae based on the appearance of the neurons, their size, orientation, and density (Figure 3.3). He numbered the laminae sequentially from dorsal to ventral. Lamina I forms a cap over the dorsal margin of the spinal gray matter and turns ventrally at its lateral edge. Because of this arrangement, this region is also called the marginal layer. Dorsomedial to lamina I lies the white matter of the dorsal columns and dorsolateral is Lissauer's tract. Lamina I contains the distinctive large flat "marginal" cells as well as many intermediate-sized neurons. It has a net-like appearance because of the numerous fiber bundles that traverse it. In fresh, unstained spinal cord, lamina II has a clear, "gelatinous" appearance that led to its original name, the substantia gelatinosa. Histological staining reveals a well-demarcated layer of very small, very tightly packed neurons. Lamina II contains relatively few glia or nerve fiber bundles. Lamina III contains neurons that are somewhat larger and less densely packed than in lamina II. The remaining laminae contain numerous cells of varying size, including some that are significantly larger than the neurons in laminae II and III. Lamina IV is the thickest in the dorsal horn. It contains some very large neurons with dendrites that spread into more superficial layers. Lamina V cells are somewhat smaller and tend to have a mediolateral orientation across the narrowest part of the dorsal horn. Lamina VI is at the base of the dorsal horn and is only present at cervical and lumbar enlargements. Lamina VII occupies an irregular area in the central part of the spinal gray matter. Lamina VIII crosses the base and middle part of the ventral horn, except in the cervical and lumbar enlargements, where it is restricted to the medial half of the ventral horn. Lamina IX is the region of the motor neuron pools and lamina X refers to the region immediately surrounding the central canal.

Terminals of Primary Afferent Nociceptors

The small-diameter afferents that enter the cord in the lateral division of the dorsal root project densely to laminae I and II of the dorsal horn (7, 34, 58). This projection includes both the unmyelinated and myelinated nociceptors as

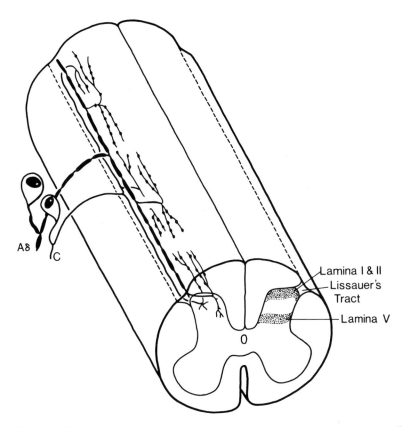

Figure 3.2 Extensive terminal field of a single small-diameter primary afferent. After bifurcating at the point of entry into Lissauer's tract (*LT*), the small-diameter fibers penetrate the spinal gray matter. Present evidence indicates that C fibers terminate predominantly in lamina II, (the substantia gelatinosa), whereas the Aδ nociceptors terminate in laminae I and V. The terminal axons of both types of small-diameter primary afferents are varicose and have a longitudinal orientation, extending for several millimeters in laminae I and II, contacting hundreds of spinal neurons.

well as some afferents that respond to innocuous thermal stimuli. Different classes of primary afferent have anatomically distinct terminal fields. It has been possible to trace the spinal terminals of single, physiologically identified myelinated afferents. One type of myelinated nociceptor has been studied in this manner, the high-threshold mechanoreceptor described in Chapter 2. The high-threshold mechanoreceptor terminates in lamina I and V but not in lamina II.

There is evidence that unmyelinated afferents project to lamina I and the outer part of lamina II (34, 38). Since most unmyelinated afferents are nociceptors, it is likely that most of the unmyelinated fibers that terminate in lamina II

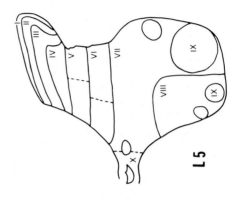

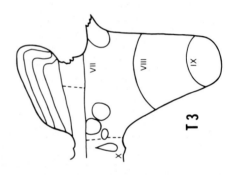

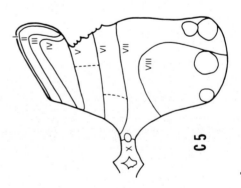

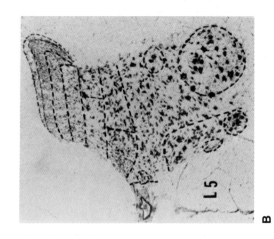

B

L5

Figure 3.3 Rexed's scheme for lamination of the spinal gray matter. (From Rexed, B.: A cytoarchitectonic atlas of the spinal cord in the cat. *J. Comp. Neurol.* **96:**415–495, 1952.) **A:** Outlines of fifth cervical (*C5*), third thoracic (*T3*), and fifth lumbar (*L5*) segments of the adult cat. The diagram of T3 shows that, in segments that innervate the trunk, laminae VII, VIII, and IX have a simple laminar relationship to each other. In contrast, in the segments that innervate the limbs (e.g., C5, L5), the cytoarchitectural divisions of the ventral horn lose their simple laminar arrangement. **B:** Photomicrograph of the L5 spinal segment that corresponds to the diagram of L5 in **A**. This is a stain for cell bodies.

are nociceptors. It is also likely, although not certain, that C fibers terminate in lamina I.

The larger diameter myelinated primary afferents (Aα and Aβ groups in peripheral nerve) that enter the cord in the medial division of the dorsal root terminate in lamina III or deeper.

Figure 3.4 summarizes the terminal patterns of the different cutaneous afferents within the superficial dorsal horn. As discussed above, myelinated nociceptors project to laminae I and V, unmyelinated nociceptors project to lamina II and possibly lamina I, and non-nociceptive myelinated afferents project only to deeper laminae.

VENTRAL ROOT AFFERENTS

A possible route for small-diameter afferents to the spinal gray matter is via the ventral roots. As many as 30 percent of ventral root axons are unmyelinated. Since motoneuron and sympathetic preganglionic axons are myelinated, this is circumstantial evidence for an afferent component in the ventral root. In fact, most of these unmyelinated ventral root axons have their cell bodies in the dorsal root ganglia. In addition, some of the ventral root unmyelinated fibers have peripheral receptive fields and a significant number appear to be nociceptive (12). Although it is possible that most of these ventral root afferents do not actually reach the cord, Light and Metz (33) were able to trace Aδ and C axons from the ventral roots to their sites of termination in laminae I and II. Their observations provide evidence that at least some nociceptive primary afferents gain entry to the spinal cord via the ventral root. On the other hand, electrical stimulation of the central end of a cut ventral root has not been shown to excite dorsal horn cells (9). Thus it is possible that many ventral root afferents do not actually enter the cord through the ventral root, but loop back out of the ventral root to enter the cord via the dorsal root (Figure 3.5).

Transmitter Substances in Nociceptive Primary Afferents

At the present time it is not possible to state with any certainty which transmitter substances mediate the excitatory effect of nociceptive primary afferents on spinal neurons. In order to prove that a substance is a transmitter for the primary afferent nociceptor it would be necessary to show that the substance is present in the primary afferent synapse on the second-order spinal neuron, that it is released by noxious stimulation, and that it has the same action on the spinal neuron as activity in the nociceptive primary afferent. Furthermore, antagonists

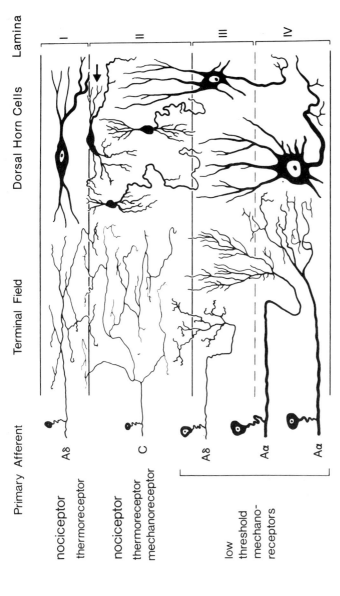

Figure 3.4 Summary of major components of the upper laminae of the spinal cord dorsal horn. (From Cervero, F., and Iggo, A: The substantia gelatinosa of the spinal cord. *Brain* **103**:717–772, 1980.)

The primary afferent nociceptor input is via Aδ fibers and C fibers. Aδ nociceptors terminate primarily in lamina I and the outermost part of lamina II. C fiber nociceptors terminate mainly in lamina II. There are some non-nociceptive Aδ and C primary afferents that also terminate in laminae I and II.

The deep part of lamina II and laminae III and IV receive input only from non-nociceptive myelinated primary afferents.

The second-order cells are of several types; there are larger neurons in laminae I, III, and IV, which include nociceptive projection neurons. The cells in lamina II are smaller, and, although some project to supraspinal sites, most make local connections.

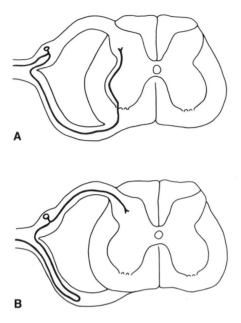

A

B

Figure 3.5 Two possible arrangements for ventral root afferent fibers. (From Coggeshall, R. E.: Afferent fibers in the ventral root. *Neurosurgery* **4:**443–448, 1979.) **A:** The central process of the dorsal root ganglion cell reaches the dorsal horn via the ventral root. **B:** The peripheral process of the dorsal root ganglion cell loops into the ventral root and then out again to join the peripheral nerve. In this case, no information actually reaches the cord through the ventral root.

of the substance should block both its action and that of the afferent on the spinal neuron. None of the present candidates for primary afferent nociceptive transmitter has met all of these criteria.

Using cytochemical techniques, a variety of peptides have been demonstrated in dorsal root ganglion cells, and all must be considered as possible transmitter candidates (3, 21, 35). Substance P, somatostatin, and vasoactive intestinal polypeptide (VIP) have been found in separate populations of small dorsal root ganglion cells. Substance P is present in dense concentration in laminae I and II (Figure 3.6). Somatostatin is most dense in lamina II and VIP in lamina I. The concentrations of all three peptides drop profoundly after cutting the dorsal roots. These observations are consistent with a role of all three in central transmission of the nociceptive message.

There is further evidence implicating substance P. As discussed in Chapter 2, some primary afferents release substance P from their peripheral terminals, where it contributes to both the nociceptive transduction process and inflammation. In addition, there is good evidence that substance P acts as a neurotransmitter in sympathetic ganglia (43). Some sympathetic postganglionic neurons receive synaptic contact from branches of substance P–containing afferents. Selective stimulation of these afferents causes substance P release and a slow depolarization that excites the postganglionic neuron. Substance P produces the same depolarizing effect as afferent stimulation. A neuron should release the same transmitter substance at all of its terminals. In fact, in second-order neurons in the spinal cord, substance P produces a slow depolarization that is similar to

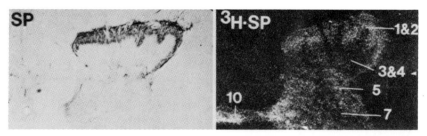

Figure 3.6 Distribution of substance P and its receptor in the spinal cord dorsal horn. On the left (*SP*) the tissue was incubated with antibody to substance P. The substance P (SP) is most densely concentrated in laminae I and II. On the right (*³H-SP*) is an adjacent tissue section that was incubated with tritiated SP to reveal the distribution of SP binding sites. The SP binding sites are quite similar in their distribution to SP. (From Mantyh, P. W. and Hunt, S. P.: The autoradiographic localization of substance P receptors in the rat and bovine spinal cord and the rat and cat spinal trigeminal nucleus caudalis and the effects of neonatal capsaicin. *Brain Res.* **332**:320, 1985.)

the depolarization produced by repetitive stimulation of the primary afferent nerves (54).

Even if substance P were an excitatory transmitter for the nociceptive primary afferent, it is unlikely to be the only transmitter. First, nociceptors comprise at least half of all primary afferents in limb nerves, and substance P is present in less than 25 percent of most dorsal root ganglion cells. Recent work on the peptide content of physiologically identified primary afferents indicates that, although some polymodal nociceptors contain substance P, most do not, and there is no consistent correlation between nociceptive response and the presence of any of the known dorsal root ganglion cell peptides. Furthermore, significant sparing of nociception is possible in the face of extensive depletion of substance P using neurotoxins (4). An intriguing possibility that might explain the conflicting evidence about substance P is that primary afferent nociceptors contain two transmitters. The two transmitters could either be coreleased from a single nociceptor afferent or represent two separate populations of nociceptors. In fact, there is physiological evidence supporting this latter idea. There are separable fast and slow components to the excitation of spinal neurons by nociceptive afferent input, but substance P only mimics the slow component. Candidates for the fast excitatory neurotransmitter include excitatory amino acids such as glutamate or aspartate, or the nucleotide adenosine triphosphate (ATP) (21).

In summary, our knowledge of the neurotransmitter for the primary afferent nociceptor is incomplete. Although the available evidence is circumstantial, it seems likely that one or more peptides, including substance P, is involved in nociceptive transmission. In addition, nonpeptide transmitters may be released concomitantly to produce fast excitatory actions.

Pain Transmission Cells in the Central Nervous System

Primary afferent nociceptors synapse directly on cells in the spinal cord dorsal horn. As illustrated in Figure 3.4, there are a variety of cells in the dorsal horn. These cells fall into three major categories: projection neurons, excitatory interneurons, and inhibitory interneurons. Each cell type plays an important role in nociception. Projection neurons relay the nociceptive message to higher brain centers. Excitatory interneurons relay the nociceptive input either to projection cells, to other interneurons, or to motor neurons that mediate spinal reflexes. Inhibitory interneurons contribute to the control of nociceptive transmission.

Identification of nociceptive projection neurons is, at least in theory, fairly straightforward. The following criteria are used (14, 46): as with the primary afferent nociceptors, the neuron should discharge maximally to noxious stimuli; manipulations that reduce the cell's discharge or block its ability to conduct impulses should reduce pain, electrical stimulation of the neurons or their axons should produce pain; and the cells should project to sites that are known to play a role in pain transmission. If a central neuron fulfills these criteria it probably plays a positive role in pain transmission.

Neurons that respond maximally to noxious stimuli are widely distributed in the spinal gray matter (58, 60). Not unexpectedly, many are concentrated in the laminae that receive direct input from primary afferent nociceptors (I, II, and V).

Most lamina I neurons respond maximally to noxious stimulation. Convergence of input from several primary afferents to a single central nociceptive neuron is the rule. Thus the receptive fields of lamina I neurons are several times larger than those of primary afferent nociceptors, and a single lamina I neuron may receive input from both myelinated and unmyelinated nociceptors. Cells that are excited only by nociceptive primary afferents are called "nociceptive-specific" or "high-threshold" neurons. Such nociceptive-specific neurons are the majority of lamina I neurons (Figure 3.7A). However, there are some lamina

---

Figure 3.7 Contrast between nociceptive-specific high-threshold and wide dynamic range cells. **A:** The nociceptive-specific or high-threshold (*NS*) cell responds minimally if at all to innocuous stimuli (brush, pressure, pinch) but discharges briskly at stimulus intensities that are above the usual pain threshold. **B:** The wide dynamic range (*WDR*) cell responds to innocuous stimuli but increases its discharge as the stimulus intensity increases into the noxious range. Wide dynamic range neurons tend to have larger receptive field areas than the nociceptive-specific neurons. (Adapted from Willis, W. D.: *The Pain System.* S. Karger, Basel, 1985.) **C:** Two examples of the complex receptive fields of cells in laminae VII, VIII, and X. *Vertical hatching,* pinch excitatory; *solid black,* pinch of subcutaneous structure excitatory; *stipple,* light touch inhibitory. The cell on the right has inputs from mirror-image areas on the two sides of the body.

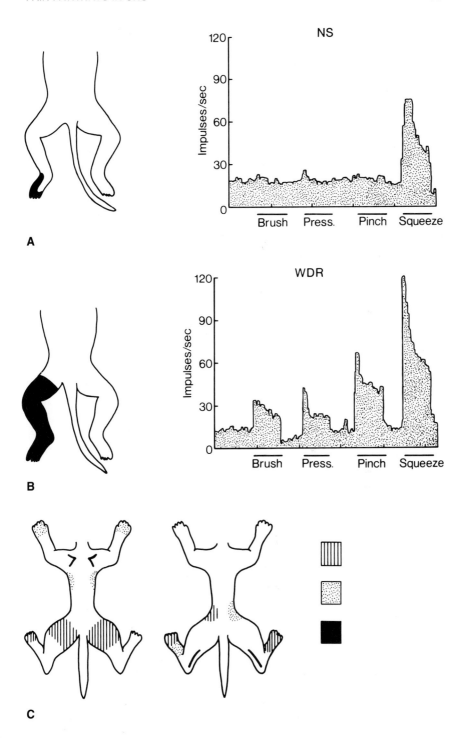

I cells that also receive input from non-nociceptive low-threshold mechanoreceptors. Such cells are called "wide dynamic range" neurons because they respond to a range of stimulus intensities from the innocuous to the noxious (Figure
3.7B). A large proportion of lamina I neurons are projection cells. A significant
number project to the thalamus. In addition, lamina I cells make local connections to other lamina I cells. It is likely that some of the same cells that give rise
to the local connections also project to higher brain areas.

Lamina II also contains cells that are excited by noxious stimulation. Although some lamina II neurons project to the brainstem and thalamus, most appear to be interneurons whose axons terminate within one or two segments of
their cell body. The bulk of the synaptic connections of lamina II neurons are
made within lamina II, probably with other lamina II neurons. In addition, many
cells in laminae I, III, IV, and V have dendrites that penetrate lamina II and may
be contacted there by lamina II–cell axon terminals.

One class of lamina II cells, the stalk cells, send their axons into lamina I.
Some stalk cells have receptive field properties very similar to those of lamina I
cells, and it has been proposed that they are excitatory interneurons that relay
nociceptive input to lamina I and IV projection cells (e.g., Figure 3.8A) (49).

There are a variety of other physiological cell types in lamina II, including
some with predominantly inhibitory inputs (7). Some of these cells are probably
inhibitory interneurons, whose function will be discussed later in this chapter.

Figure 3.8 illustrates some of the major patterns of connection in dorsal
horn. The unmyelinated primary afferent nociceptors terminate on interneurons
in lamina II. Some of these interneurons send their axons into lamina I, where
they contact projection cells. Some lamina I projection neurons also receive a
direct input from the Aδ myelinated nociceptors. Since they receive input from
both Aδ and C nociceptors, it is not surprising that most lamina I projection
neurons are excited by noxious stimuli (Figure 3.8A).

The majority of neurons in laminae III and IV respond maximally to innocuous stimuli. This is consistent with the fact that large myelinated afferents (Aα)
that respond to mild mechanical stimuli terminate most densely in these laminae.
A significant number of lamina IV neurons project to the thalamus in the primate. It is also possible (55) that the non-nociceptive cells in these laminae
project to other laminae and contribute to the responses of wide dynamic range
neurons to innocuous stimuli.

Similar to cells in lamina I, lamina V cells respond maximally to noxious
stimuli; however, lamina V cells manifest a greater degree of convergence. The
receptive fields of lamina V cells tend to be larger than those of lamina I, and
more lamina V cells are of the wide dynamic range category (Figure 3.7B).
Although some myelinated primary afferent nociceptors terminate in lamina V
(Figure 3.8B), the density of nociceptive afferent terminals is much less in lamina V than in laminae I and II. The great convergence of input could reflect

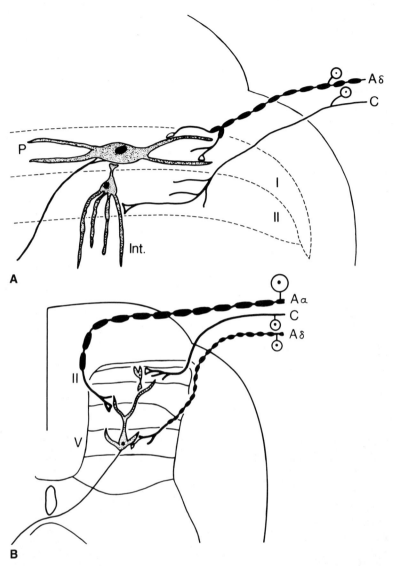

Figure 3.8 Input to dorsal horn projection cells. **A:** Lamina I neurons are predominately excited by nociceptive input. They receive direct input from myelinated (Aδ) nociceptors and indirect input from unmyelinated nociceptors (C) via stalk cell interneurons in lamina II. **B:** Lamina V neurons are predominately of the wide dynamic range type. They receive low-threshold input from large-diameter myelinated primary afferents (Aα) as well as both direct and indirect input from nociceptive afferents (Aδ and C). In this figure, the lamina V neuron is depicted as sending a dendrite up through lamina IV, where it is contacted by the terminal of the Aα primary afferent. This provides the low-threshold input. The lamina V dendrite is also contacted in lamina III by the axon terminal of a lamina II interneuron, which relays C fiber (nociceptive) input.

indirect connections via interneurons in laminae I through IV (Figure 3.8B). In addition, since wide dynamic range neurons in lamina V have dendrites that extend into laminae I and II, it is likely that they receive direct inputs from primary afferent nociceptors in those laminae (51). A large fraction of lamina V cells project to the brainstem and thalamus.

Lamina VI only exists in the cervical and lumbar enlargements. Its cells are similar to those in lamina V except that a significant number of lamina VI neurons also have proprioceptive (joint, muscle, tendon) inputs.

Laminae VII and VIII also contain significant numbers of nociceptive neurons. However, the receptive fields of cells in these laminae are much more complex than those of cells in more superficial laminae (16). Whereas the receptive fields of neurons in laminae I through V are predominantly cutaneous and have excitatory components restricted to part of a single limb, those of laminae VII and VIII neurons often consist of discontinuous cutaneous regions on both sides of the body (Figure 3.7C). The receptive fields of these cells may cover half the body and include inputs from poorly defined receptors in deep tissues such as muscle and viscera. Cells in these laminae project to the thalamus and reticular formation. The complexity of their receptive fields somewhat obscures their role in nociception.

What information there is about lamina X cells indicates that they are more like the neurons in laminae I and II than those in the deeper layers (41). They have relatively small receptive fields and are predominantly nociceptive. Some lamina X neurons project to the brainstem reticular formation.

In summary, nociceptive neurons are scattered throughout the spinal gray matter. Laminae I and II are the major receiving areas for the terminals of primary afferent nociceptors. Lamina II neurons make mainly local connections. Neurons in laminae III and IV do not appear to play a positive role in normal pain transmission, although an inhibitory contribution cannot be ruled out. Figure 3.9 summarizes the important features of spinal nociceptive relay cells. Laminae I, V, VII, and VIII are the major source of rostrally projecting nociceptive neurons. Lamina I cells show less convergence, their receptive fields are smaller, and fewer receive input from non-nociceptive afferents. In contrast, most lamina V cells have larger receptive fields and receive input from both nociceptive and non-nociceptive afferents. Thus, lamina V cells have a wide dynamic range of responses to cutaneous stimulation. Input to lamina V cells from viscera has also been demonstrated (58; see Chapter 4). Nociceptive projection cells in the deeper layers show even greater convergence. The input to these deep-lying neurons is often bilateral, and they frequently respond to receptors in deep tissues such as muscles and viscera.

The evidence that laminae I and V nociceptive neurons are crucially involved in transmitting the pain message is substantial. Both the wide dynamic range nociceptors concentrated in lamina V and the nociceptive-specific neurons concentrated in lamina I project to the thalamus (58, 59, 61). Cutting this pro-

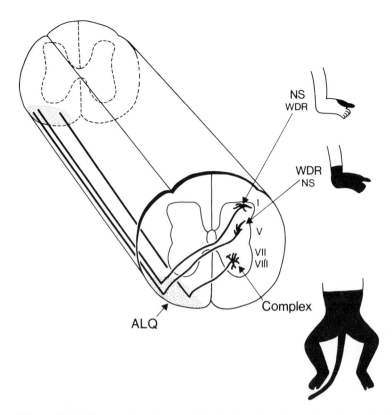

Figure 3.9 Three major classes of spinal nociceptive projection cells. The nociceptive-specific (*NS*) cell, which is the predominant class in lamina I, is also present in lamina V. The wide dynamic range (*WDR*) cell, which is present in lamina I and predominates in lamina V, typically has a larger receptive field than NS cells. Finally, cells in laminae VII and VIII, which I have termed complex, are characterized by highly convergent input that is often bilateral and includes visceral receptors.

Axons of cells of each class cross to the contralateral anterolateral quadrant (*ALQ*), the major pathway for ascending nociceptive transmission to brainstem and thalamus.

jection abolishes cutaneous pain and electrical stimulation of it produces pain (37). Using thermal stimuli, the discharge of both lamina I and V spinothalamic tract neurons increases as a function of skin temperature from 43°C to 50°C (Figure 3.10) (24). Over this same temperature range the intensity of pain reported by human subjects increases in parallel with the increase in spinothalamic tract cell discharge.

As discussed in Chapter 2, brief noxious heat pulses to human skin produce two distinct sensations: an early, sharp pain mediated by myelinated nociceptors and a later, duller pain produced by the action of unmyelinated polymodal nociceptors. Nociceptive spinothalamic neurons in laminae I and V show both an early and a late discharge in response to brief noxious heat pulses (8, 47, 48).

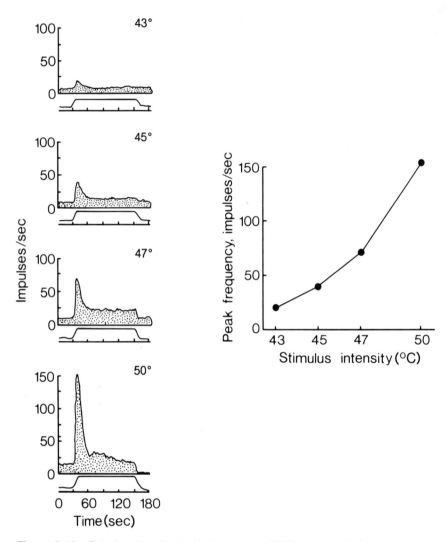

Figure 3.10 Relationship of spinothalamic tract (STT) neuron discharge to stimulus intensity. **Left:** Histograms represent averaged responses of 11 STT neurons to heating from a baseline of 35°C to progressively higher temperatures. The time of heating is indicated by vertical displacement of trace just below the histogram. The discharge clearly increases as the temperature increases across the noxious range: from top to bottom, 43°, 45°, 47°, and 50°C. **Right:** Peak discharge frequency of the same neurons is plotted against temperature. (Adapted from Kenshalo, D. R., Jr., Leonard, R. B., Chung, J. M., and Willis, W. D.: Responses of primate spinothalamic neurons to graded and to repeated noxious heat stimuli. *J. Neurophysiol.* **42:**1370–1389, 1979.)

These responses are produced by Aδ and C fiber inputs, respectively, and are a remarkable neurophysiological parallel to the human experience of first and second pain (Figure 3.11) (47).

Repetitive stimuli of constant (noxious) intensity can be shown to produce sensations of pain that progressively increase in intensity. The increase in intensity is called *summation*. Summation depends on activity in unmyelinated nociceptors because it persists (or is enhanced; see below) when myelinated axons are blocked. Summation can be observed with stimuli that do not sensitize C fibers. This indicates that the mechanism of summation is within the CNS. Price and his colleagues (47) have shown that repetitive noxious heat pulses produce parallel increases in the intensity of second pain in humans (summation) and in the C fiber–elicited discharge in primate spinothalamic neurons.

Assuming that humans have spinothalamic tract neurons resembling those described in the primate, the observations described above provide strong evidence that spinothalamic tract neurons in the dorsal horn are essential for normal pain sensation in humans.

INHIBITION OF NOCICEPTIVE RESPONSES BY AFFERENT INPUT

Injuries to the peripheral and central nervous system are often accompanied by pain and by exaggerated responses to innocuous and mildly noxious stimuli. The mechanisms of pain in nerve injury will be discussed extensively in Chapter 5. In this section, the presence of pain with nerve injury is used to emphasize the critical importance of inhibitory interactions in the normal operation of the sensory pathways that underlie pain perception. The crucial clinical observation is that pain frequently results from damage to somatosensory pathways at any point from peripheral nerve to cortex. This leads to the striking paradox that severe pain exists in the face of impaired sensation. In such patients, the initial sensation produced by pinprick or noxious heat (first pain) is often reduced in the face of ongoing pain and hyperreactivity.

These clinical observations led to the elegantly simple concept that pain can result from the removal of a normally inhibitory afferent input. This conclusion has been reinforced and extended by careful psychophysical studies. For example, in humans, when myelinated primary afferents are selectively blocked, leaving only C fibers intact, the sensations produced by noxious skin stimuli are perceived as more painful. As discussed above, brief noxious stimuli elicit an early sharp, pricking (first) pain and the later burning (second) pain. When myelinated fibers are blocked by pressure the sharp first pain disappears and the second pain is enhanced and prolonged (30, 47). Summation of second pain is strikingly enhanced when myelinated afferent fibers are selectively blocked (Figure 3.12). the simplest explanation of these observations is that myelinated nociceptor afferents have both excitatory and inhibitory actions on spinal cord no-

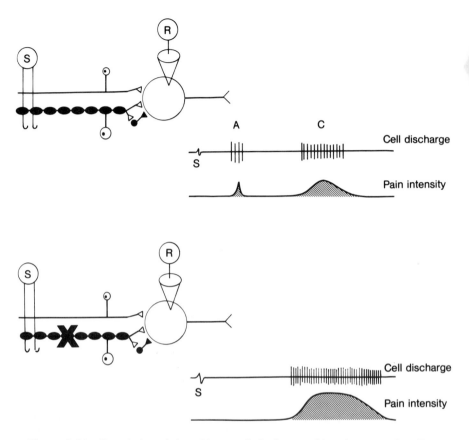

Figure 3.11 Correlation of dorsal horn cell discharge with pain perception. **Top:** A brief electrical stimulus (*S*) to the peripheral nerve excites both the large myelinated primary afferent (*lower row*) and the unmyelinated nociceptive primary afferent (*upper line*). Both types of primary afferent excite the pain transmission cell (shown with a recording electrode, *R,* in it). In addition, the myelinated afferent excites an inhibitory interneuron [the small cell (*filled*) contacting the pain transmission cell]. Because of this arrangement, the rapidly conducting myelinated afferents produce the early discharge (first pain). The myelinated afferents, by activating the inhibitory interneuron, also produce a persistent inhibition that limits the late discharge (second pain) produced by the unmyelinated afferents. **Bottom:** When myelinated afferents are blocked, no early discharge (first pain) is produced, and the inhibitory interneuron is not activated, resulting in a greater late discharge by the unmyelinated afferents.

ciceptive projection cells. Most noxious stimuli will activate both myelinated and unmyelinated nociceptors. Input from the myelinated nociceptors arrives at the spinal cord early and excites the projection cell, leading to first pain. Presumably, input from the myelinated nociceptors also activates an inhibitory interneuron (Figure 3.11). This will produce a lingering inhibition that suppresses

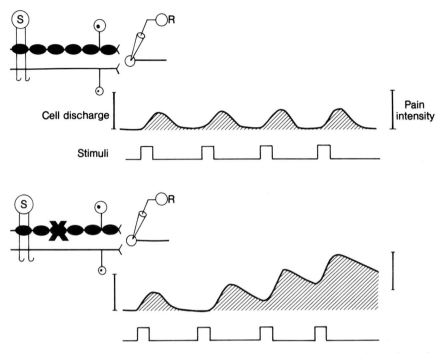

Cell discharge

Stimuli

Pain intensity

Figure 3.12 Enhancement of summation by selective blockade of myelinated fibers. When repeated electrical stimulation is delivered to a peripheral nerve at an appropriate rate (**top**), a brief response that is the same for each stimulus can be recorded in dorsal horn neurons. The pain sensation reported by human subjects also remains stable with repeated stimuli. When myelinated axons are selectively blocked (**bottom**), both the dorsal horn response and the subjective pain intensity grow larger with each successive stimulus (summation).

This phenomenon indicates that activity in myelinated axons produces a long-lasting inhibition of pain transmission neurons. When this inhibition is removed, the response to activity in unmyelinated fibers is greatly enhanced.

the response of the projection cell to the later arriving input from unmyelinated nociceptors.

In fact, studies of primate spinothalamic tract neurons reveal evidence of just such inhibitory mechanisms. In addition to excitatory inputs, spinothalamic tract neurons receive inhibitory inputs from wide areas of the body surface and from deep structures (18). Although stimulation of the large myelinated Aα mechanoreceptors is somewhat effective, the most powerful inhibition of spinothalamic tract cells is produced by activation of myelinated (Aδ) nociceptors. As mentioned above, brief heat pulses produce a biphasic response in dorsal horn nociceptive neurons: an early Aδ response and a later C fiber–evoked response. In cat dorsal horn, progressive blockade of myelinated fibers produces a concomitant increase in the C fiber–induced response of nociceptive dorsal horn cells (Figure 3.11) (20). This observation parallels the increased intensity of second (C fiber) pain when first pain transmitted by myelinated nociceptors is blocked.

At present, the physiological function of these potent inhibitory inputs to CNS pain transmission cells is unknown. They may play a role in localizing stimuli or in limiting reflex responses. It has even been proposed that, by enhancing contrast with surrounding unstimulated skin, the inhibition may actually enhance pain transmission (31). Whatever its role, it seems likely that afferent inhibition contributes to the phenomenon of counterirritation, in which mildly noxious manipulations such as needling (acupuncture), heat, mustard plasters, and deep pressure afford temporary pain relief.

Ascending Pathways for Pain: The Anterolateral Quadrant of the Spinal Cord

The location of the spinal pathway for pain transmission is in the anterolateral quadrant. This was discovered over a century ago by clinical observation (19). Since Spiller and Martin (53) first reported that severe pain in the lower body could be treated by spinal incision restricted to the anterolateral quadrant, this operation has become established as an important surgical tool for the treatment of pain. The large number of patients who have undergone this procedure have provided a wealth of clinical observations to supplement experimental studies of spinal pain pathways.

Provided a sufficiently large lesion is made, most patients who have an anterolateral cordotomy experience a profound loss of normal pain and temperature sensation that lasts for years (56, 57). The loss of sensation is on the side opposite the lesion and the upper limit of the deficit is about four segments below the level of the lesion. Cordotomy reduces the sensitivity of all tissues to noxious stimuli. Skin, musculoskeletal tissue, and viscera are all rendered hypalgesic. It is this pervasive impairment of pain transmission that makes cordotomy a clinically useful procedure. It is important to point out, however, that the effects of cordotomy are variable, incomplete, and, to some extent, transient. Isolated patches of skin may retain pain sensitivity. Furthermore, sensitivity to very intense stimuli is preserved, especially in deep tissues, although the perceived intensity is still much less than normal. Thus it is really more correct to say that cordotomy produces hypalgesia than that it produces analgesia. Curiously, over a period of months there is a partial recovery of sensitivity to noxious stimuli (29, 56, 57). The upper margin of hypalgesia drops, often by several dermatomal levels, and there is a partial recovery of sensitivity to noxious stimuli in the remaining area of deficit. Along with this partial recovery of function, there may be a return of the original pain problem. This recovery of pain sensitivity obviously limits the applicability of cordotomy for chronic pain problems.

A very instructive case reported by Noordenbos and Wall (42) relates to this issue. Their patient was a 24-year-old woman who was stabbed in the back with a knife. This injury cleanly severed the spinal cord at the third thoracic segment, sparing only the left anterolateral quadrant. Pain and temperature sensation were preserved on the right side below the lesion. On the left side, temperature sensation was lost and pinprick was felt as a dull but distinctly painful sensation. In addition to confirming the importance of the anterolateral quadrant for transmitting nociceptive and thermal information from the contralateral body, this case demonstrates that the anterolateral quadrant is capable of transmitting crude information about *ipsilateral* noxious stimuli.

These clinical observations indicate that there may be several routes by which the nociceptive message can reach higher centers. Because of this, *partial recovery of nociceptive transmission after damage to the anterolateral quadrant is the rule*. Since functional regeneration in the CNS does not occur, it seems likely that recovery of pain sensation after cordotomy involves an increased participation by pathways that may not normally contribute to pain transmission.

ROSTRAL PROJECTIONS OF AXONS IN THE ANTEROLATERAL QUADRANT

Rostrally projecting axons in the anterolateral quadrant project to a variety of target nuclei in the brainstem and thalamus (1) (Figure 3.13). Although all these nuclei are potentially involved in pain sensation, attention has focused on the thalamic projection. The major reason for this is that the thalamus is the most rostral target of anterolateral quadrant axons, and clinical observations have demonstrated that lesions of the spinothalamic tract, anywhere along its length, produce profound and lasting deficits in pain and temperature sensation (56). Furthermore, electrical stimulation of the spinothalamic tract produces sharp pain felt on the contralateral body. Thus, normal pain sensation requires an intact spinothalamic tract.

These clinical observations establishing the importance of the spinothalamic tract in pain sensation have been bolstered in recent years by electrophysiological studies of identified spinothalamic neurons. These studies have demonstrated that a large proportion of primate spinothalamic neurons are nociceptive and that their responses to noxious stimuli correlate well with human ratings of pain intensity.

THALAMIC RECEIVING AREAS AND INPUT PATHWAYS

Spinothalamic tract axons terminate in several distinct thalamic nuclei, each of which projects to a different cortical area. This raises the possibility that there are several parallel pathways to the cortex, each of which makes a distinct contribution to pain perception. Spinothalamic tract axons segregate into a medial

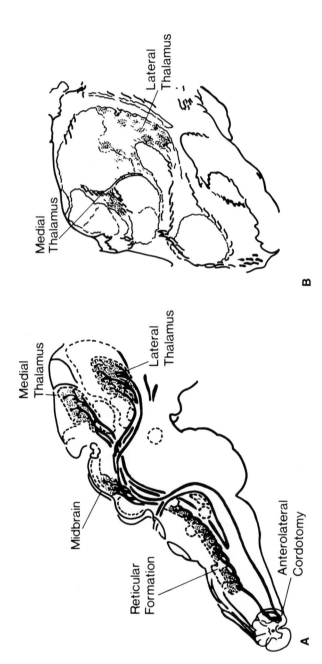

Figure 3.13 Targets of axons ascending in the anterolateral quadrant of the spinal cord. (Adapted from Mehler, W. R.: The anatomy of the so-called "pain tract" in man: An analysis of the course and distribution of the ascending fibers of the fasciculus anterolateralis. In J. D. French and R. W. Portor (eds.), *Basic Research in Paraplegia.* Charles C. Thomas, Springfield, IL, 1962.) **A:** Rostral projection sites based on tracing axons that degenerated following a successful anterolateral cordotomy in a patient for relief of severe pain. There are major projections to the medullary reticular formation, the midbrain, and both the medial and lateral thalamus. **B:** Same patient; enlarged coronal section through the posterior thalamus (right side) showing major terminal fields in the lateral thalamus (ventrobasal complex) and medial thalamus (mainly the central lateral nucleus).

and a lateral division as they approach the thalamus (1, 39). The medial division terminates most densely in the central lateral nucleus of the intralaminar complex and in the nucleus submedius (Figure 3.14). The lateral division terminates in the lateral part of the ventrobasal (VB) nucleus and the posterior nuclear group (PO).

Nociceptive inputs from the face (i.e., the trigeminal nucleus) also divide into medial and lateral components. The lateral trigeminothalamic component terminates medially in the ventrobasal nucleus.

Although the spinothalamic tract is predominantly crossed, there is also an ipsilateral component. The ipsilateral projection is primarily to the intralaminar thalamus.

Different populations of spinal cells project to the intralaminar and the VB nuclei of the thalamus. Over two-thirds of the cells projecting to the VB nucleus arise from lamina I and V of the contralateral cord. These cells have receptive fields restricted to one side of the body, usually part of a limb. Most have typical nociceptive-specific (lamina I) or wide dynamic range (lamina V) response characteristics. In contrast, most spinal cells projecting to the intralaminar thalamus are located in the deeper laminae (VI, VII, or VIII) and have large, complex receptive fields with inputs that may include nociceptors over the entire body surface (Figure 3.7C and 3.9). About 10 percent of spinothalamic tract neurons project to both the VB and the medial thalamic nuclei. Their laminar locations and receptive field properties are similar to those of the spinothalamic tract neurons which project only to the VB complex.

The nucleus submedius is a distinct subregion of the medial thalamus that is ventral to the central lateral nucleus (Figure 3.14) (1). It is of interest because, although it has a medial location, it receives a large, topographically organized projection from cells in lamina I of the spinal cord (12). In this respect, the submedius seems more like the VB complex in its organization. However, submedius neurons project to the orbitofrontal cortex, a region not known to be part of the somatosensory cortex (1). At present, the nucleus submedius should be thought of as a separate functional entity, rather than being grouped with the nearby nuclei of the intralaminar complex that receive spinothalamic input.

The thalamic termination sites for spinothalamic axons also receive input from other ascending somatosensory pathways. The most prominent of these other inputs originates in the dorsal column nuclei. Neurons of the dorsal column nuclei project to the VB complex and PO but not to the medial thalamus. The dorsal column nuclei projection cells respond maximally to mild mechanical stimulation and to changes in joint position. They show no differential response to noxious stimuli. Lesions of the dorsal columns do not impair pain transmission, and stimulation of the dorsal columns actually *inhibits* pain transmission. Thus the dorsal column pathway does not normally contribute in a positive way to pain transmission. It may, however, have a modulating influence.

The other major somatosensory input to the thalamus is via the brainstem reticular formation. Spinoreticular axons are interspersed with spinothalamic ax-

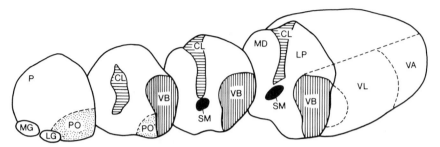

Figure 3.14   Conglomerate diagram of major thalamic nuclei that receive direct input from the spinal cord. These include the ventrobasal complex (*VB; vertical hatching*), the posterior nuclear complex (PO; *stippled*), the central lateral nucleus (*CL; crosshatched*) and the nucleus submedius (*SM; black*).
     Adjacent nuclei [dorsomedial (*MD*), lateral posterior (*LP*), ventral lateral (*VL*), ventral anterior (*VA*), medial geniculate (*MG*), lateral geniculate (*LG*), and pulvinar (*P*)] do not receive significant direct spinal input.

ons in the anterolateral quadrant, and there is reason to believe that they play a role in pain transmission. The locations and receptive field properties of spinoreticular neurons are very similar to those of the spinothalamic tract neurons that project to the medial-intralaminar thalamus. Thus they arise primarily from the deeper laminae of the spinal gray matter, including V, VI, VII, and VIII, and they have complex receptive fields that often include nociceptive inputs from both sides of the body (16, 27, 60). Spinoreticular neurons project to both sides of the brainstem reticular formation. The brainstem region that receives the largest input from the spinal cord is the medial medullary reticular formation (Figure 3.13). This region projects bilaterally to the medial thalamus (45). The terminals of the reticulothalamic projection cells overlap with those of the medial spinothalamic projection cells in the central lateral nucleus. Thus the spinoreticulothalamic "pathway" shares many anatomic and physiological properties with the medially projecting direct spinothalamic pathway.

NOCICEPTIVE THALAMIC NEURONS

The receptive field properties of thalamic neurons reflect those of their input pathways. In the primate, the VB complex is the major thalamic relay to the somatosensory cortex. Its input is via the lateral division of the spinothalamic tract and the dorsal column nuclei. Since nociceptors are only one of several types of input relayed to the cortex, it is not surprising that most VB neurons do not respond differentially to noxious stimuli. However, those that do faithfully mirror the response properties of the laterally projecting spinothalamic neurons. Thus, there are two classes of nociceptive neuron in primate VB, nociceptive specific and wide dynamic range (25). As with spinal laminae I and V cells, VB nociceptive neurons show response magnitudes that are a positively accelerating function of temperatures in the noxious range. These responses are abolished by cutting the spinal anterolateral quadrant. Nociceptive VB neurons project directly to primary somatosensory cortex.

There is not as much information available about the PO of the thalamus, which lies just caudal and ventral to the ventral posterolateral nucleus (VPL). Part of the problem may be that the boundaries of this nucleus are not well defined. Furthermore, what information there is about PO neurons comes mostly from work on cats and may not apply to primates. The PO region receives direct spinothalamic tract input and projects to a specific part of the somatosensory cortex (the retroinsular cortex). Most workers have found significant numbers of nociceptive neurons in the PO, although the receptive fields tend to be larger than is typical for VB neurons. A direct comparison of the properties of PO neurons with those of other thalamic nuclei under similar experimental conditions is not available. Thus it is difficult to say whether PO neurons differ in function from nociceptive neurons in the VPL. It does seem likely, however, that both the VB and the PO function as nociceptive relay nuclei.

Recordings in the central lateral nucleus and nearby structures of the medial thalamus reveal that well over half of the neurons there are maximally responsive to noxious stimuli (13, 44). Their receptive fields are large, often including the entire body or half of it. Furthermore, inputs from deep, musculoskeletal receptors are common. These response properties are similar to those of medial spinothalamic and spinoreticular neurons. As with the nociceptive neurons in the lateral thalamus, cutting the anterolateral quadrant of the spinal cord abolishes the responses of medial thalamic neurons to noxious stimulation. In contrast to the VB and PO, the central lateral nucleus and the other nearby medial thalamic regions are not simple somatosensory relay nuclei. Projections from this region have been shown to terminate in the basal ganglia, prefrontal and motor cortex as well as the somatosensory and visual cortices. Since a high percentage of medial thalamic neurons respond to noxious stimulation, it is likely that nociceptive neurons project to several different cortical areas. The diffuse nature of its efferent projection has suggested to some that, rather than playing any specific role in pain sensation, the medial thalamus may be part of a nonspecific arousal system, or that it is involved in motor responses produced by noxious stimuli.

In summary, the medial (central lateral) and lateral (ventrobasal) divisions of the thalamus have distinct properties (Table 3.1). Although both receive input from nociceptive spinothalamic tract cells, the lateral thalamic nuclei give rise to a dense projection restricted to the somatosensory cortex. The input to the VB complex of the thalamus is from the contralateral spinal cord and derives from spinothalamic tract cells in more superficial dorsal horn laminae, with smaller receptive fields. Nociceptive neurons in the VB complex are topographically arranged and project to somatosensory cortex. In contrast, the central lateral nucleus receives bilateral input from cells in deeper laminae of the spinal gray

Table 3.1 Thalamic Nuclei in Nociception

Nucleus	Cortical target	Spinal input cell type (predominant)[a]	Receptive field size
Ventrobasal	Primary somatosensory	Lamina I, IV, V NS, WDR, and Non-nociceptive	Contralateral restricted
Posterior	Secondary somatosensory (retroinsular)	?	Large, often bilateral
Central lateral	Frontal, somatosensory, visual	Lamina V, VII, VIII WDR, Complex	Large, often whole body
Submedius	Frontal	Lamina I NS?	Contralateral restricted?

[a]NS, nociceptive specific; WDR, wide dynamic range.

matter and from the brainstem reticular formation. The nociceptive neurons of this area have highly convergent input from large areas of skin and deep tissues. They have no obvious topographical arrangement. Neurons of the medial thalamus project to wide areas of the ipsilateral cortex (22, 23).

A further differentiation of the medial and lateral nociceptive transmission systems has been made on phylogenetic grounds. The spinoreticular pathway is present in all vertebrates, including those fish and amphibia that have no direct spinothalamic projection. The spinoreticular pathway is the major route by which the nociceptive message is transmitted to the brain in those species without a spinothalamic tract. In the lower vertebrates that do have a direct spinothalamic projection, it is to the medial thalamus. Since this medial projection is the earliest to appear phylogenetically, it is referred to as the paleospinothalamic tract. The paleospinothalamic tract has much in common with its phylogenetic precursor, the spinoreticulothalamic pathway. The spinal laminar origin and receptive fields of spinoreticular and paleospinothalamic neurons are indistinguishable, and there is significant overlap in the intralaminar thalamus between reticulothalamic and spinothalamic terminals. Furthermore, a high proportion of spinothalamic neurons in the deeper spinal laminae send collaterals into the brainstem reticular formation (28). Thus it seems justified to consider the spinoreticulothalamic and the paleospinothalamic tract as a single functional entity. Melzack and Casey (40) have referred to this entity as the paramedian pathway (Figure 3.15).

With the evolution of increased encephalization, the lateral thalamic projection made its appearance, reaching its greatest development in primates. The direct spinal projection to the VB is referred to as the neospinothalamic tract. Some of the spinothalamic neurons that project to the VB also send collateral branches to the brainstem reticular formation or to the medial thalamus, suggesting a strong functional link between the two systems. However, the striking differences in receptive field organization of the neurons in the two regions, and their distinct efferent projections, suggest that the paramedian and lateral pathways make functionally distinct contributions to nociception (Figure 3.15).

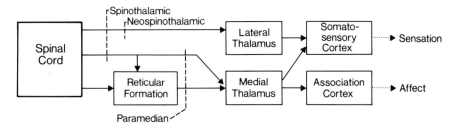

Figure 3.15   Schematic diagram of the major central nervous pathways that contribute to pain sensation.

SOMATOSENSORY CORTEX

There has been considerable controversy over the years about what role the cerebral cortex plays in normal pain sensation. There is a clear disparity between different reports of the effect of cortical lesions on pain sensation. On the one hand, many clinical studies reported that, when large areas of somatosensory cortex are damaged, two-point discrimination, position sense, and stereognosis are impaired but there is no abnormality of pain sensation. In fact, there are reports of patients with complete hemispherectomy who have almost normal pain sensation (2). Electrical stimulation of somatosensory cortex occasionally elicits reports of pain in awake human subjects, and there are well-documented cases in which the discharge of an epileptic seizure focus in the parietal cortex is associated with pain in the contralateral body (see Chapter 6). Furthermore, extensive cortical lesions usually do impair responses to noxious stimulation, and there are several convincing reports of patients in whom lesions restricted to the parietal cortex were associated with long-lasting deficits of pain and temperature sensation (15, 32, 36, 52). In some patients the only sensory deficit observed was in pain sensation.

The reason for the conflicting reports about deficits in pain sensation following cortical lesions is not clear. As discussed above, there are at least four distinct thalamic nuclei that receive nociceptive input from the spinal cord. Each of these thalamic nuclei has a distinct cortical projection pattern. It is thus possible that there are several different cortical representations for pain, each capable of independently providing normal nociceptive function. Another possibility is that, as with language representation, the cortical representation for pain is bilateral in some individuals and unilateral in others. In those individuals having bilateral representation, recovery of pain sensation following cortical injury would be rapid and complete. Those individuals with a strongly unilateral representation would have more lasting deficits following unilateral lesions.

Electrophysiological recording has demonstrated conclusively that there is a population of neurons in the primary somatosensory cortex (SI) that responds selectively to noxious stimuli (26). Although the overwhelming majority of SI neurons respond maximally to *innocuous* stimuli, both nociceptive-specific and wide dynamic range neurons are also present. In terms of receptive field size and laterality, there are two types of nociceptive neurons in the SI. One type is very much like the cortically projecting nociceptive neurons found in the lateral thalamus, with a restricted contralateral receptive field. The other type has a large receptive field more like that of cells in the intralaminar thalamus. These two types of nociceptive cortical neurons may reflect the dual input to the somatosensory cortex from the lateral and intralaminar thalamus (22).

These single-unit studies support the notion that the SI plays an important role in nociception and are consistent with the clinical studies indicating lasting deficits of pain sensation with parietal lobe lesions. However, only the lateral thalamic nuclei (VB and PO) have cortical projections restricted to the parietal lobe. The medial thalamic nuclei (central lateral and submedius) have widespread cortical projections that include a large projection to the frontal lobes. As discussed in the following section, these frontal connections from the medial thalamus may make a contribution to the pain experience that is not, strictly speaking, sensory.

Sensory-Discrimative versus Affective-Motivational Aspects of Pain

Melzack and Casey (40) divided pain into two operational components: the sensory-discriminative and the affective-motivational. The sensory-discriminative aspects refer to the processes that underly the localization and identification of the noxious stimulus. Pain threshold, that is, the intensity at which a stimulus is subjectively judged as painful, is a sensory discrimination. The assessment of stimulus intensity is also a sensory-discriminative function. As discussed in Chapter 2, the sensory-discriminative aspects of pain are relatively consistent within an individual and between different individuals. Melzack and Casey proposed that the topographically organized lateral or neospinothalamic pathway, with its discrete projection to the somatosensory cortex, subserves the sensory-discriminative aspects of pain.

In addition to its distinct identity as a somatic sensation, pain is usually associated with a characteristic unpleasant feeling tone and a desire to escape. These feelings represent the affective-motivational aspects of pain. They are largely independent of the location and nature of the stimulus but are directly related to its intensity. It might be argued that because similar unpleasant feelings can be produced by extremely bright lights, bad odors, or loud noises, they are not a necessary part of the pain experience and should be considered to be a separate phenomenon. On the other hand, it seems highly artificial to abstract pain from the very qualities that distinguish it from other somatic sensations.

In contrast to the uniformity of the sensory-discriminative aspects of pain, there is great variability in the suffering, unpleasantness, or anxiety reported by different individuals in response to apparently identical stimuli. This variability is manifested by differences between individuals in the vehemence of their complaints and in their capacity to tolerate very similar noxious stimuli (See Chapter 7).

Melzack and Casey (40) proposed that the paramedian pathway, with its diffuse projection to the limbic system and to the frontal lobe, primarily subserves the affective-motivational aspects of pain. Consistent with this idea is the well-established role of the brainstem reticular formation in behavioral arousal and in the generalized cortical arousal produced by a variety of sensory stimuli. In addition to producing arousal, the paramedian reticular formation plays an important role in escape behavior. The nucleus reticularis gigantocellularis of the medulla, which receives a dense spinal input via the anterolateral quadrant and projects to the intralaminar thalamus, contains neurons whose discharge in response to noxious stimulation is highly correlated with escape behavior. Furthermore, stimulation of the nucleus reticularis gigantocellularis or its projection target in the intralaminar thalamus produces escape behavior (5, 6). This evidence supports the idea that the paramedian pathway is essential for the motivational aspects of pain.

THE ROLE OF THE FRONTAL LOBE

Clinical observations of patients with frontal lobe lesions have provided important evidence that the affective components of pain are dependent on the integrity of the paramedian pain pathway. As mentioned above, there is a large projection from both the central lateral and submedius nuclei of the thalamus to the frontal lobe. At one time, extensive frontal lobotomies were used as a treatment of last resort in patients with otherwise intractable pain (2). The operation was successful in only about one-third of patients, and in those patients who did obtain relief the personality changes were striking. The patients became extremely apathetic about everything, including their pain. Interestingly, there was no elevation of pain threshold in the lobotomized patients (2). If anything, the pain threshold was actually lower. However, the patients only noticed their pain when their attention was called to it. When specifically asked about their pain, these patients would acknowledge its presence and often say that it was just as intense as before the operation; however, they exhibited very little behavior indicative of severe pain or anxiety and seldom complained or asked for pain medication. They had ceased to be worried about or even interested in their pain. As Freeman and Watts (17) put it, "Prefrontal lobotomy changes the attitude of the individual toward his pain, but does not alter the perception of pain."

A similar picture is produced by bilateral lesions of the medial thalamus. In contrast, lesions of the lateral thalamus, although producing a long-lasting impairment of cutaneous pain and temperature sensation, have little, if any, lasting effect on clinical pain. Lesions restricted to the lateral thalamus or somatosensory cortex do not produce apathy or other personality changes.

These clinical observations are consistent with the idea that the sensory-discriminative and affective-motivational aspects of pain have distinct neuroanatomic substrates. The paramedian pathway, with its ultimate projection to the limbic system and frontal lobes, is primarily involved with the affective-motivational aspects, whereas the lateral pathway, with its ultimate projection to the somatosensory cortex, is responsible for the sensory-discriminative aspects of pain. Despite this clear evidence of the dual nature of pain and of the central pathways that underlie it, there may be some overlap in function of the two systems. Under certain circumstances, the medial pathway is sufficient to produce both aspects of the pain experience. Thus, clinical pain, which usually arises from deep visceral or musculoskeletal structures, may be relatively unaffected by lesions of the lateral thalamus.

Summary

In summary, many of the subjective features of pain reported by human subjects are consistent with the properties of neurons in the established pain pathways. Nociceptive spinothalamic tract neurons have responses to noxious stimuli that parallel human subjective intensity ratings for the same stimuli. Such subjective phenomena as summation, first and second pain, and inhibitory interactions between different noxious stimuli are mirrored by similar responses in nociceptive spinothalamic tract cells. These observations provide compelling evidence that these neurons relay the information that underlies the perceptual event of pain. The rostrally projecting axons of these neurons enter the anterolateral quadrant, lesions of which produce profound and long-lasting deficits in pain sensation. The anterolateral quadrant, in turn, gives rise to two distinct pathways above the brainstem level. The lateral, or neospinothalamic, pathway projects to the somatosensory cortex and subserves the sensory-discriminative aspect of pain (Figure 3.15). The paramedian pathway projects to widespread cortical areas, including the frontal lobes, and underlies the affective-motivational aspects of pain.

References

1 Albe-Fessard, D., Berkley, K. J., Kruger, L., Ralston, H. J., III, and Willis, W. D., Jr.: Diencephalic mechanisms of pain sensation. *Brain Research Reviews* **9**:217–296, 1985.

2 Barber, T. X.: Toward a theory of pain: Relief of chronic pain by prefrontal leucotomy, opiates, placebos, and hypnosis. *Psychological Bulletin* **56**:430–460, 1959.

3 Basbaum, A. I.: Functional analysis of the cytochemistry of the spinal dorsal horn. In H. L. Fields et al. (eds.): *Advances in Pain Research and Therapy* (Vol. 9). Raven Press, New York, 1985.

4 Bittner, M. A., and Lahann, T. R.: Biphasic time-course of Capsaicin-induced substance P depletion: Failure to correlate with thermal analgesia in the cat. *Brain Res.* **322**:305–309, 1984.

5 Casey, K. L.: Responses of bulboreticular units to somatic stimuli eliciting escape behavior in the cat. *Int. J. Neurosci.* **2**:15–28, 1971.

6 Casey, K. L.: Escape elicited by bulboreticular stimulation in the cat. *Int. J. Neurosci.* **2**:29–34, 1971.

7 Cervero, F., and Iggo, A.: The substantia gelatinosa of the spinal cord. A critical review. *Brain* **103**:717–772, 1980.

8 Chung, J. M., Kenshalo, D. R., Jr., Gerhart, K. D., and Willis, W. D.: Excitation of primate spinothalamic neurons by cutaneous C-fiber volleys. *J. Neurophysiol.* **42**:1354–1369, 1979.

9 Chung, J. M., Lee, K. H., Kim, J., and Coggeshall, R. E.: Activation of dorsal horn cells by ventral root stimulation in the cat. *J. Neurophysiol.* **54**:261–272, 1985.

10 Coggeshall, R. E.: Afferent fibers in the ventral root. *Neurosurgery* **4**:443–448, 1979.

11 Coggeshall, R. E., Chung, K., Chung, J. M., and Langford, L. A.: Primary Afferent Axons in the tract of Lissauer in the monkey. *J. Comp. Neurol.* **196**:431–442, 1981.

12 Craig, A. D., and Burton, H.: Spinal and medullary lamina I projection to nucleus submedius in medial thalamus: A possible pain center. *J. Neurophysiol.* **45**:443–466, 1981.

13 Dong, W. K., Ryu, H., and Wagman, I. H.: Nociceptive responses of neurons in medial thalamus and their relationship to spinothalamic pathways. *J. Neurophysiol.* **41**:1592–1613, 1978.

14 Dubner, R., and Bennett, G. J.: Spinal and trigeminal mechanisms of nociception. *Annu. Rev. Neurosci.* **6**:381–418, 1983.

15 Fields, H. L., and Adams, J. E.: Pain after cortical injury relieved by electrical stimulation of the internal capsule. *Brain* **97**:169–178, 1974.

16 Fields, H. L., Clanton, C. H., and Anderson, S. D.: Somatosensory properties of spinoreticular neurons in the cat. *Brain Res.* **120**:49–66, 1977.

17 Freeman, W., and Watts, J. W.: *Psychosurgery—In the Treatment of Mental Disorders and Intractable Pain* (2nd ed.). Charles C. Thomas, Springfield, IL, 1950.

18 Gerhart, K. D., Yezierski, R. P., Giesler, G. J., Jr., and Willis, W. D.: Inhibitory receptive fields of primate spinothalamic tract cells. *J. Neurophysiol.* **46**:1309–1325, 1981.

19 Gowers, W. R.: A case of unilateral gunshot injury to the spinal cord. *Trans. Clin. Lond.* **11**:24–32, 1878.

20 Gregor, M., and Zimmermann, M.: Characteristics of spinal neurons responding to cutaneous myelinated and unmyelinated fibres. *J. Physiol. (Lond.)* **221**:555–576, 1972.

21 Jessell, T. M., and Jahr, C. E.: Fast and slow excitatory transmitters at primary afferent synapses in the dorsal horn of the spinal cord. In H. L. Fields et al. (eds.): *Advances in Pain Research and Therapy* (Vol. 9). Raven Press, New York, 1985.

22 Jones, E. G., and Leavitt, R. Y.: Retrograde axonal transport and the demonstration of non-specific projections to the cerebral cortex and striatum from thalamic intralaminar nuclei in the rat, cat and monkey. *J. Comp. Neurol.* **154**:349–378, 1974.

23 Kaufman, E. F. S., and Rosenquist, A. C.: Efferent projections of the thalamic intralaminar nuclei in the cat. *Brain Res.* **335**:257–279, 1985.

24 Kenshalo, D. R., Jr., Leonard, R. B., Chung, J. M., and Willis, W. D.: Responses of primate spinothalamic neurons to graded and to repeated noxious heat stimuli. *J. Neurophysiol.* **42**:1370–1389, 1979.

25 Kenshalo, D. R., Jr., Giesler, G. J., Jr., Leonard, R. B., and Willis, W. D.: Responses of neurons in primate ventral posterior lateral nucleus to noxious stimuli. *J. Neurophysiol.* **43**:1594–1614, 1980.

26 Kenshalo, D. R., Jr., and Isensee, O.: Responses of primate SI cortical neurons to noxious stimuli. *J. Neurophysiol.* **50**:1479–1496, 1983.

27 Kevetter, G. A., Haber, L. H., Yezierski, R. P., Chung, J. M., Martin, R. F., and Willis, W. D.: Cells of origin of the spinoreticular tract in the monkey. *J. Comp. Neurol.* **207**:61–74, 1982.

28 Kevetter, G. A., and Willis, W. D.: Collateralization in the spinothalamic tract: New methodology to support or deny phylogenetic theories. *Brain Res. Rev.* **7**:1–14, 1984.

29 King, R. B.: Postchordotomy studies of pain threshold. *Neurology* **7**:610–614, 1957.

30 Landau, W., and Bishop, G. G.: Pain from dermal, periosteal and fascial endings and from inflammation. *Arch. Neurol. Psychiatry* **69**:490–504, 1953.

31 Le Bars, D., Dickenson, A. H., and Besson, J. M.: Diffuse noxious inhibitory controls (DNIC). I. Effects on dorsal horn convergent neurones in the rat. *Pain* **6**:283–304, 1979.

32 Lewin, W., and Phillips, C. G.: Observations on partial removal of the post-central gyrus for pain. *J. Neurol. Neurosurg. Psychiatry* **15**:143–147, 1952.

33 Light, A. R., and Metz, C. B.: The morphology of the spinal cord efferent and afferent neurons contributing to the ventral roots of the cat. *J. Comp. Neurol.* **179:**501–516, 1978.

34 Light, A. R., and Perl, E. R.: Reexamination of the dorsal root projection to the spinal dorsal horn including observations on the differential termination of coarse and fine fibers. *J. Comp. Neurol.* **186:**117–132, 1979.

35 Lynn, B., and Hunt, S. P.: Afferent C-fibres: Physiological and biochemical correlations. *Trends Neurosci.* **7:**186–188, 1984.

36 Marshall, J.: Sensory disturbances in cortical wounds with special reference to pain. *J. Neurol. Neurosurg. Psychiatry* **14:**187–204, 1951.

37 Mayer, D. J., Price, D. D., and Becker, D. P.: Neurophysiological characterization of the anterolateral spinal cord neurons contributing to pain perception in man. *Pain* **1:**51–58, 1975.

38 McMahon, S. B., and Wall, P. D.: The distribution and central termination of single cutaneous and muscle unmyelinated fibres in rat spinal cord. *Brain Res.* **359:**39–48, 1985.

39 Mehler, W. R.: The anatomy of the so-called "pain tract" in man: An analysis of the course and distribution of the ascending fibers of the fasciculus anterolateralis. In J. D. French and R. W. Portor (eds.): *Basic Research in Paraplegia.* Charles C. Thomas: Springfield IL, 1962.

40 Melzack, R., and Casey, K. L.: Sensory, motivational, and central control determinants of pain. A new conceptual model. In D. Kenshalo (ed.): *The Skin Senses.* Charles C. Thomas, Springfield, IL, 1968, pp. 423–439.

41 Nahin, R. L., Madsen, A. M., and Giesler, G. J.: Anatomical and physiological studies of the gray matter surrounding the spinal cord central canal. *J. Comp. Neurol.* **220:**321–335, 1983.

42 Noordenbos, W., and Wall, P. D.: Diverse sensory functions with an almost totally divided spinal cord. A case of spinal cord transection with preservation of part of one anterolateral quadrant. *Pain* **2:**185–196, 1976.

43 Otsuka, M., Konishi, S., Yanagisawa, M., Tsunoo, A., and Akagi, H.: Role of substance P as a sensory transmitter in spinal cord and sympathetic ganglia. *Ciba Found. Symp.* **91:**13–34, 1982.

44 Peschanski, M., Guilbaud, G., and Gautron, M.: Posterior intralaminar region in rat: Neuronal responses to noxious and nonnoxious cutaneous stimuli. *Exp. Neurolog.* **72:**226–238, 1981.

45 Peschanski, M., and Besson, J. M.: A spino-reticulo-thalamic pathway in the rat: An anatomical study with reference to pain transmission. *Neuroscience* **12**:165–178, 1984.

46 Price, D. D., and Dubner, R.: Neurons that subserve the sensory-discriminative aspects of pain. *Pain* **3**:307–338, 1977.

47 Price, D. C., Hu, J. W., Dubner, R., and Gracely, R. H.: Peripheral suppression of first pain and central summation of second pain evoked by noxious heat pulses. *Pain* **3**:57–68, 1977.

48 Price, D. D., Hayes, R. L., Ruda, M. A., and Dubner, R.: Spatial and temporal transformations of input to spinothalamic tract neurons and their relation to somatic sensations. *J. Neurophysiol.* **41**:933–947, 1978.

49 Price, D. D., Hayashi, H., Dubner, R., and Ruda, M. A.: Functional relationships between neurons of marginal and substantia gelatinosa layers of primate dorsal horn. *J. Neurophysiol.* **42**:1590–1608, 1979.

50 Rexed, B.: A cytoarchitectonic atlas of the spinal cord in the cat. *J. Comp. Neurol.* **96**:415–495, 1952.

51 Ritz, L. A., and Greenspan, J. D.: Morphological features of lamina V neurons receiving nociceptive input in cat sacrocaudal spinal cord. *J. Comp. Neurol.* **238**:440–452, 1985.

52 Schuster, P.: Beitrage zur Pathologie des thalamus opticus. *Arch. Psychiatr. NervKrankh.* **105**:550–622, 1936.

53 Spiller, W. G., and Martin, E.: The treatment of persistent pain of organic origin in the lower part of the body by division of the anterolateral column of the spinal cord. *JAMA* **58**:1489–1490, 1912.

54 Urban, L., and Randic, M.: Slow excitatory transmission in rat dorsal horn: Possible mediation by peptides. *Brain Res.* **290**:336–341, 1984.

55 Wall, P. D.: The laminar organization of the dorsal horn and the effects of descending impulses. *J. Physiol. (Lond.)* **188**:403–423, 1967.

56 White, J. C., and Sweet, W. H.: *Pain and the Neurosurgeon.* Charles C. Thomas, Springfield, IL, 1969.

57 White, J. C., Sweet, W. H., Hawkins, R., and Nilges, R. G.: Anterolateral cordotomy: Results, complications and causes of failure. *Brain* **73**:346–367, 1950.

58 Willis, W. D.: *The Pain System.* S. Karger, Basel, 1985.

59 Willis, W. D., Kenshalo, D. R., Jr., and Leonard, R. B.: The cells of origin of the primate spinothalamic tract. *J. Comp. Neurol.* **188:**543–573, 1979.

60 Willis, W. D., and Coggeshall, R. E.: *Sensory Mechanisms of the Spinal Cord.* Plenum Press, New York, 1978.

61 Willis, W. D., Trevino, D. L., Coulter, J. D., and Maunz, R. A.: Responses of primate spinothalamic tract neurons to natural stimulation of hindlimb. *J. Neurophysiol.* **37:**358–372, 1974.

Chapter 4

Pain from Deep Tissues and Referred Pain

Pain from Deep Tissues

Pain-sensitive structures can be divided into three functional groups: the skin, the deep somatic (musculoskeletal), and the visceral. Although most clinically significant pains are produced by damage to deep somatic and visceral structures, our knowledge about pain transmission comes primarily from studies using cutaneous stimuli. This is because the skin is densely innervated and easily accessible to controlled, rapidly reversible noxious stimuli. The skin, however, is a highly specialized tissue and it is clear that pain from deep structures differs from that arising from the skin. For one thing, the types of stimuli required to evoke pain differ. Another difference is that the pain arising from deep structures is rarely as sharp and well localized as that produced by cutaneous stimuli.

It is likely that the function of deep pain differs from that of cutaneous pain. The skin encounters external noxious stimuli from which escape is possible and where speed of escape is crucial. For example, the rapid removal of an extremity from a hot or a sharp surface can prevent burns and lacerations. In these cases, accurate withdrawal movements require precise localization of the stimulus. For deep structures, the requirements are different. Pain from deep structures often results either from disease or from trauma that has already occurred, and it is immobilization of the structure rather than rapid escape that is required to prevent further damage. In this case, rapidity of transmission and precise localization are not crucial.

Our knowledge of the primary afferents that innervate deep structures such as muscle, joint, and gut is much less complete than that for cutaneous afferents. In contrast to cutaneous nociceptors, it is difficult to stimulate nociceptors in deep structures under conditions similar to those that "naturally" occur with tissue damage. Furthermore, although it is possible to show that there are classes of visceral afferent that respond best to intense stimuli, it is difficult to demonstrate that their activity results in pain. There have been no studies of deep receptors in humans; even in those cases where nociceptive primary afferents in a deep structure have been characterized in animals, the responses of those afferents to noxious stimuli have not been systematically compared with subjective reports in human subjects using similar stimuli.

DEEP SOMATIC AFFERENTS

In the majority of people, the most commonly occurring type of pain is of musculoskeletal origin. Both joint and muscle are innervated by Aδ and C primary afferents, which presumably include nociceptors.

In normal joints, about half of the Aδ and almost all C afferents respond only to extreme joint movements or to intense pressure around the joint capsule (12, 29, 30). Such stimuli would probably be painful. It is of interest and great importance that, when inflammation of a joint (arthritis) is experimentally induced, the Aδ and C primary afferents undergo a change similar to the sensitization of cutaneous nociceptors (8, 12). In contrast to the normal joint, when a joint is inflamed, most of the afferents in and around it can be activated by small movements well within the normal working range of the joint. The joint capsule mechanoreceptors also become much more sensitive to pressure. In addition to this increase in sensitivity, many of the Aδ and C joint afferents develop a relatively high background discharge in the absence of any joint stimulation. These changes clearly parallel the situation in patients with arthritis, whose joints are often painful, even at rest, and in whom slight movements or pressure over the joint are exquisitely painful.

Skeletal muscle is innervated by both Aδ and C primary afferent nociceptors. Some of the C fibers have properties similar to those of cutaneous polymodal nociceptors (16). They respond to high pressure, noxious heat, and certain chemicals, such as hypertonic saline, that are known to be painful when injected into human muscle (13, 14, 21, 22).

Skeletal muscle pain is particularly severe during contraction under conditions of ischemia, and there is a class of unmyelinated primary afferents that discharges maximally in response to muscle contraction under ischemic conditions (21, 23). These unmyelinated primary afferents seem likely to contribute to muscle pain. Responses to ischemia have also been demonstrated in many small-diameter afferents innervating the heart (2).

VISCERAL AFFERENTS

Our knowledge of visceral nociceptors is meagre. Although it has been possible to record from primary afferents that innervate the abdominal viscera, it has been difficult to identify them as nociceptors (5, 7). In part this is because visceral pain is relatively uncommon and the precise nature of the stimuli that produce it is not known. Surgeons report that viscera are relatively insensitive to cutting, heat, or pinching (3, 18), but twisting and distension are often effective noxious stimuli for hollow viscera such as the gut, ureter, gallbladder, and urinary bladder. Visceral pain is usually associated with inflammation or chemical irritants (such as stomach acid) and inflamed viscera are more likely to produce pain when stimulated. This suggests that, as is the case for joint afferents, visceral afferents become sensitized with inflammation. This issue has not been systematically studied.

Another complication is that the nerves that innervate many viscera run in close proximity to the blood supply. The blood vessels are invested with a dense plexus of small-diameter afferent axons (see Figure 2.11B, Chapter 2). Many blood vessels are known to be pain sensitive, and their nociceptors may make an important contribution to the pain arising from deep structures.

The best evidence relating particular receptors to abdominal visceral pain comes from studies of afferents innervating the biliary tree and the urinary bladder. Extreme distension of the urinary bladder is painful. There are Aδ and C afferents that innervate the bladder wall and respond with increasing discharge across the range of extreme bladder distension (9). In the gallbladder and bile duct, distension has been shown to be effective for producing pain in humans (32). In animal studies, using controlled pressure within the lumen, Cervero (4) showed that there are two classes of afferents. One class responds at low pressures; the other class begins to discharge only at pressures that produce blood pressure increases. Since blood pressure increases usually accompany the activation of other nociceptors, this was taken as evidence that the high-threshold class of bile-duct afferent is nociceptive.

In summary, although it is clear that deep somatic and visceral structures are pain sensitive, the primary afferent nociceptors whose activity results in pain is not definitely established for visceral organs. Animal studies have demonstrated primary afferents that discharge maximally only to apparently noxious stimuli. As is the case for skin, these visceral afferent nociceptors have either small myelinated or unmyelinated axons. In the case of joint nociceptors, prominent sensitization and spontaneous discharge accompany inflammation.

CENTRAL PATHWAYS OF VISCERAL NOCICEPTION (6, 7)

The viscera are innervated by two routes: either via the body wall through nerves that primarily innervate somatic structures or via nerves that are primarily of autonomic function, such as the splanchnics.

Most anatomic and physiological studies of the visceral sensory system have focused on the splanchnic innervation because the sensory component is devoid of somatic fibers. Afferents from the splanchnic nerve enter the spinal cord in the thoracic and upper lumbar region and terminate predominately in dorsal horn laminae I and V (Figure 4.1B). In contrast to the terminals of primary afferents in cutaneous nerves, there is very little, if any, splanchnic input to laminae II, III, and IV.

A large proportion of dorsal horn neurons receive visceral afferent input. Such neurons are found primarily in laminae I and V and in the deeper laminae (VII and VIII) (Figure 4.1A). All neurons that are excited by visceral afferent input have also been shown to receive somatic inputs. In other words, there are no spinal neurons that respond specifically to visceral stimuli. This may be one reason for the poor localization of visceral stimuli.

It is obviously difficult to know whether the visceral afferents to these spinal neurons are nociceptors. However, the weight of evidence indicates that the visceral input can elicit pain. For one thing, the overwhelming majority of dorsal horn cells that have visceral input also have a somatic input that is nociceptive (7). Furthermore, the visceral afferent input excites neurons of the ascending pathways usually implicated in pain transmission: the spinothalamic (24) and spinoreticular (6).

Referred Pain

There are important differences between the pain elicited from the skin and that arising from deep somatic and visceral tissues. One difference is in the quality of pain. Superficial pains have a sharp, pricking or burning quality, whereas the pain caused by stimulation of deep tissues, whether somatic or visceral, usually has an aching quality and is relatively dull. The ability to localize noxious stimuli is another striking difference. For example, touching the skin with a pin elicits a sharp sensation of rapid onset that is accurately localized to the site of stimulation. The accuracy of localization is best in those skin regions that have the greatest innervation density, such as the hands and face. In contrast, pain arising from deep structures is characteristically of gradual onset and is very poorly localized. In fact, the sensation produced by noxious visceral stimulation is rarely restricted to the site of stimulation. When pain is elicited experimentally or by disease of a deep visceral or somatic structure, the affected person usually

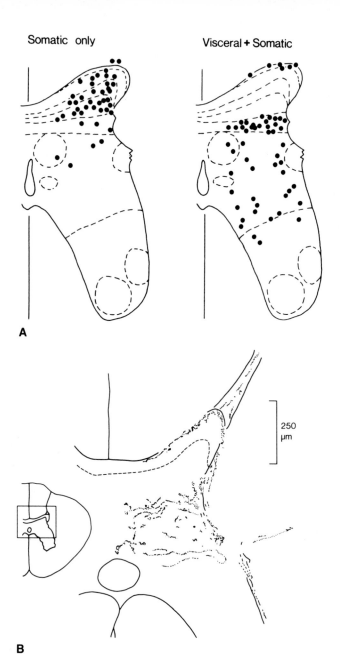

Somatic only

Visceral + Somatic

A

B

250 µm

Figure 4.1 A: Contrast between the location of cells that are activated by visceral and somatic afferents **(right)** and those activated only by somatic afferents **(left)**. (From Cervero, F.: Visceral nociception: Peripheral and central aspects of visceral nociceptive system. *Trans. R. Soc. Lond.* [*B*] **308:**325–337, 1985.) **B:** Illustration of the pattern of termination of primary afferents from the splanchnic nerve (in this case horseradish peroxidase was the marker, applied to the central end of the cut splanchnic nerve. (Adapted from Cervero, F.: Visceral nociception: Peripheral and central aspects of visceral nociceptive systems. *Trans. R. Soc. Lond.* [*B*] **308:**325–337, 1985.)

perceives pain in an area that is larger than the affected structure. For example, in the early stages of appendicitis, pain may be felt diffusely over the abdomen.

One of the most intriguing aspects of the pain that arises from a deep structure is that it may actually be felt in a body region remote from the site of pathology. This phenomenon is known as referred pain. Although somewhat variable from individual to individual, the pattern of referral has a distribution that is characteristic for a particular structure. One familiar example of this is the pain of myocardial infarction. With myocardial infarction, about 25 percent of patients report pain not only in the central chest beneath the sternum and in the upper abdomen but along the ulnar aspect of the left arm as well.

In many cases of pain from a specific deep structure, certain muscles become tender and certain areas of skin become hypersensitive, producing an exaggerated painful sensation when stimulated. In contrast to the referred pain itself, which is subjective and often has vague boundaries, the cutaneous hypersensitivity has definite margins and can be studied objectively. In a classic series of studies, Head (11) carefully recorded the patterns of referred pain and precisely mapped the zones of cutaneous hypersensitivity produced by diseases of different visceral organs. The zones of cutaneous hypersensitivity (now called Head's zones) and muscle tenderness largely overlap the areas to which pain is referred from a given organ, and are similar from patient to patient. Figure 4.2 illustrates some common patterns of cutaneous hyperalgesia elicited by disease of deep tissues. Because the boundaries of the zones of cutaneous hypersensitivity follow the margins of skin areas innervated by identified spinal segments (dermatomes), Head proposed that the zones are determined by the dorsal roots through which primary afferents from an organ gain access to the spinal cord.

The evidence for a segmental relationship between the deep structure stimulated and the region in which pain is perceived is most convincing for musculoskeletal structures. Using injection of hypertonic saline into muscle and the region around joints and periosteum, extensive maps have been constructed (13, 15) showing the consistent segmental patterns of pain referral for these structures (e.g., Figure 4.3). Although localization of noxious stimuli is not nearly as accurate for deep structures as for cutaneous stimuli, the correspondence between the site stimulated and the location of the perceived pain is best when the structure stimulated is near the body surface. For example, when the knee is injected, there is a reasonably good correlation between the site of stimulation and the location of perceived pain (Figure 4.4). When a muscle is injected, the pain is felt in a region that may or may not even include the injected muscle (Figure 4.5). The pain is generally referred to muscles innervated by the spinal segment that innervates the injected muscle. The same phenomenon is seen when ligaments and periosteum are stimulated with hypertonic saline (13).

When more deeply situated structures such as the deep abdominal or thoracic viscera are stimulated, the degree of mislocalization tends to be greater. The general rule is that the further the stimulated structure is from the body

Esophagus

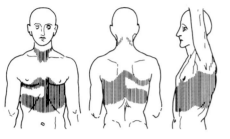

Angina

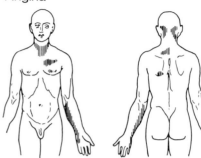

Left Ureter

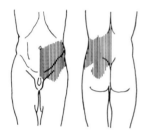

Urinary Bladder

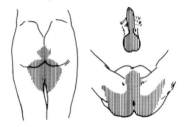

Labor Pain

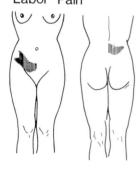

Right Lobe Prostate

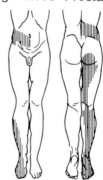

Figure 4.2 *Stippled regions* illustrate zones of cutaneous hyperalgesia produced by disease of different viscera. (Adapted from Head, H.: On disturbances of sensation with especial reference to the pain of visceral disease. *Brain* **16**:1–132, 1893.)

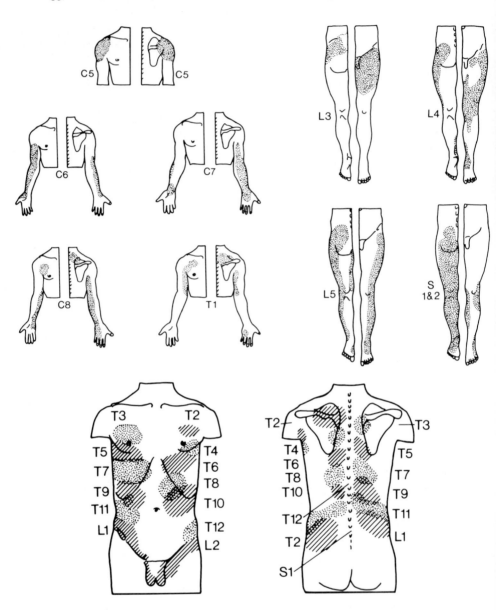

Figure 4.3 Patterns of referred pain and muscle tenderness produced by injecting 0.1–0.3 ml of 6% saline into the ligament between the spinous processes of
adjacent vertebrae. The injections were made just off the midline at the specified
spinal levels. (Adapted from Kellgren, J. H.: On the distribution of pain arising from
deep somatic structures with charts of segmental pain areas. *Clin. Sci.* **4:**35–46,
1939–1942.)

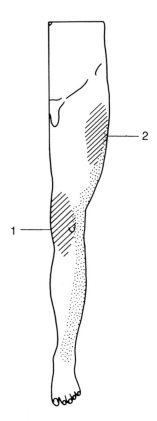

Figure 4.4 Distribution of pain produced by injecting hypertonic saline into different structures around the knee. Medial collateral ligament, (1) *hatching*; lateral part of the capsule, *stipple*; posterior part of capsule, (2) *hatching*. (From Kellgren, J. H.: On the distribution of pain arising from deep somatic structures with charts of segmental pain areas. *Clin. Sci.* **4**:35–46, 1939–1942.)

Kellgren reported that these injections produce a deep aching sensation. The pain is perceived at a distance from the site of injection (in the back). With this method, it is uncertain what structure is activated; however, the small volume would limit it to the ligament, the adjacent periosteum, or the paraspinous muscle. It is important to point out that, in the limbs, the distribution of pain is somewhat different than the classic dermatomal pattern. Occasionally the injections stimulated a nearby spinal nerve, which instances gave rise to a distinctive tingling and burning sensation.

Romboids   Serratus Anterior

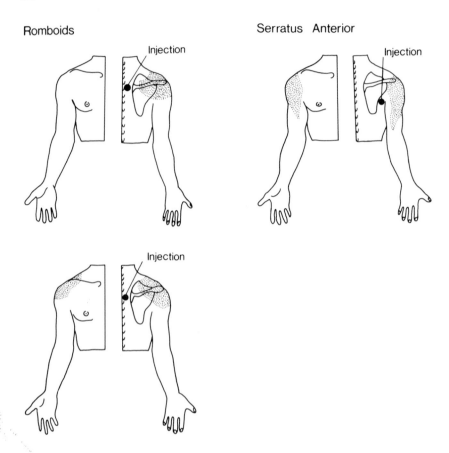

Figure 4.5   Mislocalization following muscle injection of hypertonic saline. (From Kellgren, J. H.: Observations on referred pain arising from muscle. *Clin Sci* **3:**175–190, 1937–1938.) **Left:** The rhomboids are located in the back, in the paraspinous region. When they are injected, the pain (*stippled zone*) is felt in the shoulder (deltoid, trapezius, and supraspinatus) and not near the injected muscle. **Right:** Pain from the serratus anterior, which is primarily located over the chest wall and under the scapula, is referred to the outer shoulder and arm, at a distance from the injected muscle.

surface the more distant is the site to which pain is referred. However, the pain tends to be referred to a somatic region that is innervated by the spinal segment(s) that innervate the stimulated visceral organ.

One of the most striking examples of the importance of the spinal segment in determining the site to which pain from a deep structure is referred is the diaphragm. The central region of the diaphragm is innervated by the third and fourth cervical spinal segments via the phrenic nerve. These spinal segments also innervate the skin and muscles of the neck and shoulder. When the central diaphragm is mechanically stimulated, pain is not perceived anywhere near its

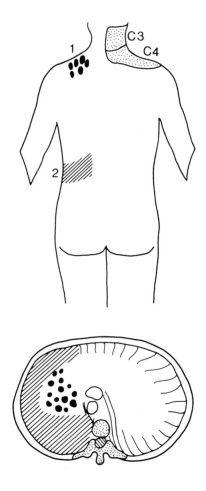

Figure 4.6 Referral patterns of pain from the diaphragm. Data collected by clinical examination and by mechanical stimulation of the diaphragm in patients with diseases affecting the nearby pleura and peritoneum. (Adapted from Capps, J. A. and Coleman, G. H.: *An Experimental and Clinical Study of Pain in the Pleura, Pericardium and Peritoneum.* Macmillan, New York, 1932.)

Mechanical stimulation of the pleural surface of the left side of the diaphragm (intrathoracic) produces sensation at two sites. If the central region of the diaphragm (*black dots*, **bottom**) is stimulated, a sharp pain is felt in the shoulder (at *1*, **top**). When the stimulus is applied to the outer region (*diagonal hatching*, **bottom**), the pain is felt in the adjacent lower chest and upper abdominal wall (at *2*, **top**).

The central region of the diaphragm is innervated by the phrenic nerve, which originates from the third and fourth cervical spinal segment. The site of referral of pain and the location of hyperalgesia is approximately the C3 and C4 dermatome (**top**).

A similar arrangement is found when the underside of the diaphragm (peritoneal surface) is stimulated.

actual thoracolumbar location, but is felt in the neck and shoulder regions innervated by the same spinal segments (Figure 4.6) (3). In contrast, when the outer edge of the diaphragm is stimulated, the pain is felt locally, presumably because this region of the diaphragm is innervated by intercostal nerves (T6–T10).

THEORIES OF THE MECHANISM OF REFERRED PAIN

Branched Primary Afferents

The clinical and experimental studies of referred pain have clearly established the importance of the gathering of afferents from widespread tissues into the dorsal root of a single spinal segment. A number of theories have been put forward to explain how this segmental convergence of primary afferents results in

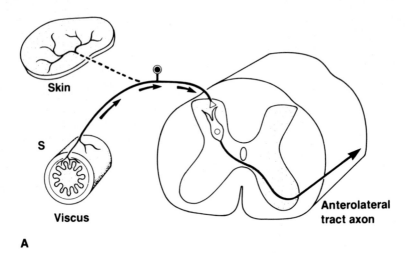

Skin

S

Viscus

**Anterolateral
tract axon**

A

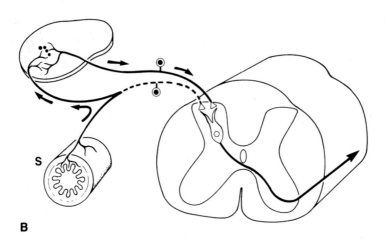

S

B

Figure 4.7 Theories of referred pain. **A:** Branched primary afferent. According to this theory, a single primary afferent branches to supply both the deep structure stimulated (S) and the structure in which the pain is perceived. **B:** Referred pain caused by antidromic activation of receptors at a distant secondary site. According to this theory, the misperception is due to antidromic conduction of impulses in a peripheral branch of the stimulated structure (S). Pain-producing substances are released from the peripheral terminals of the branch to the site of pain referral. Other nociceptors are activated and conduct the message to the CNS. In this case, the brain correctly localizes the site of origin of the nociceptive message but not the site of the original pathological process.

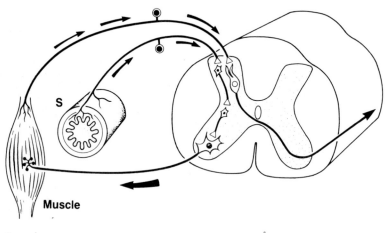

C

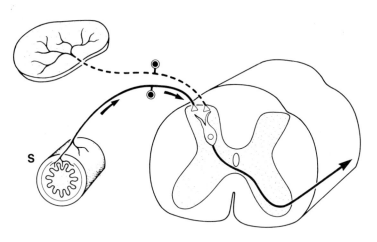

D

Figure 4.7C (*Continued*). Referred pain resulting from reflex muscle contraction that causes activation of a distant secondary site. In this situation, impulses originating in the stimulated structure (*S*) cause the reflex activation of motoneurons, which produces muscle contraction and activation of muscle nociceptors. As in the process described in **B**, the brain correctly localizes the active muscle nociceptor but not the site of the original pathology. **D:** The convergence-projection hypothesis of referred pain. According to this hypothesis, visceral afferent nociceptors (*S*) converge on the same pain-projection neurons as the afferents from the somatic structures in which the pain is perceived. The brain has no way of knowing the actual source and mistakenly "projects" the sensation to the somatic structure.

the mislocalization of sensory input from deep structures. According to one theory (31), a single primary afferent fiber branches to supply two structures, one visceral and one somatic (Figure 4.7A). This arrangement could contribute to referred pain in at least two ways. First, because the sensory messages from two different locations arrive over the same channel, there is the obvious problem of confusion as to their source. Since there is no nociceptive input from the site that is felt to be painful, we say that the brain has referred the sensation to the unstimulated site or structure.

Another mechanism by which branched axons could contribute to faulty localization would be through antidromic release of sensitizing chemicals such as substance P (31) (Figure 4.7B). This could occur in the following way. Impulses elicited in the branch of the nociceptor innervating the stimulated structure could antidromically invade the other branch, which innervates the unstimulated structure. The nociceptors in that structure could be sensitized by the chemicals released by the antidromic impulses in the branch. Those sensitized nociceptors could then respond to innocuous stimuli, and pain would be produced.

Recent anatomic studies have actually demonstrated that a very small percentage (approximately 1 percent) of dorsal root ganglion cells have two branches supplying two anatomically remote structures such as the shoulder and the diaphragm (17) or the arm and the pericardium (1). It is possible that this anatomic arrangement contributes to referred pain, but it is not known whether such branched afferents are present in other parts of the body.

Reflex Activation of Nociceptors

There is evidence that spinal reflex mechanisms contribute to the remote pain that is often produced by pathological processes in deep structures. One potentially important factor is muscle contraction. Input from visceral nociceptors is known to produce a powerful and sustained reflex muscle contraction (19) that is often associated with muscle tenderness (11, 18, 31). In this way, continued input from visceral nociceptors could lead to the development of a secondary source of nociceptive input from the contracting muscles (Figure 4.7C).

In addition to muscle contraction, a secondary locus of nociceptive input may be produced by activity in the sympathetic nervous system. There is no question that noxious input can elicit a significant increase in sympathetic outflow. This is usually manifested by increases in blood pressure, pupillary dilatation, piloerection, and sweating. There is also evidence that sympathetic efferent activity can produce pain. This is most apparent in patients with reflex sympathetic dystrophy, in whom sympathetic blockade produces immediate and sustained pain relief and raises the cutaneous pain threshold (26, 27). Furthermore, as will be discussed in Chapter 6, sympathetic efferent activity can sensitize and/or activate a variety of cutaneous afferents. These clinical and experimental observations support the concept that noxious input can reflexly induce sympathetic activity that in turn activates or sensitizes peripheral nociceptors.

The reflex activation of somatic motor and sympathetic outflow could contribute to the muscle tenderness and cutaneous hypersensitivity observed by Head in patients with visceral disease. In addition to contributing to referral of pain, such reflex outflow may sustain and intensify pain.

Perceptual Projection

According to either the antidromic release, muscle contraction, or sympathetic outflow mechanisms discussed above, activation of afferents from one region could lead to the secondary activation of distant nociceptors. Under these circumstances, the referral of pain is due to the accurate localization of input from peripheral nociceptors that are at a distance from the original pathological process. However, there are clinical conditions that cannot be explained by activation of nociceptors in the location where the pain is felt. The most striking of these conditions is phantom limb pain, in which the sensation is perceived as arising in a body part that no longer exists. In this condition, the mislocalization of the offending stimulus is apparently due to the activation of cells in the brain that are normally activated by receptors in the missing limb.

The mislocalization that occurs with phantom limb illustrates an important process that is part of normal perception. Somatic sensations are mental phenomena that are produced by activity in the brain but are usually perceived as occurring at the site where the stimulus is applied (i.e., in the body). This mental "displacement" of the perceived sensation to the body from the brain is called *projection*. Perhaps the clearest illustration of this process is what happens when the somatosensory cortex is electrically stimulated during a neurosurgical procedure. Stimulation applied to the hand area of the somatosensory cortex elicits a sensation that is perceived as if the stimulation were being applied to the hand (25).

The brain has a topographically arranged neuronal representation, or map, of the body. It seems likely that this map is the anatomic correlate of the mental image of the body. This neuronal map of the body persists, even when parts of the body are lost. The phantom limb is a projected mental image that depends on the persistence of the neuronal map of the missing body part. The important point is that, once the map is acquired, sensory input from a particular part of the body is no longer required for the brain to form and project a mental image. This conclusion is supported by studies of normal subjects. When the nerves to the arm are blocked with a local anesthetic, subjects still feel that the arm is there (20), although the perceived position of the arm may be incorrect (if the subjects' eyes are closed). The effect of sensory input is to modify rather than produce the mental image.

These observations indicate that the sensation elicited by a noxious stimulus is a projected image determined by the interplay of the sensory input with a preexistent spatial representation of the body in the brain. With this background it is somewhat easier to understand referred pain.

At present, the most widely accepted explanation of referred pain is the "convergence-projection" theory of Ruch (28) (Figure 4.7D). This theory also takes into account the fact that nociceptive primary afferent fibers innervating visceral organs enter the same spinal segment as the nociceptive somatic afferents innervating the body region to which pain from that organ is referred. According to the convergence-projection theory, the two types of afferents entering that spinal segment converge onto the same sensory projection cells (e.g., spinothalamic tract cells). Since the same projection cell could be activated by either the visceral or the somatic afferent, the message arriving at the brain could be due to stimulation at either site. However, because of the protected location of the viscera, the spinothalamic neuron is more frequently activated by somatic stimulation and consequently, over time, the brain comes to associate activity in that spinothalamic tract cell with somatic stimulation. The mental image elicited by activity in the spinothalamic cells receiving convergent input reflects this disparity. Subsequently, when visceral afferents activate the spinothalamic tract cell, the brain misinterprets the message and localizes the source of activity as the somatic structure. The sensation is said to be "projected" to the somatic site.

For example, part of the afferent input from the heart enters the first thoracic segment. This segment also receives afferent input from the skin of the first thoracic dermatome (the chest and the ulnar side of the left arm) as well as musculoskeletal structures innervated by that segment. With myocardial ischemia, spinothalamic tract cells in the first thoracic segment are activated by cardiac afferents instead of the usual input from the skin, joints, and muscles of the arm. The brain "projects" the sensation to the chest wall and arm because they are the usual source of the input.

In support of this theory, spinothalamic tract cells have been identified that receive convergent input from both visceral structures and cutaneous nociceptors (7). Furthermore, there is evidence for a specific segmental relationship between the visceral and somatic nociceptive input that converges upon spinal neurons. For example, there are cells in the cat thoracic spinal cord that respond both to cardiac ischemia and to cutaneous stimulation of the left shoulder and forelimb (10).

In summary, according to the convergence-projection theory, the mislocalization of sensations arising from stimulation of deep structures results from both their sparse innervation and the fact that their afferent innervation converges onto sensory projection neurons that also receive input from segmentally related somatic structures. The sensation is referred to the somatic structures because they are more commonly the source of the input that activates the projection cell.

Summary

It is likely that several mechanisms contribute to referred pain. In many instances, muscle contraction, tenderness, and cutaneous hyperalgesia are produced by pathology in visceral organs. In these cases it is possible that there are secondary peripheral sites of nociceptive input that account for the spread of pain. Consistent with this idea is the observation that local anesthetic injected into the site of referral provides significant relief. In other situations, local anesthetic injected at the site of referral has no effect on referred pain (31). In these latter cases, the mislocalization of pain is clearly due to a process in the central nervous system because there is no nociceptor input from the site in which the pain is felt.

Whatever the explanation, referred pain is an important phenomenon to be aware of in patients with puzzling pain problems. Pain of visceral and musculoskeletal origin is commonly projected to a distant, unstimulated structure and this is a potential source of confusion in patients whose diagnosis is in doubt. Obviously, if the cause of the pain is not within the area that hurts, the clinician may be misled when looking for objective evidence of disease. Although spatial patterns of referral are somewhat variable from patient to patient, the spinal segmental relationship between the diseased structure and the site of pain referral provides a basis for a systematic clinical examination.

References

1 Alles, A., and Dom, R. M.: Peripheral sensory nerve fibers that dichotomize to supply the brachium and the pericardium in the rat: A possible morphological explanation for referred cardiac pain? *Brain Res.* **342**:382–385, 1985.

2 Brown, A. M.: Excitation of afferent cardiac sympathetic nerve fibres during myocardial ischemia. *J. Physiol.* (Lond.) **190**:35–53, 1967.

3 Capps, J. A., and Coleman, G. H.: *An Experimental and Clinical Study of Pain in the Pleura, Pericardium and Peritoneum.* Macmillan, New York, 1932.

4 Cervero, F.: Afferent activity evoked by natural stimulation of the biliary system in the ferret. *Pain* **13**:137–151, 1982.

5 Cervero, F.: Mechanisms of visceral pain. *Pain* **4**:1–19, 1983.

6 Cervero, F.: Supraspinal connections of neurons in the thoracic spinal cord of the cat: Ascending projections and effects of descending impulses. *Brain Res.* **275**:251–261, 1983.

7 Cervero, F.: Visceral nociception: Peripheral and central aspects of visceral nociceptive systems. *Trans. R. Soc. Lond.* [*B*] **308**:325–337, 1985.

8 Coggeshall, R. E., Hong, K. A. P., Langford, L. A., Shaible, H. G., and Schmidt, R. F.: Discharge characteristics of fine medial articular afferents at rest and during passive movements of inflamed knee joints. *Brain Res.* **272:**185–188, 1983.

9 Floyd, K., Hick, V. E., and Morrison, J. F. B.: Mechanosensitive afferent units in the hypogastric nerve of the cat. *J. Physiol. (Lond.)* **259:**457–471, 1976.

10 Foreman, R. D., and Ohata, C. A.: Effects of coronary occlusion on thoracic spinal neurones receiving viscerosomatic inputs. *Am. J. Physiol.* **238:**667–674, 1980.

11 Head, H.: On disturbances of sensation with especial reference to the pain of visceral disease. *Brain* **16:**1–132, 1893.

12 Iggo, A., Guilbaud, G., and Tegner, R.: Sensory mechanisms in arthritic rat joints. In L. Kruger and J. C. Liebeskind (eds.): *Neural Mechanisms of Pain.* Advances in Pain Research and Therapy (Vol. 6). Raven Press, New York, 1984.

13 Inman, V. T., and Saunders, J. B. deC. M.: Referred pain from skeletal structures. *J. Nerv. Ment. Dis.* **99:**660–667, 1944.

14 Kellgren, J. H.: Observations on referred pain arising from muscle. *Clin. Sci.* **3:**175–190, 1937–1938.

15 Kellgren, J. H.: On the distribution of pain arising from deep somatic structures with charts of segmental pain areas. *Clin. Sci.* **4:**35–46, 1939–1942.

16 Kumazawa, T., and Mizumura, K.: Thin fibre receptors responding to mechanical, chemical and thermal stimulation in the skeletal muscle of the dog. *J. Physiol. (Lond.)* **273:**179–194, 1977.

17 Laurberg, S., and Sorensen, K. E.: Cervical dorsal root ganglion cells with collaterals to both shoulder skin and the diaphragm. A fluorescent double labelling study in the rat. A model for referred pain? *Brain Res.* **331:**160–163, 1985.

18 Lewis, T.: *Pain.* Macmillan, New York, 1942.

19 Lewis, T., and Kellgren, J. H.: Observations relating to referred pain, visceromotor reflexes and other associated phenomena. *Clin. Sci.* **4:**47–71, 1939–42.

20 Melzack, R., and Bromage, P. R.: Experimental phantom limbs. *Exp. Neurol.* **39:**261–269, 1973.

21 Mense, S., and Meyer, H.: Different types of slowly conducting afferent units in cat skeletal muscle and tendon. *J. Physiol. (Lond.)* **363:**403–417, 1985.

22 Mense, S., and Schmidt, R. F.: Activation of group IV afferent units from muscle by algesic agents. *Brain Res.* **72:**305–310, 1974.

23 Mense, S., and Stahnke, M.: Responses in muscle afferent fibres of slow conduction velocity to contractions and ischaemia in the cat. *J. Physiol. (Lond.)* **342:**383–397, 1983.

24 Milne, R. J., Foreman, R. D., Giesler, G. J., Jr., and Willis, W. D.: Convergence of cutaneous and pelvic visceral nociceptive inputs onto primate spinothalamic neurones. *Pain* **2:**163–183, 1981.

25 Penfield, W., and Boldrey, E.: Somatic motor and sensory representation in the cerebral cortex of man as studied by electrical stimulation. *Brain* **60:**389–443, 1937.

26 Procacci, P., Francini, F., Maresca, M., and Zoppi, M.: Cutaneous pain threshold changes after sympathetic block in reflex dystrophies. *Pain* **1:**167–175, 1975.

27 Procacci, P., Francini, F., Maresca, M., and Zoppi, M.: Skin potential and EMG changes induced by cutaneous electrical stimulation. *Appl. Neurophysiol.* **42:**125–134, 1979.

28 Ruch, T. C.: Pathophysiology of pain. In T. C. Ruch and H. D. Patton (Eds.): *Physiology and Biophysics.* Saunders, Philadelphia, 1965, pp. 345–363.

29 Schaible, H. G., and Schmidt, R. F.: Activation of groups III and IV sensory units in medial articular nerve by local mechanical stimulation of knee joint. *J. Neurophysiol.* **49:**35–44, 1983.

30 Schaible, H. G., and Schmidt, R. F.: Responses of fine medial articular nerve afferents to passive movements of knee joint. *J. Neurophysiol.* **49:**1118–1126, 1983.

31 Sinclair, D. C., Weddell, G., and Feindel, W. H.: Referred pain and associated phenomena. *Brain* **71:**184–211, 1948.

32 Zollinger, R.: Observations following distention of the gallbladder and common duct in man. *Proc. Soc. Exp. Biol. Med.* **30:**1260–1261, 1933.

Chapter 5

Central Nervous System Mechanisms for Control of Pain Transmission

In Chapters 2 and 3 the pain message was traced along neural pathways from the peripheral receptor to the cortex. Neurons in the dorsal horn, thalamus, and cortex showed responses to noxious stimuli that were seen to be well correlated with the intensity of the stimulus applied. Furthermore, the psychophysical studies described demonstrated a similar correlation between stimulus intensity and the intensity of pain reported by human experimental subjects. By themselves, these observations would suggest that the relationships among stimulus intensity, activity in pain transmission cells, and the perceived intensity of pain are simple and reproducible.

Despite the appealing simplicity of this conclusion and the elegance of the studies supporting it, clinical observations indicate that such an excellent correlation between stimulus intensity and reported pain is unusual outside the psychophysical laboratory. In fact, the severity of pain may range from minimal to unbearable in different individuals with apparently similar injuries, and it is obvious that the subjectively experienced intensity of pain depends not only on the stimulus intensity but to a very large extent on psychological factors. For example, Beecher (8) and later Carlen et al. (16) observed that a high proportion of soldiers with severe battle wounds reported little or no pain. Many of the wounded expressed surprise at the painlessness of the injury. In contrast, civilian

patients with equivalent injuries complained of severe pain (8). Another example
of how perception can be modified by situational factors is the susceptibility of
pain to placebo administration (31). Thus, if subjects in pain are led to believe
that they have received an effective therapy, many will report significant relief
even if the therapy is an inert substance (placebo). This indicates that psychological factors can have a major influence on the intensity of perceived pain.
How do such factors modify pain perception? Although we are far from understanding all the complexities of the human mind, we now know that there are
specific pathways in the central nervous system (CNS) that control pain transmission, and there is evidence that these pathways can be activated by psychological factors. This chapter outlines the anatomy, physiology, and pharmacology of the systems that control pain transmission and reviews the evidence that
they contribute to the variability of the pain experience in humans.

The neuronal systems that modify pain are fundamentally different from the
more familiar sensory systems. Stimulation of a sensory system produces sensation, whereas stimulation of a sensory modulatory system will either reduce
or enhance the effect of activity in a sensory system. It will have no perceptual
or behavioral effect unless there is concomitant activity in the sensory system
that it modulates. Thus, in the absence of nociceptor activity the pain modulatory
system has no behavioral effect. When there is a noxious input, activation of
this system selectively reduces pain intensity.

Stimulation-Produced Analgesia (27, 56)

Although the variability of pain had been appreciated for many years, the concept of an independent and specific CNS network that modified pain sensation
was first suggested by the observation that electrical stimulation of the midbrain
in rats selectively suppressed responses to painful stimuli. The inhibition was
apparently selective for pain because the rats were able to ambulate and to respond to innocuous stimuli. The importance of this phenomenon, termed *stimulation-produced analgesia* (SPA), was confirmed when neurosurgeons placed
electrodes in homologous midbrain sites in humans (Figure 5.1) and demonstrated that stimulation produced a striking and selective reduction of severe
clinical pain (7, 45, 64). Although not all patients respond, there have since
been a sufficient number of cases successfully treated by different surgical
groups to warrant confidence that midbrain stimulation does relieve pain. The
observations of SPA in humans are particularly revealing because they indicate
that the neural system activated by the stimulation specifically modulates pain
sensation. There are no consistent objective or subjective phenomena that accompany the analgesia. Patients report a fading of their pain over a period of
minutes. Occasionally there is a feeling of warmth or relaxation, but nothing to
indicate that sensory impairment or distraction is the cause of the relief. The

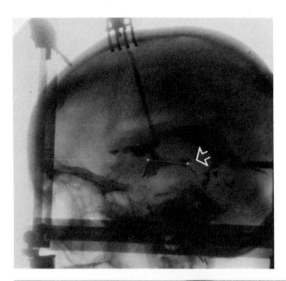

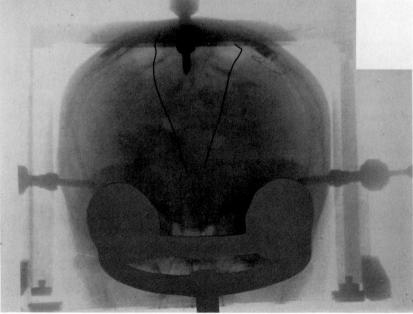

Figure 5.1 Stereotaxic method of electrode implantation in a human subject with chronic pain. **Top:** Lateral view of radiograph of patient's cranium in the stereotaxic frame. Radiopaque medium is used to reveal the ventricular system. The target for placement of the electrodes is lateral to the point where the cerebral aqueduct meets the caudal end of the third ventricle (*arrow*). **Bottom:** AP view of same patient, showing electrodes in place. (Radiographs courtesy of Professor John E. Adams.)

specificity of the analgesic effect constitutes powerful evidence for the existence of a neural network that can selectively control pain.

The behavioral similarity of SPA in humans and in experimental animals and the fact that it is elicited from anatomically homologous sites in several species (rat, cat, nonhuman primate, and human) are important for several reasons. First, this reduces the likelihood that human SPA is a placebo effect and, second, it indicates that the blockade of nociceptive responses in animals is a correlate of reduced pain intensity rather than a reflection of decreased motor responsiveness. Furthermore, it indicates that some of the neural mechanisms underlying pain modulation are similar in all species. We now know that the analgesic effect of midbrain stimulation is due to activation of a pain-modulating circuit that projects via the medulla to the spinal cord dorsal horn. This descending pain-modulating circuit, which contains high concentrations of endogenous opioid peptides, can also be activated by opiate analgesics such as morphine and by certain kinds of stress.

Anatomy of Descending Pain-Modulating Circuits (5, 6, 27, 73)

In humans, SPA is elicited by stimulation of the midbrain in the region of the periaqueductal gray matter (PAG) (Figure 5.2). SPA can also be elicited from contiguous but slightly more rostral sites in the periventricular gray matter of the hypothalamus. More lateral sites have not been systematically explored, so the exact boundaries of the effective areas for SPA are not known. In animals, SPA can also be elicited from the midbrain and the periventricular hypothalamus. At the midbrain level the most effective sites are ventral to the cerebral aqueduct and include areas lateral to the PAG (Figure 5.3). These midbrain and hypothalamic analgesia-producing areas are interconnected anatomically (1, 10, 54). In addition, the midbrain region receives major inputs from the rostral medulla, the spinal cord, and the frontal lobe (41). It is likely that the spinal inputs play an important role in pain modulation because noxious somatic stimuli consistently activate the modulatory network under physiological conditions. The cortical contribution to pain modulation has not yet been systematically studied.

In addition to the midbrain sites, the rostroventral medulla (RVM) is another region in which electrical stimulation is highly effective for suppressing nociceptive responses in animals (80). This region (Figure 5.3) includes the midline serotonin-containing nucleus raphe magnus and the adjacent reticular formation. The behavioral effects of RVM stimulation are similar to those of PAG stimulation. This is not surprising since the RVM receives its major input from the PAG and the adjacent midbrain reticular formation.

A third region that is effective in inhibiting nociceptive responses is the lateral and dorsolateral pontine tegmentum (Figure 5.4) (43, 57). This area, which contains many noradrenergic neurons, has not been as extensively studied as have the PAG and RVM. Some of the neurons in this area project to the PAG, and some to the RVM. There is also a large direct projection to the spinal cord from this area.

Since PAG and RVM stimulation inhibit the spinal withdrawal reflexes that are commonly used to assess "analgesia" in animals, a descending pathway to the spinal cord must be involved. In fact, lesions of the dorsolateral white matter of the spinal cord block the PAG- or RVM-induced inhibition of spinal withdrawal reflexes. Thus there is a pathway in the dorsolateral funiculus (DLF) that modulates nociceptive responses.

The major brainstem projections to the spinal cord via the DLF arise from the RVM and dorsolateral pons (Figure 5.4). Since there is only a minor direct projection from the PAG to the spinal cord via the DLF, the pain-inhibiting effect of PAG stimulation must be relayed to the spinal cord through the RVM. In fact, the major input to the RVM is from cells located in the PAG and the immediately adjacent midbrain areas that are most effective for SPA. Stimulation of the PAG has a predominately excitatory effect on RVM cells that project to the spinal cord (30). Furthermore, either lesions of or injection of local anesthetic into the RVM block the spinal effects of PAG stimulation (9, 35).

Thus, the RVM gives rise to a major projection to the spinal cord via the DLF. The terminals of this projection are concentrated in those dorsal horn laminae (I, II, and V) that contain both the terminals of nociceptive primary afferents and cell bodies of spinothalamic tract neurons (Figure 5.5). Stimulation of either the PAG or RVM inhibits nociceptive neurons in these laminae, including identified spinothalamic tract neurons in primates (28, 73). Cells in lamina IV (which do not respond differentially to noxious stimuli) are not inhibited by RVM stimulation. The concentration of the terminals of the descending RVM projection in laminae I, II, and V, and the specificity of the RVM's inhibitory action for nociceptive neurons in these laminae, may explain the selectivity of PAG stimulation in modifying pain sensation.

In summary, there is a nociceptive modulatory network with major anatomic components at midbrain, pontine, and medullary levels. Electrical stimulation at these sites produces behavioral analgesia and inhibits dorsal horn nociceptive neurons.

BIOGENIC AMINE TRANSMITTERS (1, 5, 13, 22, 65)

As mentioned above, there is one projection to the spinal cord that originates in the dorsolateral pons and another that arises from the rostral ventral medulla (Figures 5.4 and 5.5). The former includes noradrenergic and the latter serotonergic neurons.

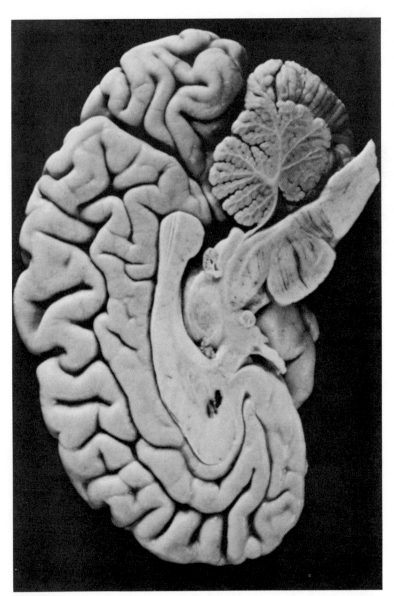

Figure 5.2A Anatomic structures underlying stimulation-produced analgesia in humans. **Top:** Sagittal section of human brain. (From Gluhbegovic, N., and Williams, T.: *The Human Brain.* Harper & Row, Philadelphia, 1980.) **Bottom:** Key to structures: *A,* cerebral aqueduct connecting third (3) and fourth ventricles; *C.C.,* corpus callosum; *P,* pineal; *S,* superior colliculus.

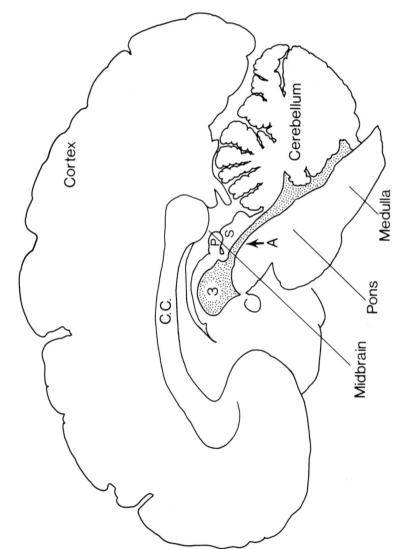

Figure 5.2A (*Continued*)

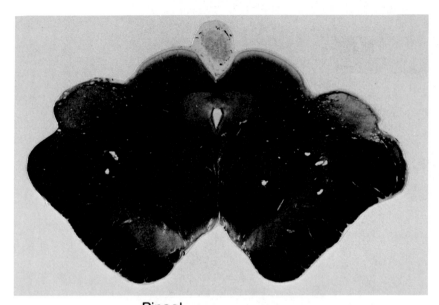

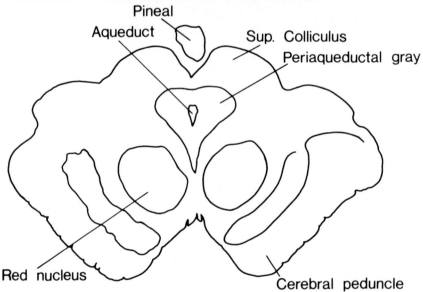

Pineal
Aqueduct   Sup. Colliculus
                                  Periaqueductal gray

Red nucleus

Cerebral peduncle

Figure 5.2B. (*Continued*).   **Top:** Coronal section, at level of midbrain.
Bottom: Key to structures.

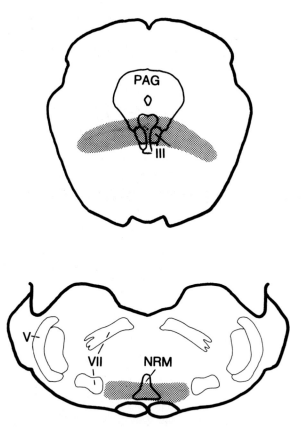

Figure 5.3 Most effective brainstem regions for SPA in the rat. **Top:** The midbrain level. The best sites are ventral to the cerebral aqueduct and extend both lateral and ventral to the periaqueductal gray (*PAG*). *III*, oculomotor nucleus. **Bottom:** At the medullary level, the most effective region lies between the facial nerve nuclei (*VII*) and includes the nucleus raphe magnus (*NRM*). *V*, trigeminal nucleus. (Adapted from Fields, H. L., and Heinricher, M. M.: Anatomy and physiology of a nociceptive modulatory system. *Phil. Trans. R. Soc. Lond.* [*B*] **308:**361–374, 1985.)

A significant number of the spinally projecting neurons located in the lateral and dorsolateral pons contain noradrenaline (71, 72). It is likely that some of these neurons project to the superficial dorsal horn. Application of norepinephrine directly to the spinal cord blocks behavioral responses to noxious stimuli (63) and selectively inhibits nociceptive dorsal horn neurons (11, 22). The noradrenergic inhibition of nociceptive transmission at the level of the spinal cord is mediated by an α_2 adrenergic receptor. There is a high concentration of α_2 binding sites in the superficial layers of the dorsal horn (70). The α_2 agonist clonidine inhibits nociceptive dorsal horn neurons (32) and produces analgesia

Pons

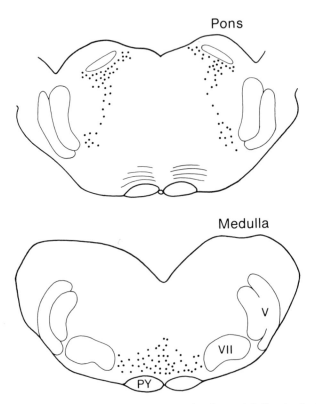

Medulla

Figure 5.4 Locations of proposed pain-modulating brainstem neurons that project to the spinal cord via the dorsolateral funiculus. **Top:** Cells in the lateral and dorsolateral pontine tegmentum. A high percentage of these cells contain norepinephrin, a biogenic amine implicated in pain modulation. **Bottom:** The rostroventral medulla (RVM), which contains a high proportion of serotonergic neurons. Serotonin has also been implicated in pain modulation. *V,* trigeminal nucleus; *PY,* pyramid; *VII,* facial nucleus.

when directly applied to the spinal cord (76). Furthermore, α_2 antagonist drugs such as yohimbine partially block the antinociceptive action of brainstem stimulation (4).

There is also a large body of evidence implicating serotonin in pain modulation (2, 12, 15, 65). The RVM contains a high percentage of spinally projecting serotonergic neurons (14). In fact the RVM is the major, if not the sole, source of serotonin in the dorsal horn (20). Nociceptive spinothalamic tract neurons in the dorsal horn receive a direct serotonergic input. Serotonin inhibits dorsal horn nociceptive neurons, including spinothalamic tract cells (47), and the inhibition of nociceptive spinothalamic tract neurons by RVM stimulation is partially blocked by serotonin antagonists (79). Consistent with these anatomic and physiological studies, direct application of serotonin to the spinal cord produces analgesia (77), and serotonergic antagonists or neurotoxins that selectively destroy

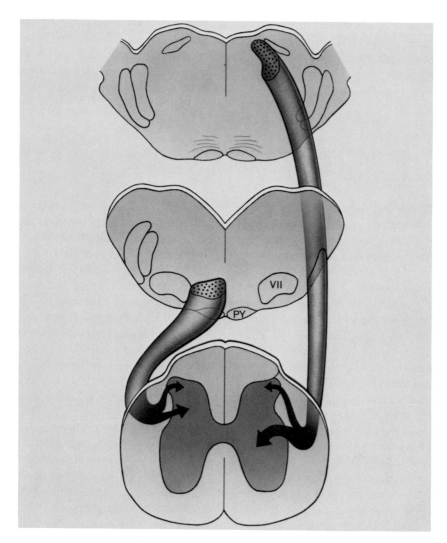

Figure 5.5 Descending axons of cells in the dorsolateral pons (*top right*) and rostroventral medulla (*middle left*). They run via the dorsolateral funiculus to terminate in the dorsal horn (most densely in laminae I and II). *PY,* pyramid; *VII,* facial nucleus.

serotonergic neurons reduce the analgesic actions of brainstem stimulation. Thus, spinally projecting serotonergic neurons in RVM contribute to analgesia by inhibiting dorsal horn pain transmission neurons.

In addition to the spinal projections of brainstem biogenic amine neurons, which clearly play an important role in control of nociception, there are major noradrenergic and serotonergic connections within the brainstem. The brainstem nuclei that are known to be part of the nociceptive modulating systems are densely innervated by biogenic amine terminals. The ventrolateral PAG, the RVM, and the dorsolateral pontine noradrenergic cell groups all receive both noradrenergic and serotonergic inputs. The contributions of these intrinsic brainstem biogenic amine connections to nociceptive modulation are presently unknown.

Opiate Activation of Pain-Modulating Networks (23, 26, 30, 74)

Opium derivatives are the most powerful analgesic agents presently available. Although the opiates produce many effects, including sedation, constipation, and respiratory depression, their analgesic potency is prominent enough so that over the centuries they have remained the preferred treatment for severe acute pain.

Opiates produce analgesia by a direct action on the CNS. The injection of small amounts of opiates directly into the brain can produce potent analgesia. For example, as little as 2 mg of morphine injected into the lateral ventricle can relieve severe pain in human patients (50, 60). The usual systemic dose to produce the same effect would be at least 5 to 10 times greater. In animals, where injections can be made directly into the substance of the brainstem, extremely sensitive sites have been found. The most extensive mapping of opiate sensitivity has been carried out in the rat. Both the PAG and the RVM are highly sensitive to morphine. Although the anatomic resolution of microinjection studies does not approach that of electrical stimulation, the brainstem regions that produce analgesia when electrically stimulated largely overlap those at which opiate microinjection produces analgesia. These data suggest that systemically administered opiates such as morphine produce analgesia in part by activation of the nociceptive modulating system. This concept is supported by the observation that the narcotic antagonist naloxone, when injected into either the PAG or the RVM, reverses the analgesic action of systemically administered opiates.

Although an action at the brainstem clearly contributes to pain inhibition, it does not entirely account for the analgesic potency of systemically administered opiates. First of all, the tissue levels of opiate produced at the microinjection site in the PAG or RVM are much higher than would be achieved by the systemic dose needed to produce the same level of analgesia. Furthermore, Yaksh and his colleagues have clearly demonstrated in rats and primates that application of opiates directly to the spinal cord produces a profound, selective, and local analgesic effect (75), an observation that has been amply confirmed in the clinical setting (18). At first, this observation called into question the importance of the brainstem contribution. However, it now seems clear that opiate-sensitive systems at both spinal cord and brainstem levels contribute to morphine analgesia. Thus, rats that are either spinalized or have bilateral DLF lesions require a higher dose of morphine to suppress withdrawal reflexes. Furthermore, when morphine is simultaneously injected at spinal and brainstem levels a much lower total dose is required, suggesting that a multiplicative interaction of the two levels contributes to the sensitivity of the nervous system to the effects of systemically administered opiates (78). In other words, when opiates are administered systemically, they act simultaneously at widely distributed sites in the CNS that interact to produce the analgesic effect.

OPIATE RECEPTOR (17, 55, 68)

The analgesia produced by opiate drugs depends on their action at a specific site on neuronal cell membranes, the opiate receptor. This receptor can be thought of as a common molecular site of action for different opiate analgesics. The receptor has two distinct functions: chemical recognition and biological action. These functions are thought to occur in different subregions of the receptor complex. The recognition site of the opiate receptor is highly specific. One indication of this is that the analgesic action of opiate alkaloids (plant derived or synthetic) is stereospecific; only the levo-isomers have biological activity. Opiates attach (bind) to the recognition site with varying strength. The strength of attachment is termed binding affinity. Binding sites are usually characterized by determining the rank order of binding affinity of a group of compounds. In order to relate opiate binding to analgesia it is necessary to demonstrate, for a group of drugs, that the rank order of analgesic potency is the same as the rank order of binding affinity. Figure 5.6 illustrates that this relationship holds for the opiate alkaloids and provides the basis for defining an opiate analgesia receptor.

The concept of a distinct and specific opiate receptor is also supported by the existence of highly specific opiate antagonists. Opiate antagonists were produced by synthesis of compounds that are slightly altered forms of the opiate agonist alkaloids. Figure 5.7 illustrates two such antagonists, nalorphine and naloxone, which were made by substitution of an allyl group for a methyl on the nitrogen of the agonists of morphine and oxymorphone, respectively. Naloxone has a high affinity for the receptor but it does not produce the biological effect produced by agonists such as morphine. It presumably works by displacing agonists from the receptor recognition site. Naloxone blocks the analgesic effect of all opiate agonists and precipitates withdrawal in individuals who are tolerant to opiates.

With continued exposure of tissues to high concentrations of opiate agonists, the potency of the drug declines so that progressively higher concentrations are required to produce the same degree of analgesia. This phenomenon, called tolerance, is characteristic of opiates. All opiate analgesic drugs produce tolerance, and when tolerance develops there is cross-tolerance to the other opiate analgesics.

In summary, a drug is said to produce analgesia by an action at the opiate receptor if its effect is stereospecific, is reversed by naloxone, and shows cross-tolerance to other opiates.

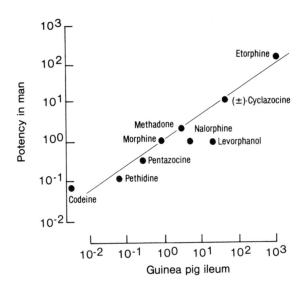

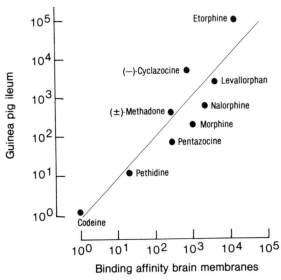

Figure 5.6 **Top:** Opiate alkaloids ranked on the basis of their clinical analgesic potency relative to morphine. For each compound, the clinical analgesic potency is plotted against its efficacy in inhibiting contraction of the guinea pig ileum. The close similarity in the rank order of potency of compounds in these two biological assays indicates that a similar receptor is involved. Both effects are reversed by naloxone. **Bottom:** A similar relationship of rank-order potencies holds for binding affinity to certain rat brain membranes. This is consistent with the idea that the binding sites on these brain membranes are associated with the opiate receptor that mediates analgesia. (Adapted from Kosterlitz, H. W. Opiate actions in Guinea Pig ileum and mouse vas deferens. In S. H. Snyder and S. Matthysse (eds.), Opiate Receptor Mechanisms. *Neurosci. Res. Program Bull.* **13:**68–73, 1975.)

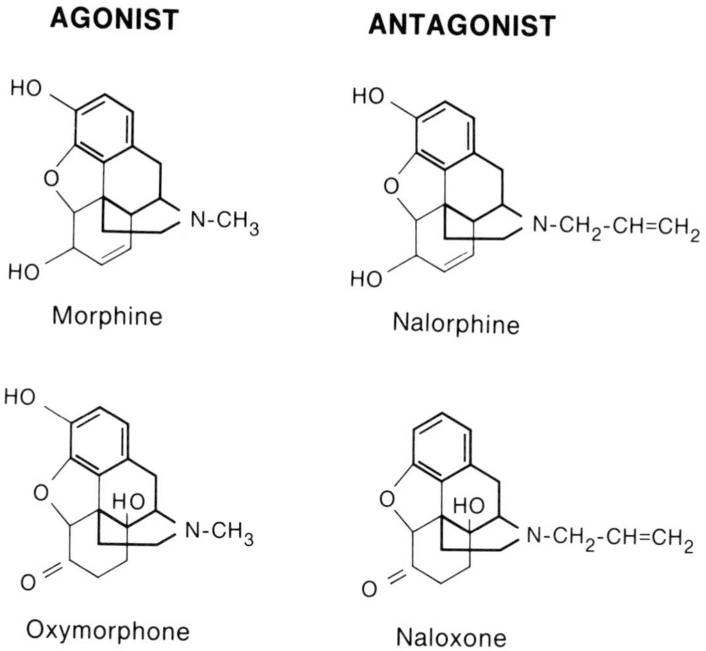

AGONIST

ANTAGONIST

Morphine

Nalorphine

Oxymorphone

Naloxone

Figure 5.7 The structures of some common opiate agonists and antagonists. The structure common to both agonists and antagonists is indicated by the heavy lines. In the antagonists an allyl group replaces the methyl group on the nitrogen.

This definition of the opiate receptor paved the way for two important advances: the characterization and localization of opiate receptors within the brain, and the isolation and purification of endogenous opioid compounds.

It has been possible to map the distribution of opiate receptors in the brain using radioactive opiates (either high-affinity agonists or antagonists). Such receptors are widely distributed in the CNS. As expected, the PAG and the superficial dorsal horn of the spinal cord, which are highly sensitive to opiate application, contain relatively dense concentrations of opiate binding sites. The RVM, which is also extremely sensitive to the analgesic effect of opiates, has not yet been carefully studied for receptor density.

Clearly, opiate agonists produce a variety of biological actions. In addition to analgesia, opiates produce respiratory depression, pupillary constriction and decreases in body temperature and gut motility. Part of this functional diversity is due to the presence of opiate receptors in tissues that are not involved in analgesia. For example, dense concentrations of opiate receptors are found in regions of the CNS such as the caudate nucleus and hippocampus, where opiate microinjection does not produce analgesia.

Another factor that may contribute to the diversity of opiate action is the existence of multiple receptor types (17, 55). Several distinct classes of opiate receptor have been defined based on binding characteristics and in vitro biological actions. Three types have been reasonably well characterized: μ, δ, and κ. In general, opiate alkaloids have a higher affinity for the μ (for morphine) binding site. Since the original description of the μ site was based, in part, on clinical analgesic potency, it is no surprise that the relative affinity of opiates for the μ site parallels their analgesic potency. Furthermore, recently developed synthetic compounds that are more selective than morphine for the μ site retain analgesic potency (25).

It is not clear whether receptors other than μ play a role in analgesia. Animal studies indicate that δ and κ ligands have a range of analgesic efficacy that is distinct from that of the μ ligands. There is some evidence from animal studies to suggest that δ- and κ-selective compounds may be particularly effective when applied directly to the spinal cord. However, at present there are no convincing clinical data to support the idea that opiates can produce analgesia by an action at the δ or κ receptor.

Endogenous Opioid Peptides

Once the actions and properties of the opiate receptor had been clearly defined, the hunt for endogenous ligands for the receptor intensified. Researchers reasoned that the brain itself ought to synthesize molecules that would act at these highly specific receptor sites. The first major breakthrough occurred when Hughes and his colleagues (46) reported that they had isolated two endogenous opioids from the brain, the pentapeptides leucine- and methionine-enkephalin (Table 5.1). These compounds have actions that are pharmacologically similar to morphine, are reversed by naloxone, and show cross-tolerance to morphine. The enkephalins are relatively weak analgesic agents, but this may be due to their rapid degradation by tissue enzymes. Appropriate inhibitors of these enzymes enhance the analgesic action of enkephalins (21, 69). Furthermore, metabolically stable analogs of met- and leu-enkephalin are much more potent in producing analgesia (58).

Since the discovery of the enkephalins, a number of other endogenous opioid peptides have been discovered. Table 5.1 illustrates the major groups. As with other peptide neurotransmitters and hormones, the endogenous opioid peptides are derived by cleavage from much larger precursor molecules that give rise to multiple biologically active fragments. Although all endogenous opioid peptides so far characterized contain the amino acid sequence tyr-gly-gly-phe-, there are at least three different precursor molecules (Figure 5.8): proenkephalin A, pro-opiomelanocortin (POMC), and proenkephalin B (prodynorphin).[1]

---

[1]*Endogenous opioid peptide* is a generic term that refers to naturally occurring peptides that contain the tyr-gly-gly-phe-sequence and are derived by metabolic breakdown

Table 5.1 Major Groups of Endogenous Opioid Peptides

Name	Amino acid sequence
Leucine-enkephalin	Tyr-Gly-Gly-Phe-Leu-OH
Methionine-enkephalin	Tyr-Gly-Gly-Phe-Met-OH
β-Endorphin	*Tyr-Gly-Gly-Phe-Met*-Thr-Ser-Glu-Lys-Ser-Gln-Thr-Pro-Leu-Val-Thr-Leu-Phe-Lys-Asn-Ala-Ile-Val-Lys-Asn-Ala-His-Lys-Gly-Gln-OH
Dynorphin	*Tyr-Gly-Gly-Phe-Leu*-Arg-Arg-Ile-Arg-Pro-Lys-Leu-Lys-Try-Asp-Asn-Gln-OH
α-Neoendorphin	*Tyr-Gly-Gly-Phe-Leu*-Arg-Lys-Tyr-Pro-Lys

From the standpoint of analgesia, the proenkephalin A–derived peptides are presently the most interesting. Proenkephalin A gives rise to multiple copies of met-enkephalin and one leu-enkephalin. In addition, longer fragments of 7, 8, 12, and 22 amino acids that include the met-enkephalin sequence are natural cleavage products of proenkephalin A (Figure 5.8). In some animal studies, the longer enkephalin fragments have been reported to produce more potent analgesic effects than leu- or met-enkephalin (44). Although the larger enkephalin fragments are released in significant amounts from adrenal medullary chromaffin cells, it is not yet clear which peptides are released by proenkephalin A–containing neurons of the CNS.

POMC gives rise to β-endorphin, the most potent endogenous opioid peptide yet discovered. Prodynorphin gives rise to the dynorphins. So far, the prodynorphin-derived fragments have not been proven to be very potent in producing analgesia.

Soon after these endogenous opioid peptides were identified, their anatomic distribution was studied. The enkephalins are found in the gut, sympathetic nervous system, and adrenal medullary chromaffin cells as well as being widely distributed in the CNS. Of particular interest in the context of this discussion is the close association of the enkephalins with structures involved in nociceptive control (48, 62). There is a high concentration of enkephalin-containing cell bodies and nerve terminals in the PAG, the RVM, and laminae I, II, V, and X of the spinal cord (Figures 5.9 and 5.10). The dynorphin peptides are also found in these locations, but in different cells whose locations do not completely overlap those containing the enkephalins (e.g.(19)). β-Endorphin has a much more restricted distribution in the brain. β-Endorphin-containing cells are present in the arcuate nucleus of the basal hypothalamus and the nucleus of the solitary tract. The axons of the hypothalamic β-endorphin neurons course along the wall of the third ventricle and terminate in the PAG and the locus ceruleus.

---

of any one of the three large precursor peptides. *Endorphin* refers to the endogenous opioid peptides derived from POMC.

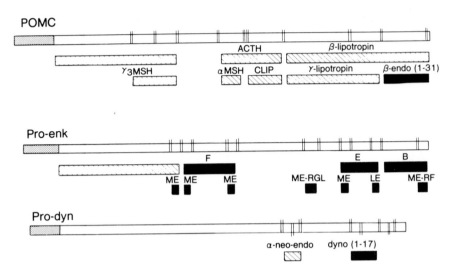

Figure 5.8 The three families of endogenous opioid peptides. Each of the precursor molecules gives rise to multiple biologically active peptide fragments, about half of which are shown in this diagram. The *double vertical lines* indicate common cleavage sites. The *horizontal bars* indicate some of the naturally occurring peptide fragments; *stipple,* signal peptide; *diagonal hatching,* cleavage product not analgesic; *black,* peptide with demonstrated analgesic potency. **Top:** Pro-opiomelanocortin (*POMC*), so named because it gives rise to β-endorphin (β-*endo*), melanocyte-stimulating hormone (*MSH*), adrenocorticotropic hormone (*ACTH*), and corticotropin-like intermediate lobe peptide (*CLIP*). **Middle:** Proenkephalin (*Pro-enk*) gives rise to multiple copies of met-enkephalin (*ME*), a leu-enkephalin (*LE*), and several "extended" enkephalins including ME-arg-gly-leu (*ME-RGL*), ME-arg-phe (*ME-RF*), and peptides E, F, and B. Peptide E is further broken down into a family of "large enkephalins" that appear to be the most potent analgesic fragments derived from proenkephalin. **Bottom:** Prodynorphin (*Pro-dyn*) gives rise to dynorphin (*dyno*), which contains the LE sequence, and neoendorphin (*neo-endo*). It is not clear whether prodynorphin-derived fragments have analgesic activity.

In summary, there are three families of endogenous opioid peptides, each derived from a different precursor and having a somewhat different anatomic distribution. The enkephalins, derived from proenkephalin A, β-endorphin from POMC, and the dynorphins from prodynorphin are all present in the PAG. The enkephalins and dynorphins are also present in the RVM and in regions of the spinal dorsal horn involved in nociception. Thus all of the known opioid peptide families are present in structures identified with nociceptive modulation. The fact that opiates are so highly effective in producing analgesia when microinjected into the PAG, RVM, and superficial dorsal horn strongly supports the conclusion that the endogenous opioid peptides normally function to relieve pain. These observations also indicate that narcotic analgesics, when adminis-

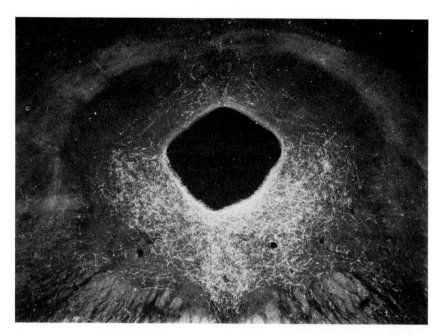

Figure 5.9A   Darkfield photomicrograph illustrating the distribution of β-endorphin immunoreactivity at the level of the midbrain. With this technique, the immunoreactivity is bright. The β-endorphin is concentrated within the ventral and ventromedial periaqueductal gray matter. (Photograph courtesy of Professor A. Basbaum.)

tered systemically, produce analgesia by mimicking the action of endogenous opioid peptides in the PAG, RVM, and spinal cord.

Physiological Properties of Brainstem Pain-Modulation Neurons (30)

In order to understand how neurons in the brainstem nuclei inhibit nociception, it is necessary to study how their activity is altered by noxious stimuli and by manipulations that produce analgesia (e.g., morphine administration). Neurons in both the PAG and the RVM have been studied under these conditions. When tested with noxious stimuli, cells in brainstem pain-modulating regions fall into three categories: those whose firing increases, those whose firing decreases, and those that are unaffected. On close examination, these neuronal "responses" are quite distinct from those of the pain transmission cells. First, changes in activity of pain-modulating neurons can usually be elicited by noxious stimuli anywhere on the body surface. Second, the changes in cell firing have a closer temporal association with the withdrawal reflex than with the noxious stimulus that elicits

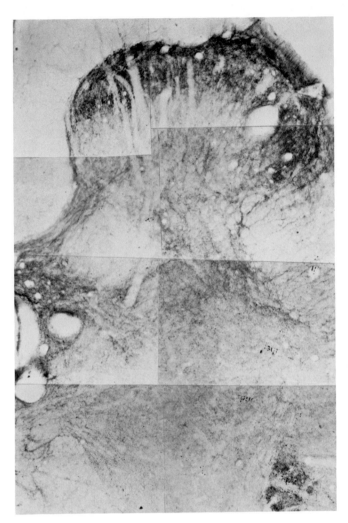

Figure 5.9B *(Continued).* Brightfield photomicrograph of leucine-enkephalin-like immunoreactivity (*dark material*) in the dorsal horn of the spinal cord. Note the dense enkephalin staining in the superficial dorsal horn and laminae I and II. (Photograph courtesy of Professor A. Basbaum.)

withdrawal. In other words, the change in cell firing is more closely related to the response than to the stimulus.

One type of pain-modulating cell, the "off–cell," pauses just prior to withdrawal (Figure 5.11). Such cells are located in PAG and RVM regions where electrical stimulation is particularly effective for inhibiting pain transmission. Since electrical stimulation excites all cells, the RVM and PAG output cells that inhibit nociceptive transmission will be active during electrical stimulation. In other words, sustained activity in pain-modulating brainstem neurons blocks no-

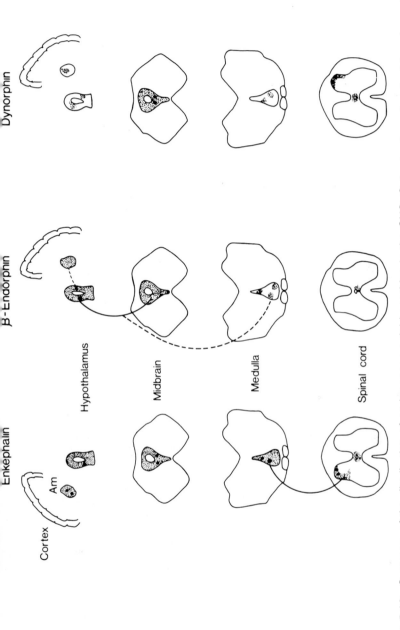

Figure 5.10 Summary of the distribution of endogenous opioid peptides in the CNS. Only structures involved in pain modulation or transmission are included. **Left:** Proenkephalin-derived peptides have the most extensive distribution. They are present in cells and terminals in the amygdala (*Am*), the hypothalamus, the midbrain PAG, the RVM, and the spinal cord dorsal horn and lamina X. **Middle:** β-Endorphin in the CNS. It is largely derived from cells in the arcuate nucleus of the hypothalamus. There is a significant amount in the PAG, and much less in the medulla and cord. **Right:** Dynorphin-related peptides. These roughly parallel the distribution of proenkephalin peptides, but there is less dynorphin in the hypothalamus and RVM.

119

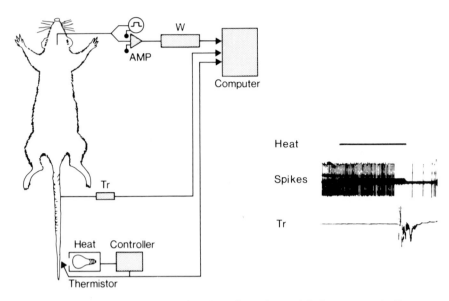

Figure 5.11A Physiological properties of a pain-modulating neuron in the medulla. **Left:** Recording set-up. A microelectrode was placed in a region of the medulla (RVM) from which "analgesia" could be produced by very low stimulation currents. Noxious stimuli (heat) were applied to the rat's tail. The heat-induced withdrawal reflex was recorded using a transducer (*Tr*). **Right:** One of the cell types in RVM. *Top trace:* duration of heat stumulus. *Middle trace:* action potentials. *Bottom trace:* tail withdrawal elicited by noxious heat. Activity in this cell stops just prior to withdrawal. This pattern defines it as an "off–cell," which has been proposed as the RVM cell that inhibits pain transmission (30). The pause in its firing would "permit" transmission of the pain message.

ciceptor-induced reflexes. If maintained activity of the inhibitory output cell inhibits the reflex, *the inhibitory output cell should reduce its firing to permit the withdrawal to occur.* The off–cell fulfills this expectation. During electrical stimulation of the RVM the off–cell cannot pause, and the withdrawal reflex is inhibited. There are several other observations that are consistent with the idea that the off–cell is the RVM output neuron that inhibits spinal nociceptive transmission. First, some off–cells project to the spinal cord. Second, all off cells are excited by PAG stimulation at the threshold for inhibiting withdrawal reflexes. Finally, off cells are the only RVM neurons that are excited by morphine when given systemically or microinjected into the PAG (Figure 5.11). These observations suggest that morphine produces its analgesic effect in part by activating off–cells in the PAG and RVM (30).

Another type of cell shows a burst of firing just prior to the occurrence of withdrawal. Because of its firing pattern, this cell, the "on–cell," is unlikely to be inhibitory at the spinal level. The presence of such a cell, however, raises the

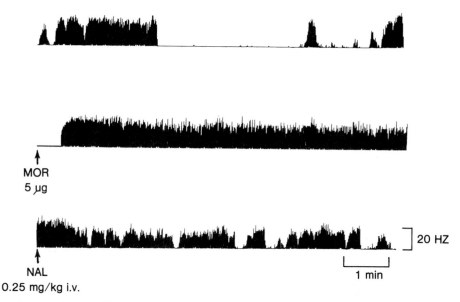

Figure 5.11B (*Continued*). Morphine excitation of an RVM off–cell. Vertical scale is spikes per second, horizontal scale is time. *Top trace:* control period. *Middle trace:* morphine (*MOR*), given at the arrow, causes a shift from intermittent to continuous firing. During this time, withdrawal reflexes are inhibited and there is no off–cell pause. This effect is reversed (*bottom trace*) by the opiate antagonist naloxone (*NAL*).

intriguing possibility that the pain-modulating system includes networks that enhance as well as inhibit pain transmission.

Spinal Mechanisms for Inhibition of Pain (67, 73)

At the present time our knowledge of how these descending pathways inhibit nociceptive transmission at the spinal level is sketchy. The problem is the great functional diversity of the neurons and neuronal connections within the dorsal horn. Much of what we do understand about the circuitry comes from studies that identify neural elements by the type of transmitter they contain. For example, virtually all serotonin in the superficial dorsal horn originates from brainstem neurons, primarily those in the RVM. There are direct contacts from these serotonergic descending neurons to spinothalamic cells in lamina I. Both RVM stimulation (36) and serotonin iontophoresis (47) have an inhibitory action on nociceptive spinothalamic tract neurons. Figure 5.12 illustrates the direct inhibitory connection to dorsal horn pain transmission cells.

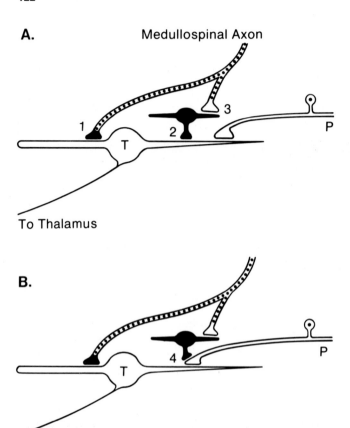

A.

Medullospinal Axon

To Thalamus

B.

Figure 5.12   Spinal circuits underlying descending inhibition of pain transmission.
A: Descending medullospinal axons, some of which are serotonergic, can inhibit
spinothalamic tract neurons (*T*) by either direct postsynaptic inhibition (*1*) or by
activating an inhibitory interneuron (*3*) that then postsynaptically inhibits the T cell
(*2*). Some of these inhibitory interneurons contain endogenous opioid peptides.
B: Alternatively, the inhibitory interneuron may presynaptically inhibit (*4*) the spinal
terminal of the nociceptive primary afferent, *P.*

There are connections from serotonin neurons to enkephalin-containing
cells in the substantia gelatinosa (37). Spinal enkephalinergic cells project heav-
ily to nearby spinothalamic neurons (66). Since opiates are inhibitory to nociceptive dorsal horn cells, it is assumed that these enkephalinergic cells are inhibitory interneurons. Presumably, serotonin would excite the enkephalinergic
interneuron. Figure 5.12 illustrates this indirect inhibitory connection.

Both of the mechanisms illustrated in Figure 5.12A are postsynaptic, that
is, the nociceptive transmission cell itself is directly inhibited by a synapse on
its cell soma or dendrite. There is also evidence for a presynaptic inhibitory
action upon the terminals of nociceptive primary afferents (Figure 5.12B). Pri-

mary afferents are known to have opiate receptors on their central branches (29, 42) and opiates reduce the release of transmitter from primary afferents (59). It is possible that locally released or circulating endogenous opioid peptides act on the spinal terminals of primary afferent nociceptors to block transmitter release.

In addition to the circuitry outlined above, it is virtually certain that other transmitter systems contribute to the control of nociceptive transmission in the dorsal horn. Norepinephrine and γ-aminobutyric acid are important inhibitory transmitters in the superficial layers of the dorsal horn (15); however, the details of their anatomic connections have not yet been worked out. In addition, there are numerous peptides in the superficial dorsal horn whose function is mysterious. A complete understanding of the interactions and connections of neurons with these different neurotransmitters is a prerequisite for decoding dorsal horn physiology.

Physiological Activation of Opioid-Mediated Analgesia Systems (5, 30, 34)

The close anatomic association of the endogenous opioid peptides with pain-modulating networks provided very powerful support for the concept that these peptides actually contribute to analgesia under physiological conditions. This idea has received some support from studies showing that SPA can be partially reduced by the narcotic antagonist naloxone (3, 45). Furthermore, there is a circadian or diurnal variation of pain sensitivity (Figure 5.13). Since naloxone dramatically attenuates the periodic reduction of pain responsivity, it probably involves endogenous opioid peptides (33).

Given that there is an opioid-mediated analgesia system, what are the conditions under which it is brought into play? The most reliable way to activate the analgesia network is by noxious stimulation. Noxious stimuli that are relatively intense and long lasting can reduce the responses of animals to subsequent noxious stimuli. Such analgesia can be reversed by naloxone or by lesions of the pain-modulating network. It seems likely that stress is actually more important than pain as an activator of the analgesia system. Analgesia can be produced by a variety of stressors that are not painful, including restraint, hypoglycemia, and fear. For example, exposing a rat to a cat causes a marked, naloxone-reversible reduction in withdrawal from noxious stimuli. In addition, if a cue, such as a tone or light, is repeatedly presented prior to a noxious stimulus, rats will become "analgesic" when the cue alone is presented (6).

Thus, in laboratory animals, pain, stress, fear, and conditioning all contribute to activation of the opioid-mediated analgesia system. However, the source and identity of the opioid peptides involved in this analgesic effect are presently unknown. In some cases, the analgesia can be blocked by adrenalectomy. This observation, plus the high concentrations of enkephalins demonstrated in the

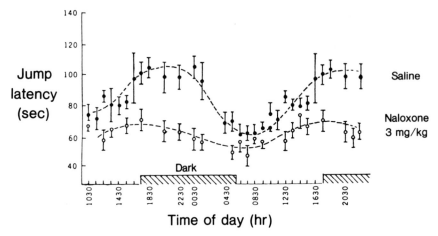

Figure 5.13   Circadian rhythm of pain sensitivity in the mouse. Sensitivity to noxious stimuli tested by measuring the time for mice to jump off a hot plate. The sensitivity drops significantly during the night. This nocturnal "analgesia" is markedly reduced by naloxone, suggesting that it is mediated by endogenous opioid peptides. (Adapted from Frederickson, R. C. A., Burgis, V., and Edwards, J. D.: Hyperalgesia produced by naloxone follows diurnal rhythm in responsivity to painful stimuli. Science **199**:756–758, 1977.)

adrenal medullary chromaffin cells, raise the possibility that, during stress, enkephalins are released along with adrenaline and reach the nervous system through the circulation. In addition to the possibility of their release from the adrenal medulla, the close anatomic association of the opioid peptides with brainstem pain-modulating nuclei makes it likely that release of opioid peptides within the CNS also contributes to stress induced analgesia. Opioid peptides thus could act either as hormone or neurotransmitter or both.

Do Endogenous Opioid Peptides Produce Analgesia in Humans?

Although there is little question about the variability of pain perception in/humans, it has been difficult to prove that the opioid-mediated pain-modulating system described above is responsible. Opiate receptors (49) and endogenous opioid peptides (24, 38) are present in human brain. The peptides are present in human spinal fluid (61), and intrathecal microinjection of opiates into supraspinal (50, 60) or spinal sites (18) produces analgesia in humans. It is not certain whether the anatomy of pain-modulating circuits is the same in humans as in animals; however, the pathway from the PAG to the spinal cord via the RVM has been demonstrated in all species studied to date, including the rat, cat, opossum, and monkey. Furthermore, the demonstration of SPA from the PAG in humans provides an important anatomic link between human and animal studies. There is controversy over whether SPA in humans is naloxone reversible. If it were, it would provide important support for the idea that opioid peptides contribute to human analgesia.

Another approach to this question is to administer naloxone to subjects who have not received opiates. The rationale is that, since naloxone ordinarily has little effect unless opiates are present, any effect produced by naloxone in subjects who have not had an exogenous opiate must be due to its antagonism of an endogenous opioid. Interestingly, naloxone usually has little effect on experimental pain (39), but clinical pain, especially if severe, is consistently worsened by naloxone (31, 53). This is particularly intriguing since stress seems to be a major factor in activating opioid-mediated pain-modulating systems in animals.

Also of interest in this regard is the observation that placebo administration can produce striking relief of postoperative pain in humans. This relief is, in large part, blocked by naloxone (40, 51, 52). In certain painful situations, the suggestion of relief seems to trigger opioid release.

Summary

There is a network within the central nervous system that can selectively inhibit pain. This network has important brainstem components, including the midbrain periaqueductal gray matter and adjacent reticular formation, which project to the spinal cord via the rostroventral medulla. This pathway inhibits spinal neurons that respond to noxious stimuli. There is also a pain-modulating pathway from the dorsolateral pons to the cord. The pathway from the rostral medulla to the cord is partly serotonergic, whereas that from the dorsolateral pons is at least partly noradrenergic. In addition to these biogenic amine–containing neurons, endogenous opioid peptides are present in all the regions so far implicated in pain modulation. This opioid-mediated analgesia system can be activated by electrical stimulation or by opiate drugs such as morphine. It can also be activated by pain, stress, and suggestion. Although by no means proven, it seems probable that this pain-modulating system contributes to the well-known variability of perceived pain in people with apparently similar injuries.

References

1 Abols, I. A., and Basbaum, A. I.: Afferent connections of the rostral medulla of the cat: A neural substrate for midbrain-medullary interactions in the modulation of pain. *J. Comp. Neurol.* **201**:285–297, 1981.

2 Akil, H., and Liebeskind, J. C.: Monaminergic mechanisms of stimulation-produced analgesia. *Brain Res.* **84**:279–296, 1975.

3   Akil, H., Mayer, D. J., and Liebeskind, J. C.: Antagonism of stimulation-produced analgesia by naloxone, a narcotic antagonist. *Science* **191**:961–962, 1976.

4   Barbaro, N. M., Hammond, D. L., and Fields, H. L.: Effects of intrathecally administered methysergide and yohimbine on microstimulation-produced antinociception in the rat. *Brain Res.* **343**:223–229, 1985.

5   Basbaum, A. I., and Fields, H. L.: Endogenous pain control systems: Brainstem spinal pathways and endorphin circuitry. *Annu. Rev. Neurosci.* **7**:309–338, 1984.

6   Basbaum, A. I., and Fields, H. L.: Endogenous pain control mechanisms: Review and hypothesis. *Ann. Neurol.* **4**:451–462, 1978.

7   Baskin, D. S., Mehler, W. R., Hosobuchi, Y., Richardson, D. E., Adams, J. E., and Flitter, M. A.: Autopsy analysis of the safety, efficacy and cartography of electrical stimulation of the central gray in humans. *Brain Res.* **371**:231–236, 1986.

8   Beecher, H. K.: *The Measurement of Subjective Responses.* Oxford University Press, New York, 1959.

9   Behbehani, M. M., and Fields, H. L.: Evidence that an excitatory connection between the periaqueductal grey and nucleus raphe magnus mediates stimulation-produced analgesia. *Brain Res.* **170**:85–93, 1979.

10   Beitz, A. J.: The organization of afferent projections to the midbrain periaqueductal grey of the rat. *Neuroscience* **7**:133–159, 1982b.

11   Belcher, G., Ryall, R. W., and Schaffner, R.: The differential effects of 5-hydroxytryptamine, noradrenaline and raphe stimulation on nociceptive and non-nociceptive dorsal horn interneurons in the cat. *Brain Res.* **151**:307–321, 1978.

12   Berge, O.-G., Hole, K., and Ogren, S.-O.: Attenuation of morphine-induced analgesia by *p*-chlorophenylalanine and *p*-chloroamphetamine: Test-dependent effects and evidence for brainstem 5-hydroxytryptamine involvement. *Brain Res.* **271**:51–64, 1983.

13   Bloom, F. E.: Neurohumoral transmission and the central nervous system. In A. G. Gilman et al. (eds.): *The Pharmacological Basis of Therapeutics.* Macmillan, New York, 1985.

14   Bowker, R., Westlund, K. N., and Coulter, J. D.: Origins of serotonergic projections of the spinal cord in rat: An immunocytochemical-retrograde transport study. *Brain Res.* **226**:187–199, 1981.

15   Brownstein, M. J., and Palkovitz, M.: Catecholamines, serotonin, acetylcholine, and γ-aminobutyric acid in the rat brain: biochemical studies. In A. Bjorklund and

T. Hökfelt (eds.): *Handbook of Chemical Neuroanatomy*, Vol. 2: *Classical Transmitters in the CNS*. Amsterdam, Elsevier, 1984.

16 Carlen, P. L., Wall, P. D., Nadvorna, H., and Steinbach, R.: Phantom limbs and related phenomena in recent traumatic amputations. *Neurology* **28**:211–217, 1978.

17 Chang, K.-J.: Opioid receptors: Multiplicity and sequelae of ligand-receptor interactions. In P. M. Conn (ed.): *The Receptors* (Vol. I). Academic Press, Orlando, 1984, pp. 1–81.

18 Cousins, M., and Mather, L.: Intrathecal and epidural administration of opioids. *Anesthesiology* **61**:276–310, 1984.

19 Cruz, L., and Basbaum, A. I.: Multiple opioid peptides and the modulation of pain: Immunohistochemical analysis of dynorphin and enkephalin in the trigeminal nucleus caudalis and spinal cord of the cat. *J. Comp. Neurol.* **240**:331–348, 1985.

20 Dahlstrom, A., and Fuxe, K.: Evidence for the existence of monoamine neurons in the central nervous system. II. Experimental demonstration of monoamines in the cell bodies of brain stem neurons. *Acta Physiol. Scand. Suppl.* **232**:1–55, 1964.

21 Dickenson, A. H.: A new approach to pain relief? *Nature* **320**:681–682, 1986.

22 Duggan, A. W.: Pharmacology of descending control systems. *Phil. Trans. R. Soc. London [B]* **308**:375–391, 1985.

23 Duggan, A. W., and North, R. A.: Electrophysiology of opioids. *Pharmacol. Rev.* **35**:219–281, 1984.

24 Emson, P. C., Arregui, A., Clement-Jones, V., Sandberg, B. E. B., and Rossor, M.: Regional distribution of methionine-enkephalin and substance P-like immunoreactivity in normal human brain and in huntington's disease. *Brain Res.* **199**:147–160, 1980.

25 Fang, F., Fields, H. L., and Lee, N. M.: Action at the mu receptor is sufficient to explain the supraspinal analgesic effect of opiates. *J. Pharmacol. Exp. Ther.* **238**:1039–1044, 1986.

26 Fields, H. L.: Neural mechanisms of opiate analgesia. *Adv. Pain Res. Ther.* **9**:479–486, 1985.

27 Fields, H. L., and Basbaum, A. I.: Brain stem control of spinal pain transmission neurons. *Annu. Rev. Physiol.* **40**:217–248, 1978.

28 Fields, H. L., Basbaum, A. I., Clanton, C. H., and Anderson, S. D.: Nucleus raphe magnus inhibition of spinal cord dorsal horn neurons. *Brain Res.* **126**:441–453, 1977.

29 Fields, H. L., Emson, P. C., Leigh, B. K., Gilbert, R. F. T., and Iversen, L. L.:
    Multiple opiate receptor sites on primary afferent fibres. *Nature* **284:**351–353, 1980.

30 Fields, H. L., and Heinricher, M. M.: Anatomy and physiology of a nociceptive
    modulatory system. *Phil. Trans. R. Soc. Lond.* [*B*] **308:**361–374, 1985.

31 Fields, H. L., and Levine, J. D.: Placebo analgesia—a role for endorphins? *Trends
    Neurosci.* **7:**271–273, 1984.

32 Fleetwood-Walker, S., Mitchell, R., Hope, P. J., Molony, V., and Iggo, A.: An α_2
    receptor mediates the selective inhibition by noradrenaline of nociceptive responses
    of identified dorsal horn neurones. *Brain Res.* **334:**243–254, 1985.

33 Frederickson, R. C. A., Burgis, V., and Edwards, J. D.: Hyperalgesia produced by
    naloxone follows diurnal rhythm in responsivity to painful stimuli. *Science* **198:**756–
    758, 1977.

34 Frederickson, R. C. A., and Geary, L. E.: Endogenous opioid peptides: Review of
    physiological, pharmacological and clinical aspects. *Progr. Neurobiol.* **19:**19–69,
    1982.

35 Gebhart, G. F., Sandkuhler, J., Thalhammer, J. G., and Zimmerman, M.: Inhibition
    of spinal nociceptive information by stimulation in midbrain of the cat is blocked by
    lidocaine microinjected in nucleus raphe magnus and medullary reticular formation.
    J. Neurophysiol. **50:**1446–1459, 1983.

36 Giesler, G. J., Gerhart, K. D., Yezierski, R. P., Wilcox, T. K., and Willis, W. D.:
    Postsynaptic inhibition of primate spinothalamic neurons by stimulation in nucleus
    raphe magnus. *Brain Res.* **204:**184–188, 1981.

37 Glazer, E. J., and Basbaum, A. I.: Axons which take up [³H] serotonin are presyn-
    aptic to enkephalin immunoreactive neurons in cat dorsal horn. *Brain Res.* **298:**389–
    391, 1984.

38 Gramsch, C., Hollt, V., Mehraein, P., Pasi, A., and Herz, A.: Regional distribution
    of methionine-enkephalin- and beta-endorphin-like immunoreactivity in human brain
    and pituitary. *Brain Res.* **177:**261–270, 1979.

39 Grevert, P., and Goldstein, A.: Endorphins: Naloxone fails to alter experimental pain
    or mood in humans. *Science* **199:**1093–1095, 1978.

40 Grevert, P., Leonard, H. A., and Goldstein, A.: Partial antagonism of placebo an-
    algesia by naloxone. *Pain* **16:**129–143, 1983.

41 Hardy, S. G. P.: Projections to the midbrain from the medial versus lateral prefrontal
    cortices of the rat. *Neurosci. Lett.* **63:**159–164, 1986.

42 Hiller, J. M., Simon, E. J., Crain, S. M., and Peterson, E. R.: Opiate receptors in culture of fetal mouse dorsal root ganglia (DRG) and spinal cord: Predominance in DRG neurites. *Brain Res.* **145**:396–400, 1978.

43 Hodge, C. J., Jr., Apkarian, A. V., Stevens, R. T., Vogelsang, G. D., Brown, O., and Frank, J. I.: Dorsolateral pontine inhibition of dorsal horn cell responses to cutaneous stimulation: Lack of dependence on catecholaminergic system in the cat. *J. Neurophysiol.* **50**:1220–1235, 1983.

44 Hollt, V., Tulunay, C., Woo, S. K., Loh, H. H., and Herz, A.: Opioid peptides derived from pro-enkephalin A but not that from proenkephalin B are substantial analgesics after administration into brain of mice. *Eur. J. Pharmacol.* **83**:355–356, 1982.

45 Hosobuchi, Y., Adams, J. E., and Linchitz, R.: Pain relief by electrical stimulation of the central gray matter in humans and its reversal by naloxone. *Science* **197**:183–186, 1977.

46 Hughes, J., Smith, T. W, Kosterlitz, H. W., Fothergill, L. A. Morgan, B. A., and Morris, H. R.: Identification of two related pentapeptides from the brain with potent opiate agonist activity. *Nature* **258**:577–579, 1975.

47 Jordan, L. M., Kenshalo, D. R., Martin, R. F., Haber, L. H., and Willis, W. D.: Depression of primate spinothalamic tract neurons by iontophoretic application of 5-hydroxytryptamine. *Pain* **5**:135–142, 1978.

48 Khachaturian, H., Lewis, M. E., and Watson, S. J.: Enkephalin systems in diencephalon and brainstem of the rat. *J. Comp. Neurol.* **220**:310–320, 1983.

49 Kuhar, M. J., Pert, C. B., and Snyder, S. H.: Regional distribution of opiate receptor binding in monkey and human brain. *Nature* **245**:447–450, 1973.

50 Leavens, M. E., Hill, C. S., Jr., Cech, D. A., Weyland, J. B., and Weston, J. S.: Intrathecal and intraventricular morphine for pain in cancer patients: Initial study. *J. Neurosurg.* **56**:241–245, 1982.

51 Levine, J. D., and Gordon, N. C.: Method of administration determines the effect of naloxone on pain. *Brain Res.* **365**:377–378, 1985.

52 Levine, J. D., Gordon, N. C., and Fields, H. L.: The mechanism of placebo analgesia. *Lancet* **2**:654–657, 1978.

53 Levine, J. D., Gordon, N. C., and Fields, H. L.: Naloxone dose-dependently produces analgesia and hyperalgesia in postoperative pain. *Nature* **278**:740–741, 1979.

54 Mantyh, P. W.: The ascending input to the midbrain periaqueductal gray of the primate. *J. Comp. Neurol.* **211**:50–64, 1982.

55 Martin, W. R.: Pharmacology of opioids. *Pharmacol. Rev.* **35**:283–323, 1984.

56 Mayer, D. J., and Price, D. D.: Central nervous system mechanisms of analgesia. *Pain* **2**:379–404, 1976.

57 Mokha, S. S., McMillan, J. A., and Iggo, A.: Descending control of spinal nociceptive transmission. Actions produced on spinal multireceptive neurones from the nuclei locus coeruleus (LC) and raphe magnus (NRM). *Exp. Brain Res.* **58**:213–226, 1985.

58 Morley, J. S.: Structure-activity relationships of enkephalin-like peptides. *Annu. Rev. Pharmacol. Toxicol.* **20**:81–110, 1980.

59 Mudge, A. W., Leeman, S. E., and Fischbach, G. D.: Enkephalin inhibits release of substance P from sensory neurons in culture and decreases action potential duration. *Proc. Natl. Acad. Sci. (USA)* **76**:526–530, 1979.

60 Nurchi, G.: Use of intraventricular and intrathecal morphine in intractable pain associated with cancer. *Neurosurgery* **15**:801–803, 1984.

61 Nyberg, F., Nylander, I., and Terenius, L.: Enkephalin-containing polypeptides in human cerebrospinal fluid. *Brain Res.* **371**:278–286, 1986.

62 Palkovits, M.: Distribution of neuropeptides in the central nervous system: A review of biochemical mapping studies. *Progr. Neurobiol.* **23**:151–189, 1984.

63 Reddy, S. V. R., and Yaksh, T. L.: Spinal noradrenergic terminal system mediates antinociception. *Brain Res.* **189**:391–402, 1980.

64 Richardson, D. E., and Akil, H.: Pain reduction by electrical brain stimulation in man. *J. Neurosurg.* **47**:178–183, 1977.

65 Roberts, M. H. T.: 5-Hydroxytryptamine and antinociception. *Neuropharmacology* **23**:1529–1536, 1984.

66 Ruda, M. A.: Opiates and pain pathways: Demonstration of enkephalin synapses on dorsal horn projection neurons. *Science* **215**:1523–1525, 1982.

67 Ruda, M. A., Bennett, G. J., and Dubner, R.: Neurochemistry and neural circuitry in the dorsal horn. *Progr. Brain Res.* **66**:219–268, 1986.

68 Snyder, S. H., and Matthysse, S. (eds.): Opiate Receptor Mechanisms. *Neurosci. Res. Program Bull.* **13**:1–166, 1975.

69 Schwartz, J.-C.: Metabolism of enkephalins and the inactivating neuropeptidase concept. *Trends Neurosci.* **6**:45–48, 1983.

70 Unnerstall, J. R., Kopajtic, T. A., and Kuhar, M. J.: Distribution of α₂ agonist binding sites in the rat and human central nervous system: Analysis of some functional, anatomic correlates of the pharmacologic effects of clonidine and related adrenergic agents. *Brain Res. Rev.* **7**:69–101, 1984.

71 Westlund, K. N., Bowker, R. M., Ziegler, M. G., and Coulter, J. D.: Descending noradrenergic projections and their spinal terminations. In H. G. J. M. Kuypers and G. F. Martin (eds.): Descending Pathways to the Spinal Cord. *Progr. Brain Res.* **57**:219–238, 1982.

72 Westlund, K. N., Bowker, R. M., Ziegler, M. G., and Coulter, J. D.: Origins and terminations of descending noradrenergic projections to the spinal cord of the monkey. *Brain Res.* **292**:1–16, 1984.

73 Willis, W. D.: *Control of Nociceptive Transmission in the Spinal Cord.* Springer-Verlag, New York, 1982.

74 Yaksh, T. L.: Narcotic analgesics: CNS sites and mechanisms of action as revealed by intracerebral injection techniques. *Pain* **4**:299–359, 1978.

75 Yaksh, T. L., and Noueihed, R.: The physiology and pharmacology of spinal opiates. *Annu. Rev. Pharmacol. Toxicol.* **25**:433–462, 1985.

76 Yaksh, T. L., and Reddy, S. V. R.: Studies in the primate on the analgetic effects associated with intrathecal actions of opiates, α-adrenergic agonists and baclofen. *Anesthesiology* **54**:451–467, 1981.

77 Yaksh, T. L., and Wilson, P. R.: Spinal serotonin system mediates antinociception. *J. Pharmacol. Exp. Ther.* **208**:446–453, 1979.

78 Yeung, J. C., and Rudy, T. A.: Multiplicative interaction between narcotic agonisms expressed at spinal and supraspinal sites of antinociceptive action as revealed by concurrent intrathecal and intracerebroventricular injections of morphine. *J. Pharmacol. Exp. Ther.* **215**:633–642, 1980.

79 Yezierski, R. P., Wilcox, T. K., and Willis, W. D.: The effects of serotonin antagonists on the inhibition of primate spinothalamic tract cells produced by stimulation in nucleus raphe magnus or periaqueductal gray. *J. Pharmacol. Exp. Ther.* **220**:266–277, 1982.

80 Zorman, G., Hentall, I. D., Adams, J. E., and Fields, H. L.: Naloxone-reversible analgesia produced by microstimulation in the rat medulla. *Brain Res.* **219**:137–148, 1981.

Chapter 6

Painful Dysfunction of the Nervous System

In most instances, the pain sensory and modulatory systems operate effectively to protect the body from injury. Pain is normally temporary. It subsides rapidly if no irreversible damage has occurred, or, if there has been damage, it persists until the healing process is complete. However, there are patients who experience persistent pain. In some of these patients, for example, those with cancer, healing does not occur because active tissue destruction continues. In such cases the pain can be explained in terms of the normal operation of the pain sensory system. In other cases, there is ongoing pain but no active tissue-damaging process to explain it. In such patients the pain may be associated with disruption of normal nerve connections and/or abnormal hyperactivity at some level of the pain sensory system.

Various terms have been used for the pain that results from nerve dysfunction: for example, deafferentation, which implies a mechanism; or dysesthetic, referring to an unfamiliar unpleasant sensation. I prefer to use the more general term *neuropathic*, which implies only that the pain is due to functional abnormalities of the nervous system.

The severity of neuropathic pain can be extreme, and it often totally disrupts the patient's life. Curiously, neuropathic pain may begin days or weeks after the termination of the destructive process that initiated it. Like referred pain, neuropathic pain may spread extensively to include sites remote from the initiating

Table 6.1   Clinical Features of Neuropathic Pain

Pain occurs in the absence of a detectable ongoing tissue-damaging process.

Abnormal or unfamiliar unpleasant sensations (dysesthesiae), frequently having a burning and/or electrical quality.

Delay in onset after precipitating injury.

Pain is felt in a region of sensory deficit.

Paroxysmal brief shooting or stabbing component.

Mild stimuli painful (allodynia).

Pronounced summation and after-reaction with repetitive stimuli.

injury. Furthermore, there may be muscle tenderness and cutaneous hypersensitivity in regions that have a segmental relation to the injured neural tissue. Neuropathic pain differs, however, from ordinary cases of referred pain in that it is not sustained by ongoing tissue damage. It persists long after the damaging and healing processes have stopped.

Table 6.1 summarizes the major clinical features that are common in patients with neuropathic pain. Because there are many different types of neuropathic pain it is rare for a patient to manifest all of the listed features. On the other hand, any of the features listed should raise the suspicion that a patient's pain is neuropathic.

There are a variety of possible mechanisms by which nerve dysfunction could cause pain. Available evidence suggests that neuropathic pains are sustained by one or more of the following factors: hyperactivity in primary afferent or central nervous system (CNS) nociceptive neurons, loss of central inhibitory connections, and increased activity in sympathetic efferents. In this chapter these factors will be discussed in relation to certain clinical problems to which they may be relevant.

Deafferentation and Hyperactivity of Central Neurons

When there is damage to the neural pathways that transmit nociceptive information there is usually a deficit of pain sensation. This is manifested as an elevation of pain threshold and a reduction in the perceived intensity of a given noxious stimulus. In some cases of damage to sensory pathways, however, a paradoxical situation ensues: in these patients, in addition to the expected impairment of sensibility for noxious stimuli, there is spontaneous pain. The pain may actually be perceived by the patient as arising from an area that is anesthetic. This pain is often severe and refractory to treatment.

One of the simplest explanations for the pain of nerve injury is that the injury causes deafferentation of a spinal pain transmission neuron and this deafferentation somehow *raises* the neuron's level of activity. Although seemingly paradoxical, this idea is not without an experimental basis. In fact, hyperactivity of CNS neurons following experimental denervation has been demonstrated. For example, in the rat, cutting the dorsal roots that innervate a section of spinal cord produces high-frequency discharge of many dorsal horn cells in the denervated segment (31). The hyperactive cells are concentrated in lamina V, which, in the intact animal, contains many nociceptive cells, some of which project to higher centers. This denervation hyperactivity begins about 6 hours after cutting the dorsal roots and continues for weeks. In most animals, the hyperactivity subsides after about 3 months.

The potential for anatomic deafferentation to produce clinically significant pain is most clearly shown in patients with brachial plexus injuries. Wynn-Parry (68) has studied over 400 patients with injuries to the brachial plexus. Such patients fall into two groups. In one group there is stretch or laceration of the plexus but the spinal roots are intact. In the other group the injury actually pulls one or more dorsal roots completely out of the dorsal root entry zone (brachial plexus avulsion). In the former group, peripheral connections are interrupted but the central processes of the dorsal root ganglion cells remain more or less intact (Figure 6.1). In the brachial plexus avulsion group the central processes are cleanly removed, producing an anatomically complete deafferentation. Severe persistent pain is rare with traumatic injury of the brachial plexus without avulsion, but it is common when avulsion (i.e., complete deafferentation of at least one spinal segment) is present.

The pain of brachial plexus avulsion is usually described as burning, and there is an associated "pins and needles" or "electricity-like" sensation. Such abnormal sensations, called *paresthesiae* or, if definitely unpleasant, dysesthesiae, are common with injury to sensory pathways in either the peripheral or central nervous system. The pain in avulsion injury is perceived in the dermatome of the segments that are denervated and therefore at least partially anesthetic. In addition to this continuous pain, patients often have brief paroxysms of pain that have a sharp and shooting quality. The paroxysms tend to shoot up the arm and into the shoulder. In many patients the pain begins only after a delay of 1 to 12 weeks. In some patients, the pain subsides somewhat with time.

The presence of this severe, persistent spontaneous pain arising from a deafferented spinal segment in humans is consistent with the finding, in animals, that dorsal horn pain transmission neurons in a deafferented segment of spinal cord become hyperactive. The delay in onset of the pain in patients is consistent with the neurophysiological studies.

Evidence consistent with the concept that hyperactive dorsal horn pain

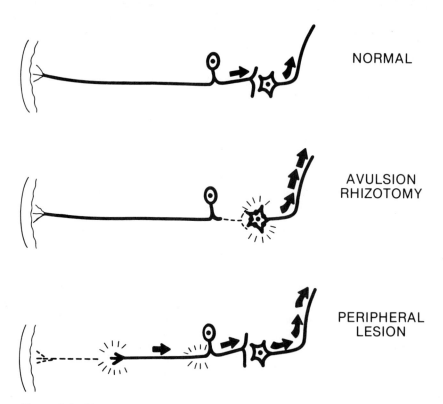

NORMAL

AVULSION
RHIZOTOMY

PERIPHERAL
LESION

Figure 6.1 Hyperactivity due to damage of primary afferents. **Top:** The normal primary afferent innvervating the skin and terminating on a second-order pain-transmitting neuron in the spinal cord. In the absence of a stimulus, there is no activity in either cell and no pain. **Middle:** With damage to the central process of the primary afferent (*dashed line*) the second-order cell becomes hyperactive, producing spontaneous pain that requires no peripheral stimulus. **Lower:** Damage to the peripheral process (*dashed lines*) leads to regeneration. There is spontaneous activity and increased mechanosensitivity in the regenerating axonal sprouts of nociceptors. In addition, the damaged primary afferents may develop secondary sites of spontaneous activity and increased mechanosensitivity near their cell bodies in the dorsal root ganglion. These changes produce increased activity in second-order cells and pain.

transmission neurons play a role in deafferentation pain comes from the results of surgical procedures for relief of brachial plexus avulsion pain. Nashold and Ostdahl (41) reasoned that if spontaneously active dorsal horn neurons produce the pain of brachial plexus avulsion, destruction of these neurons should eliminate the pain. They developed the so-called dorsal root entry zone (DREZ) operation. In this operation, lesions are made that destroy a significant region of the dorsal horn. Although some patients obtain only limited or transient pain relief, in the majority of patients, including those whose pain is refractory to other forms of treatment, DREZ lesions are reported to be remarkably effective.

The clinical and experimental evidence discussed above indicates that complete sensory deafferentation of a spinal segment places an individual at high risk for developing severe pain in the region made anesthetic. A noxious peripheral stimulus is not required to produce this pain. The pain may be due to spontaneous hyperactivity in dorsal horn pain transmission neurons, and there is evidence that the pain can be eliminated if these neurons are destroyed.

Loss of Segmental Inhibition

A certain percentage of individuals who suffer traumatic injury of peripheral nerve have persistent pain. However, in contrast to brachial plexus avulsion, where pain is the rule, it is the exceptional patient with peripheral nerve injury who has significant pain. As with avulsion, the pain experienced by patients with peripheral nerve injury is often described as burning, and paresthesias are the rule.

The pain of peripheral nerve injury cannot be completely explained by the hyperactivity of deafferented central neurons. In contrast to brachial plexus avulsion, the pain that accompanies peripheral nerve damage depends on input from the periphery. The point is illustrated by the observation that local anesthetic block of the peripheral nerve at or distal to the site of injury will temporarily relieve the pain in most cases (24, 29).

In addition to spontaneous pain, patients with nerve injury report a variety of other sensory disturbances. Both hyperalgesia (an exaggerated response to a noxious stimulus) and allodynia (a painful sensation produced by a stimulus that would ordinarily be innocuous) are present. When noxious stimuli of identical intensity are repeatedly applied to the area of skin innervated by the damaged nerve, the intensity of pain increases with successive stimuli (summation) and the pain persists after the stimulus has stopped (after-reaction). Summation and after-reaction are present to a certain extent in normally innervated skin, but are exaggerated in patients with pain due to nerve injury.

A strikingly similar picture can be produced experimentally in human subjects by applying pressure to a peripheral nerve that is sufficient to block conduction in myelinated axons but that does not affect unmyelinated axons. As discussed in Chapter 3, in subjects with such partial nerve blocks, summation and after-reaction become much more prominent (Figure 3.13). In addition, both noxious and innocuous thermal and mechanical stimuli are reported to produce a delayed, unpleasant, tingling, burning sensation that is poorly localized. Thus not only do the myelinated afferents transmit the information required for accurate localization and identification of a stimulus, but their activity usually has a net inhibitory effect on pain transmission.

Neurophysiological observations that parallel these psychophysical studies have also been made. As discussed in Chapter 2, myelinated primary afferents, including Aδ nociceptors and A-α mechanoreceptors, inhibit spinal dorsal horn pain transmission neurons that are activated by unmyelinated nociceptors. Thus when the myelinated fibers are blocked, activity in the unmyelinated fibers produces a greater discharge in the dorsal horn cells (Figures 3.12 and 6.2). Presumably, the increased discharge of the dorsal horn cell would be perceived as more intense pain.

These studies raise the possibility that, in some cases, peripheral nerve injury produces selective damage to myelinated primary afferents with relative sparing of the unmyelinated nociceptive primary afferents. Under these conditions, loss of the inhibition normally produced by the myelinated afferents results in an exaggerated response of spinal pain transmission neurons to activity in unmyelinated nociceptors. In fact, when peripheral nerves are subjected to chronic pressure, such as occurs in ligamentous entrapment, there is often damage to myelinated axons with sparing of the unmyelinated afferents (14, 22, 47, 48, 58). Such entrapment neuropathies frequently produce dysesthesias and may become quite painful. Meralgia paresthetica of the lateral femoral cutaneous nerve and carpal tunnel syndrome are two of the most common painful entrapment neuropathies.

Support for the idea that large fiber loss contributes to the pain of traumatic neuropathies comes from the clinical observation that selective electrical stimulation of large-diameter myelinated primary afferents can give striking relief of the burning pain caused by peripheral nerve injury (38, 42, 64). Relief is particularly effective if the nerve can be stimulated proximal to the lesion site.

The idea that primary afferents responsible for fine discrimination of cutaneous stimuli inhibit the central actions of nociceptive primary afferents was first proposed by Head and his colleagues in the early 20th century (18). It was determined later that myelinated primary afferents subserve fine somatosensory discrimination, whereas small-diameter myelinated and unmyelinated primary afferents subserve pain, crude touch, and heat. The awareness of these two distinct afferent systems and their distinct central actions led to the later proposal that selective damage to large-diameter afferents is causally related to the pain of peripheral nerve injury (44).

The first attempt to incorporate these clinical observations into a detailed hypothesis of the neural mechanisms underlying pain sensation was the gate control hypothesis of Melzack and Wall (34). According to this theory, the interaction between myelinated and unmyelinated inputs to the spinal cord occurs at two sites: inhibitory interneurons in the substantia gelatinosa (lamina II) and dorsal horn pain transmission neurons. Both myelinated and unmyelinated primary afferents were proposed to have a direct excitatory action on the pain transmission neurons (T cells). The substantia gelatinosa neurons were proposed to inhibit transmitter release from both classes of primary afferent, thus presynapti-

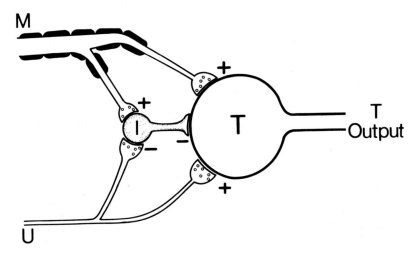

Afferent Input	I Cell Effect	T Cell Effect	T-Cell Output (T-I)
M	+	+	0
U	−	+	+ +
M + U	0	+	+

Figure 6.2 Revised version of the gate control hypothesis (35). This hypothesis focuses upon interactions in the dorsal horn of the spinal cord. **Top:** The four important types of neural element: the unmyelinated, nociceptive primary afferent (*U*), the myelinated non-nociceptive primary afferent (*M*), the transmission cell (*T*), whose activity usually results in the sensation of pain, and an inhibitory interneuron (*I*), which is spontaneously active and whose activity inhibits the T cell, thus reducing perceived pain intensity. The inhibitory interneuron is excited by the myelinated non-nociceptive afferent. The other crucial point is that the unmyelinated nociceptor inhibits the inhibitory interneuron secondarily exciting the T cell. The unmyelinated primary afferent thus has both direct and indirect excitatory effects on the T cell. **Bottom:** The table shows how perceived pain (T cell output) is the result of a balance of input from myelinated (*M*) and unmyelinated (*U*) primary afferents. For example, a stimulus that activates only the M afferents has both a direct excitatory and an indirect inhibitory effect on the T cell. There is no net increase in T cell activity and no pain. A stimulus that activates only the U afferents produces a very large increase in T cell firing because there are both direct and indirect excitatory actions and no inhibition. Most stimuli activate both M and U afferents, producing intermediate levels of pain intensity.

cally inhibiting all afferent input to the pain transmission cells. The myelinated afferents were proposed to excite the inhibitory substantia gelatinosa neuron, thereby reducing input to the T cell and consequently inhibiting pain. This point is supported by the clinical observation that selective stimulation of large-diameter myelinated fibers produces analgesia. In contrast, activity in unmyelinated nociceptors was proposed to *inhibit* the inhibitory substantia gelatinosa cells, resulting in an enhancement of transmission from primary afferents to the T cells and consequently increasing pain intensity. In this way, the unmyelinated afferents were proposed to have two distinct excitatory effects on dorsal horn pain transmission cells: a direct synaptic excitation and an indirect excitation resulting from the inhibition of the inhibitory substantia gelatinosa cell.

The gate control hypothesis emphasized that the perceived intensity of pain is the result of a balance of input from myelinated and unmyelinated fibers. Under normal conditions stimuli activate both types of afferent, and the sensation produced by brief noxious stimuli is of rapid onset and short duration. In this case, both the intensity and duration of the pain are reduced by the inhibitory input from the myelinated afferents.

Subsequent physiological studies have established that at least part of the inhibitory effect produced in spinal pain transmission neurons is postsynaptic (19). Furthermore, neither presynaptic inhibition of myelinated cutaneous afferents nor presynaptic disinhibition of unmyelinated fibers has been established experimentally. Thus, although the theory as originally proposed remains possible, the weight of present evidence suggests that it is incomplete and perhaps wrong in some details. Accordingly, Melzack and Wall (35) have incorporated numerous changes in a revised version of the hypothesis. The strength of the theory is that it offers an explanation of otherwise puzzling and apparently paradoxical clinical findings, for example, summation and the production of pain by stimuli that would be innocuous if applied to normally innervated skin (allodynia).

The exaggerated summation seen after nerve injury was explained as follows. When the myelinated input and its inhibitory effect are reduced, the unopposed action of the unmyelinated afferent results in an excitation of the T cell that is both greater in magnitude and prolonged. The unopposed action of the unmyelinated afferent also results in greater inhibition of the substantia gelatinosa neuron. The inhibition of this inhibitory interneuron adds to the excitation of the T cell. Under these conditions, subsequent impulses in the unmyelinated afferent sum with the lasting excitatory effect of previous input, producing a progressive increase in T cell discharge and pain that builds in intensity (Figure 3.13). The explanation of summation is important because it suggests how a stimulus of constant intensity can, when repeated, produce a pain that grows in intensity over time. That loss of input from myelinated fibers can enhance summation is indicated by the psychophysical studies discussed in Chapter 3, which demonstrate that, when myelinated afferents are blocked in a peripheral nerve, repeated C fiber inputs produce a sensation that progressively builds in intensity.

Allodynia, or the production of pain by mild, normally innocuous stimuli, is another phenomenon that can be explained by the gate control hypothesis. As discussed in Chapter 1, repeated noxious stimuli will sensitize both myelinated and unmyelinated nociceptors. Thus, allodynia could be at least partially explained by sensitization of nociceptors, which would lower their thresholds enough so that they respond to very mild stimuli. Sensitization, however, cannot completely account for allodynia. For one thing, even when sensitized, nociceptor thresholds are still too high to allow them to be activated by the lightest stimuli that can produce allodynia. Furthermore, in some patients, allodynia is abolished by selective blockade of large-diameter myelinated afferents (39), which include few if any nociceptors. This indicates that large-diameter myelinated afferents can contribute to pain under pathological conditions. If this is the correct explanation of allodynia, it requires that nerve injuries that produce it spare at least some large-diameter primary afferents.

According to the gate control hypothesis, myelinated afferents have a direct excitatory and an indirect inhibitory effect on the pain transmission cell (Figure 6.2). Thus myelinated afferents have the potential either to *produce or inhibit* pain. Activity in non-nociceptive myelinated afferents would produce pain when the inhibitory substantia gelatinosa neuron is maximally inhibited by activity in unmyelinated nociceptors. The indirect inhibitory effect of the myelinated fibers is then blocked, and their direct excitatory action on the T cells would predominate.

In summary, it seems likely that a relative loss of myelinated primary afferents contributes to the painfulness of some nerve injuries. The loss of their inhibitory effect is associated with spontaneous pain; summation, due to the unopposed action of unmyelinated afferents; and allodynia, in which surviving non-nociceptive myelinated axons, which usually inhibit pain transmission cells, now excite them, thus permitting mild stimuli to produce pain.

Ectopic Impulse Generation in Primary Afferents

Despite its importance, clinical observations indicate that loss of central inhibition from myelinated afferents does not account for all pain resulting from pathological processes affecting peripheral nerve. Thomas (60) has pointed out that some neuropathies, such as those associated with Friedreich's ataxia and uremia, predominantly affect large fibers and are rarely associated with pain. Furthermore, in the neuropathy of Fabry's disease and that of the diabetic sensory neuropathy, it is predominantly small fibers that are affected, and these neuropathies are characteristically painful.

Studies of experimentally injured peripheral nerves have indicated how damage to unmyelinated primary afferents can lead to pain. When the axon of a peripheral nerve is damaged it will sprout new extensions that grow out toward the peripheral structure that it formerly innervated. If the original connective tissue sheath of the distal part of the nerve is intact and nearby, the axon will enter it and continue to grow toward the target structure. If the distal sheath is removed, the sprouting axons end blindly in a tangled ball called a neuroma. The histological appearance of axonal sprouts that enter a neuroma differ from their parent axons in normal segments of peripheral nerve. Most are of very small diameter (<0.5 µm) and are derived from unmyelinated parent axons. About 80 percent of unmyelinated axons are primary afferents and the rest are sympathetic postganglionic efferents. There are many sprouts for each parent axon (Figure 6.3), and the Schwann cell sheath around the sprout is incomplete, so that the sprouts are much closer to each other than are normal unmyelinated axons (2, 48).

The physiological properties of regenerating primary afferents also differ from those of normal afferents in several respects (9, 55, 63). First, the area of sprouting becomes sensitive to direct mechanical stimulation. This is presumably the basis of Tinel's sign, in which light tapping of the growing tip of a regenerating peripheral nerve elicits a tingling sensation. It may also account for the shooting pains that are occasionally elicited by movements that stretch or compress the nerve. A second property acquired by regenerating axons is spontaneous activity. This begins within a week of transection and, in rat sciatic nerve, reaches a peak in about 3 weeks. It then subsides slowly over a period of months.

"Spontaneous" discharge and increased mechanosensitivity in damaged primary afferents are present in at least two different sites: the regenerating sprout near the site of injury, and near the cell body in the dorsal root ganglion (5, 20, 62) (Figure 6.4). The mechanical sensitivity of the region near the dorsal root ganglion may contribute to the radiation of pain into the dermatome that is produced when nerve roots are compressed by a protruding intervertebral disc (e.g., the radicular pain of sciatica).

Evidence that ectopic impulse generation can contribute to clinically signif-

Figure 6.3 Appearance of sprouting in damaged peripheral nerve. Electronmicrographs of medial popliteal nerve of baboon. **A:** Normal axons, mostly unmyelinated. The unmyelinated axons have fairly uniform diameters (0.5–3.0 µm) (*m, myelinated axon; u, unmyelinated axon*). **B:** Region of regenerating sprouts in previously damaged nerve. An individual Schwann cell may surround many more unmyelinated axons (same magnification as part A). The unmyelinated axons have smaller diameters, in some cases only one-fifth of normal (e.g., *arrows*). In addition, in contrast to the normal nerve where individual unmyelinated axons are separated by Schwann cell cytoplasm, neighboring regenerating sprouts often come into direct apposition, with no intervening Schwann cell cytoplasm (*arrows with stars*). (From Fowler, T. J., and Ochoa, J.: Unmyelinated fibers in normal and compressed peripheral nerves of the baboon: A quantitative electron microscopic study. *Neuropathol. Appl. Neurobiol.* **1**:247–265, 1975.)

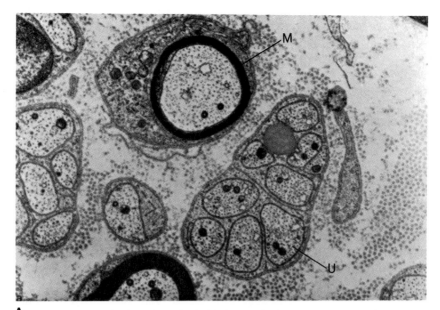

A

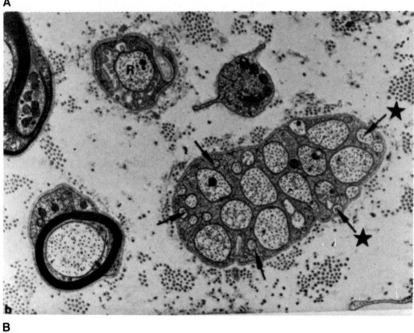

B

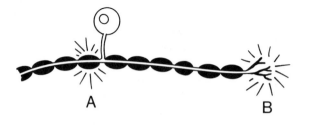

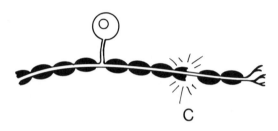

Figure 6.4 Sites of ectopic discharge in damaged primary afferent nociceptors. **Top:** A transected nerve begins to regenerate, sending out sprouts (*B*) that are mechanically sensitive, sensitive to α-adrenergic agonists, and spontaneously active. In addition, a secondary site of hyperactivity (*A*) develops near the cell body in the dorsal root ganglion. **Bottom:** Ectopic impulses may arise from a short patch of demyelination on a primary afferent (*C*).

icant pain comes from recent studies of C fibers innervating stump neuromas in two patients (46). Both patients had phantom limb pain following traumatic limb amputation. In both, heightened mechanosensitivity of neuromas in the stump contributed to their pain. Furthermore, there was evidence that in some of the unmyelinated afferents innervating the neuroma, there was spontaneous activity arising *proximal to the neuroma*, suggesting a second site for ectopic impulse generation.

In addition to sites of sprouting and the dorsal root ganglion region, ectopic impulses can be generated from demyelinated patches of myelinated axons (4, 5, 70) (Figure 6.4). Under these conditions a single impulse arriving at the demyelinated patch can elicit multiple spikes propagated in the same direction. If the demyelinated axon is a nociceptor, the burst of repetitive firing might result in a brief stab of pain. Such a mechanism has been proposed for the distinctive syndrome of tic douloureux, which is characterized by repeated brief stabs of intense pain (4, 5). There is evidence that the trigeminal nerves of such patients have areas of focal demyelination (23). Patients with tic douloureaux have normal sensation in the region of pain, except for discrete trigger zones in which a very slight mechanical stimulus will result in a brief but intense stab of pain.

The idea that patchy loss of myelination might be the cause of pain in tic douloureaux is supported by the increased frequency of pain identical to tic douloureaux in patients with multiple sclerosis, a disease that produces patchy demyelination of axons within the CNS (33). A further parallel is that repetitive ectopic impulses in experimentally demyelinated axons can be reduced by treatment with anticonvulsants such as phenytoin (4). These drugs are useful for the treatment of tic douloureux and the paroxysmal pains of multiple sclerosis (57) (see Chapter 10).

Efferent Activity and Pain: The Reflex Sympathetic Dystrophy Syndrome

Among the most curious and dramatic of clinical problems is that of patients whose pains are maintained by efferent activity in the sympathetic nervous system. The existence of this condition has been unequivocally demonstrated by the clinical observation that regional blockade of the sympathetic nervous system in such patients can produce immediate and complete relief of pain (29). Furthermore, in patients with such sympathetically maintained pain, electrical stimulation of the sympathetic outflow exacerbates their pain (61). It is important to stress that in normal people sympathetic blockade does not impair pain sensation, nor does electrical stimulation of the sympathetic outflow evoke pain. Thus sympathetic activity is neither necessary for normal pain sensation nor sufficient to produce pain. However, it is clear that, under certain poorly understood circumstances, primary afferents become capable of eliciting pain in response to activity in the sympathetic efferent.

The following case, abstracted from Livingston's classic book (29), is fairly typical of patients with sympathetically maintained pains. This case illustrates many of the characteristics of pain associated with traumatic injury to peripheral nerve, including the abnormal burning quality, the hypersensitivity to light touch, and the focus on the distal extremity (in this case the hand). There were obvious signs of sympathetic hyperfunction, including coldness (cutaneous vasoconstriction) and sweating. Complete relief was obtained by sympathetic block. Local block of the nerve either proximal or distal to the site of injury also gave complete relief. The pain returned even after complete section of the nerve proximal to the injury.

Case 6.1

Mr. C. S., a 35-year-old worker in a lumber mill, was struck by a flying belt on November 25, 1935, and thrown against a timber. The upper third of the right humerus was fractured transversely. From the time of the accident, he complained bitterly of pain. There was an aching pain in the upper arm and a burning pain in the hand. The ring and little fingers felt "numb" and "half asleep," subjectively, but at the same time were extremely sensitive to the lightest touch. Several times each day the forearm muscles would go into a cramp so that the fingers, particularly the ring and little fingers, would be drawn tightly into the palm and the patient "had to work them loose with the other hand." It was noted that these two fingers sweated excessively and were constantly discolored and cold.

I examined this man for the first time more than two years after his injury. He kept the hand carefully guarded from any contact and was reluctant to have it examined. The ring and little fingers, particularly the distal two joints of the ring finger, were red and shiny and the nails were opaque and long. He dared not cut these two nails because it so aggravated his pain, but at times they were accidentally broken off. The ulnar side of the hand was glistening wet with perspiration and when he hung the hand down the drops of sweat dripped from the end of the ring finger every few seconds. In spite of the subjective sensation of burning in the hand, it was colder than the left hand; the ring and little fingers measuring 2°C. colder than the same fingers of the left hand. The fractured humerus had never united. . . . There was some fibrous union present, but movement at the fracture site or any pressure on the arm in this region aggravated his pains to an intolerable degree. The man looked thin and pain-worn and had lost 22 pounds since his accident. He stated: "My whole right side seems to be affected; my right eye blurs when I try to read; my chest and neck on that side hurt most of the time and my right leg is weak and often gives way under me."

Examination of the arm showed an enlargement of the ulnar nerve trunk at the level of the ununited fracture. A small amount of novocaine solution injected into the trunk above this lump gave him relief from pain for several hours. There were two other methods by which temporary relief could be conferred. One was to inject the upper thoracic sympathetic ganglia (2nd, 3rd and 4th) with novocaine. The other was a similar injection of the ulnar nerve at the elbow. This last is of interest because the injection was several inches *distal* to the irritative lesion. On May 18, 1938, the nerve was exposed in the upper arm and found to be partially divided and the protruding lateral mass of fibers imbedded in a highly vascular scar tissue. This segment of the nerve was excised and an end-to-end suture carried out. There was, of course, the usual change in the hand that follows an interruption of the ulnar nerve. But the relief from pain was complete and the change in the patient himself was dramatic. But after two months some of the pain began to recur and by October it was as bad as ever.

. . .

A second resection of the nerve and a new anastomosis not only failed to confer relief, but seemed to aggravate the whole pain picture. Thereafter a combination of injections of the stellate ganglion and of the anastomotic area were sufficient to hold his pain under reasonable control until early in 1940. . . . In July 1940, a third resection of the nerve was done, and this time he again experienced complete relief. In September he reported a gain of twelve pounds in weight and was sleeping and eating well. There was less local sensitiveness in the

Table 6.2   Some of the Many Terms Applied to the Reflex Sympathetic Dystrophy Syndrome

1	Causalgia
2	Acute atrophy of bone
3	Sudeck's atrophy or osteodystrophy
4	Peripheral acute trophoneurosis
5	Traumatic angiospasm
6	Post-traumatic osteoporosis
7	Traumatic vasospasm
8	Reflex dystrophy of the extremities
9	Minor causalgia
10	Post-infarctional sclerodactyly
11	Shoulder hand syndrome
12	Reflex neurovascular dystrophy

Adapted from Kozin, F., McCarty, D. J., Sims, J., and Genant, H.: The reflex sympathetic dystrophy syndrome. 1. Clinical and histologic studies: Evidence for bilaterality, response to corticosteroids and articular involvement. *Am. J. Med.* **60:**321–331, 1976.

operative area than at any time previously. He remained quite comfortable until the middle of October, when he caught a cold, and hard coughing spells brought back the pain in the chest, axilla and upper arm and within a few weeks his pain was again as bad as ever, with the entire right side affected. At his request the nerve was exposed again, and this time permanently sacrificed, the cut end being buried in the deltoid muscle well away from the scar tissue area. The relief conferred by the operation was only partial and in the next few months the pain gradually returned to its full force.

Before resorting to a high chordotomy or a resection of the posterior roots of the brachial plexus, two more attempts were made to secure bony union at the fracture site, acting on the theory that irritation caused by slight movement there might be keeping active the pain process. The first attempt failed because he simply could not tolerate his cast. The second attempt, carried out late in 1941, resulted in a solid union and since then there has been a progressive diminution of all of his complaints.[1]

The terminology that has been applied to painful conditions associated with sympathetic activity is confusing and somewhat misleading (Table 6.2). Part of

[1]Reprinted by permission from Livingston, W. K.: *Pain Mechanisms.* Macmillan, New York, 1943, pp. 91–93.

Table 6.3   Precipitating Factors for Reflex Sympathetic Dystrophy

Precipitating factor	Approximate incidence (%)
Soft tissue trauma (e.g., cuts, sprains)	30
Fracture	30
Myocardial infarction	10
Surgery	5
Nerve injury	5
Tendinitis	< 5
Cervical spondylosis	< 5
Cerebrovascular disease	< 5

Data from refs. 49, 50.

the confusion is due to the large number of precipitating events that can produce it (see Table 6.3). When it is produced by nerve injury, as in the case described above, the pain usually has a burning quality and it is called causalgia ("heat-pain"). Causalgia is by far the most dramatic form of the condition and was the first of the sympathetically maintained pain syndromes to be described (40). However, it is not necessary to have a lesion of the nerve trunk to initiate a sympathetically maintained pain syndrome. A more general term that has come into widespread use is the reflex sympathetic dystrophy syndrome (RSDS) (8). This term is useful because it refers to a specific group of painful disorders initiated by an injury to peripheral tissues and sustained by neural mechanisms that include sympathetic efferent activity.

RSDS is important to understand, not only because it is a treatable syndrome that is severely painful but because it illustrates that the sympathetic nervous system can play an important role in the development and maintenance of pain. In addition to persistent pain, which is its most consistent feature, RSDS is characterized by painful hypersensitivity (hyperalgesia) of the skin, muscle tenderness, swelling of soft tissues, and smooth, glossy skin with a mottled appearance. In addition, there may be muscle atrophy, osteoporosis, and arthritis. The evidence of sympathetic hyperactivity is increased sweating and decreased skin temperature resulting from vasoconstriction. Regardless of the site of the precipitating injury or disease, the abnormalities are most pronounced on the distal extremities, most often in the distribution of the median or sciatic nerves.

Although the mechanism of the pain in RSDS is not understood, clinical observations implicate certain factors. The most obvious factor is efferent sympathetic activity. The pain relief following sympathetic blockade in patients with RSDS is immediate, and it occurs whether the block is done by locally anesthetizing the sympathetic chain or by regional infusion of the affected area with drugs, such as guanethidine or resperine, which deplete peripheral catecholamines (3, 17). One of the more curious aspects of the relief produced by sympathetic block is that it usually outlasts the expected duration of action of the blocking drug. For example, despite the fact that the local anesthetic effect of xylocaine lasts only 2–3 hours, it is not unusual for a patient with RSDS pain of the upper extremity to have more than 12 hours of relief after a xylocaine block of the stellate ganglion (which supplies sympathetic efferents to the upper extremity).

In some cases, with repeated sympathetic blocks, the relief lasts for progressively longer periods, finally resolving for weeks, months, or even permanently. I have had several patients whose pain resolved permanently after a single block.

The observations that pain relief outlasts the duration of sympathetic block and that sympathetic activity does not produce pain in normal subjects indicate that, although a peripheral action of sympathetic efferent activity is necessary to produce and sustain the pain in RSDS, other factors must also be involved.

One important possibility is that damaged primary afferent nociceptors become sensitive to sympathetic efferent activity. The earliest proposal along these lines was that, following nerve damage, regenerating sprouts of sympathetic efferent and nociceptive primary afferents form an artificial electrical junction, called an *ephapse* (12, 16) (Figure 6.5). According to this hypothesis, impulses traveling toward the periphery in sympathetic efferents would directly excite the nociceptors at the site of damage. Subsequent experiments have established that ephaptic connections do occur in a neuroma between motor axons and sensory axons (56), but whether sympathetic efferents make ephaptic connections with primary afferent nociceptors is unknown.

Another variation on the peripheral connection theme is the idea that regenerating nociceptors become sensitive to noradrenaline released by the sympathetic efferents (Figure 6.5). This hypothesis is supported by studies showing that regenerating afferents in an experimental neuroma can be activated both by sympathetic efferent activity (10) and by local application of noradrenaline (55). Furthermore, in this model, treatments with guanethidine and α adrenergic antagonists reduce the spontaneous activity and mechanical sensitivity of the regenerating primary afferents. It is possible that in causalgia the sensitivity of damaged and regenerating nociceptors to sympathetic efferent activity contributes to the severe pain that characterized the syndrome.

There are features of sympathetically maintained pains that cannot be explained by a functional sympathetic efferent–to–nociceptor afferent connection at the site of damage in a peripheral nerve. For one thing, local anesthetic block distal to the site of nerve injury often stops the pain (24) (Figure 6.6). Furthermore, in patients with nerve damage, sympathetic activity appears to sensitize afferents in the skin, distant from the injury. Application of norepinephrine directly to the *skin* reproduces causalgic pain that had been relieved by recent

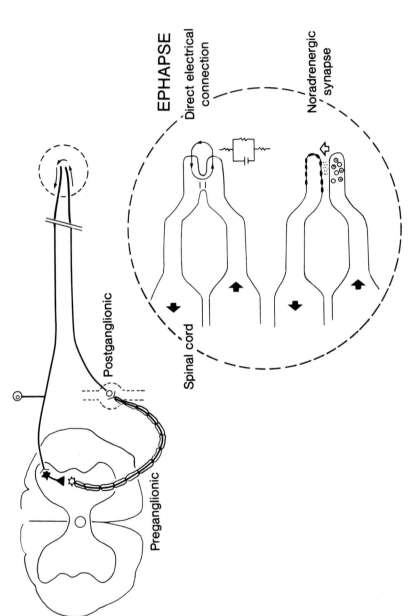

EPHAPSE

Direct electrical connection

Noradrenergic synapse

Spinal cord

Postganglionic

Preganglionic

Figure 6.5 Aberrant neuronal connections in the periphery giving rise to pain. Regenerating sprouts in a peripheral nerve come into close apposition (see Figure 6.3). This sets up the conditions for abnormal connections between axons. Enlargement illustrates two types of abnormal connection. One type (upper) is a direct electrical connection between apposed axons (an ephapse). Under these conditions, a sensory axon could be activated by another sensory axon, a motor axon, or a sympathetic axon.

Another possibility (lower) is that there is a connection between a noradrenergic sympathetic postganglionic axon and a nociceptive

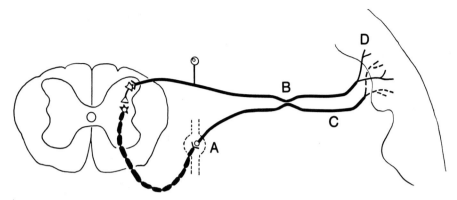

Figure 6.6 Sites in the peripheral nervous system where local anesthetic block-ade can relieve pain (see text). **A:** The sympathetic chain, a relatively specific block of sympathetic efferents. **B:** Site of ectopic impulse generation, either from a neuroma, an aberrant neuronal connection, or a demyelinated patch of axon. **C:** Distal to a neuroma. This indicates that in some pains due to peripheral nerve injury, impulses arising distal to the site of damage can produce pain. **D:** Peripheral terminals of sensitized primary afferents. There is also evidence in reflex sympa-thetic dystrophy that primary afferents have increased sensitivity to noradrenaline.

sympathetic block (39, 65). Finally, many patients with RSDS have no clinical evidence of peripheral nerve damage. These observations indicate that, whatever may be going on at the site of nerve damage, there is also a process involving sympathetic activation or sensitization of receptors in the skin that contributes to sympathetically maintained pain.

Direct activation of cutaneous primary afferent nociceptors would be an attractive explanation for the pain in RSDS. In fact, sensitized myelinated mech-anothermal nociceptors can be activated by sympathetic efferent activity (53). In contrast, animal studies indicate that unmyelinated fibers are only sensitive to sympathetic efferent activity when they are damaged and regenerating. It is pos-sible, however, that in humans undamaged unmyelinated nociceptors are sensi-tive to sympathetic activity or become so following injury to nearby tissues.

One of the most striking findings in causalgia and other types of RSDS is the extreme allodynia. There is evidence that allodynia is partly due to activity in large-diameter myelinated afferents (39). The stimuli that produce allodynia are too mild to activate nociceptors even if they were sensitized by repeated noxious stimuli. Furthermore, allodynia is abolished by selective blockade of large-diameter myelinated afferents, the activity of which normally does not elicit pain. Allodynia can also be eliminated by sympathetic efferent blockade, suggesting that, in patients with sympathetically maintained pains, allodynia is due in part to sensitization (or activation) of low-threshold mechanoreceptors by sympathetic efferents (e.g., at site D, Figure 6.6). Sympathetically induced sensitization of low-threshold mechanoreceptors has been demonstrated in experimental studies of undamaged nerve (54).

It is important to point out that, although the allodynia associated with causalgia involves a peripheral sympathetic process, it may not be completely explained by a peripheral mechanism (52). As discussed in the previous section, if allodynia depends on activity in larger diameter myelinated afferents there must be some additional change in the central pain pathways, because activity in large myelinated primary afferents normally does not produce pain.

The ongoing burning pain in causalgia certainly depends on activity in peripheral primary afferents, but it is not clear whether changes in central pathways also play a role in its maintenance. It is also unclear whether normal levels of sympathetic activity are sufficient to sensitize or activate the afferents that produce pain or increased sympathetic activity is required. From a clinical standpoint, it may not matter since, in either case, sympathetic blockade abolishes the pain. From a theoretical standpoint, however, it is important since a process involving the CNS would be required to explain an increase in sympathetic efferent outflow. Nerve damage does produce changes in central autonomic reflexes, which could increase sympathetic efferent outflow (1, 21), and there is evidence that nociceptor input excites some sympathetic efferents. Thus there is a potential mutually excitatory influence between sympathetic efferents and primary afferent nociceptors.

Efferent Activity and Self-Sustaining Pains: The Vicious Circle

Whatever its mechanism, RSDS illustrates that pain can be sustained by efferent activity arising from sympathetic preganglionic fibers. This efferent activity can activate or sensitize primary afferents by an action in the periphery. The primary afferents, in turn, feed back and excite the efferents in the spinal cord, thus creating a positive feedback loop, or "vicious circle."

The idea of a vicious circle for pain was put forth most clearly by Livingston (29), who based it on a wealth of clinical experience with patients with RSDS, including many such as the one described above (Case 6.1). Livingston was struck by certain features of the pain that cannot be completely explained by the passive transmission of activity in primary afferent nociceptors. These extraordinary features are:

1 Undamaged tissues become painful and hyperalgesic.

2 The pain builds in intensity and, over a period of days to weeks, it spreads spatially.

3 Brief local anesthetic block of sympathetic efferents, nociceptive afferents, or muscle trigger points can give prolonged relief.

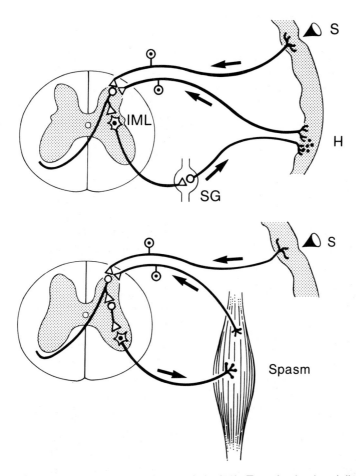

Figure 6.7 Livingston's vicious circle (29). **Top:** A stimulus delivered at *S* activates a primary afferent nociceptor that, in turn, activates the sympathetic preganglionic neuron in the intermediolateral column (*IML*). The preganglionic neuron activates the noradrenergic postganglionic neuron in the sympathetic ganglion (*SG*), which sensitizes, and can activate primary afferent nociceptors (*H*) that feed back to the spinal cord, maintaining the pain. **Bottom:** Nociceptive input may also set in motion another reflex nociceptive input by activating motoneurons that cause muscle spasm. Prolonged muscle spasm activates muscle nociceptors that feed back to the spinal cord to sustain the spasm.

In both situations, the original noxious stimulus sets in motion a spreading and potentially self-sustaining process. In some cases the precipitating noxious input may be trivial and short lasting. In such cases, blocking the spasm or interruption of the reflex loops may provide long-lasting relief.

The spread of pain and hyperalgesia to undamaged skin and muscle is a regular feature of referred pain and can be reproduced experimentally in normal subjects by injection of hypertonic saline into deep tissues (see Chapter 4, pp. 83–88). With referred pain there is often muscle contraction and tenderness. This suggests that motoneurons contribute to pain by activating sensitized muscle nociceptors. In addition, as described above, sympathetic efferent activity can activate or sensitize primary afferents at their peripheral terminals. These two mechanisms may explain how pain elicited by tissue damage in one part of the body can lead to the activation of nociceptors in nearby undamaged muscle and skin. According to the vicious circle concept, as muscle contraction and sympathetic activation of cutaneous nociceptors proceeds, the pain will build in intensity and spread spatially (Figure 6.7). These processes clearly have the potential to produce pain, and it is even conceivable that the neurally generated spread could create independent foci of pain at sites distant from the precipitating injury. The pain originating from these new independent foci could persist after the input from the original site of injury has ceased. In fact, Livingston described patients who, after having pain in an injured part of the body for a period of time, developed a "mirror-image" pain in the same structure on the opposite (uninjured) side of the body. In some of those cases the mirror-image pain persisted after the original pain was relieved. Consistent with these clinical observations, Levine and his colleagues (27) have demonstrated that hyperalgesia develops in an unstimulated rat paw that is contralateral to a paw injured by saline injection. This mirror-image hyperalgesia depends on afferent fibers from the injured extremity and on the sympathetic nervous system.

The available evidence is thus consistent with the idea that efferent activity from the spinal cord, by activating peripheral nociceptors, can play an important role in the development and maintenance of certain pains. Because such efferent activity does not produce pain in normal subjects, some other change in either the primary afferents, the CNS, or both must be postulated to explain the pain. Whatever the change, it must be sustained by ongoing impulse activity in either the efferent or afferent neuron (or both), because brief blockade of either can produce prolonged (in some cases permanent) reversal of the condition. These observations provide strong support for the concept of the vicious circle; a pathological reflex loop maintained by activity in primary afferents and sympathetic or motor efferent neurons.

Long-Term Changes in CNS Pain Pathways

In this chapter I have reviewed several mechanisms that could contribute to persistent neuropathic pain following damage to peripheral tissues. These have included deafferentation-induced hyperactivity of dorsal horn pain transmission cells, loss of central inhibition by loss of myelinated primary afferents, ectopic impulse generation in damaged nociceptive primary afferents, sympathetic ef-

Table 6.4   Possible Mechanisms of Neuropathic Pain (with clinical examples)

Spontaneous hyperactivity of deafferented spinal pain transmission neurons (brachial plexus avulsion)

Plasticity: development or activation of aberrant inputs to deafferented central pain transmission neurons (stump neuroma, central pain syndromes)

Loss of afferent inhibition: nociceptive inputs produce an exaggerated response (entrapment neuropathies, postherpetic neuralgia)

Ectopic impulse generation in damaged nociceptive primary afferents: at the regenerating tip, near the dorsal root ganglion, or in demyelinated regions (tic douloureux, diabetic neuropathy)

Ephaptic transmission: to primary afferents from motor or sympathetic efferents or from other primary afferents

Sympathetic activation or facilitation of primary afferents (causalgia, reflex sympathetic dystrophy syndrome)

Reflex muscle spasm

Epileptic discharge of cortical nociceptive neurons

ferent activation of damaged or intact primary afferents, and changes in autonomic reflexes (Table 6.4). Up to this point, it has been assumed that activation of central pain transmission cells to which primary afferent nociceptors normally project is required for pain to develop. An unstated assumption was that central pain transmission pathways are stable anatomic entities. In fact, there is evidence that central somatosensory pathways have a certain inherent plasticity and that, when the normal input to a central pain transmission neuron is removed, it will begin to respond to inputs to which it formerly did not respond. For example, a cell that formerly responded only to stimulation of a region of the foot may, after removal of its normal afferent input from the foot, begin to respond to stimuli applied to an area of the leg adjacent to the foot (11, 36). It is not clear whether this acquisition of new inputs is due to sprouts from undamaged afferents, to activation of normally present but ineffective connections, or to activation of indirect pathways in the CNS (Figure 6.8). This acquisition of inputs from nearby structures by cells that have lost their normal input is a general property of cells in the somatosensory pathway (37).

In addition to this reorganization of inputs to central neurons, there is also evidence that denervation induces sprouting at the peripheral terminals of intact nearby primary afferents. When a peripheral nerve is cut, nerves that supply the adjacent skin area send sprouts into the denervated area (43) (Figure 6.8). In the rat, by 3 weeks after cutting the sciatic nerve, the intact saphenous nerve, which supplies adjacent skin, can mediate responses to stimuli from the denervated

PERIPHERAL
FIELD

SPINAL
CORD

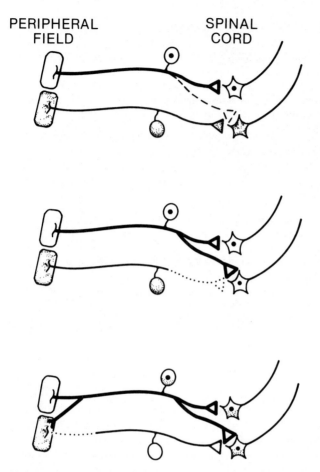

Figure 6.8 Functional plasticity of primary afferent nociceptors. **Top:** Normal connectivity of primary afferent. Primary afferents innervate a defined peripheral region and activate a specific set of spinal cord neurons. In addition, the primary afferent has central connections that are normally ineffective (*dashed line*). In the normal situation, each spinal cord cell responds only to stimulation of its own peripheral field. **Middle:** When the *central* process of a primary afferent that innervates an adjacent peripheral field (*stipple*) is interrupted (*dotted line*), the formerly ineffective central connection of the intact primary afferent (*heavy line*) becomes effective. Both spinal cord cells now respond only to stimulation of the innervated peripheral field (*not stippled*). **Lower:** When the *peripheral* process of the adjacent primary afferent is cut (*dotted line*), changes occur in the spinal cord that are similar to those produced by cutting the central process. In addition, the peripheral process of the intact primary afferent (*heavy line*) sprouts and grows into the denervated peripheral region (*stipple*). In this case, both spinal cord cells respond to stimulation of both peripheral fields.

sciatic territory (32). In addition, these rats become hyperresponsive to mildly noxious stimuli within the intact saphenous nerve region. The presence of the normal sciatic nerve actively inhibits central responses to noxious stimuli within the saphenous territory. Similar evidence of hyperalgesia adjacent to a denervated region of skin has also been observed in the primate (25).

Deafferentation is thus associated with two processes that may be related to neuropathic pain. One is the growth of nociceptive primary afferents into a denervated patch of skin and the other is the activation of aberrant connections to pain transmission neurons in the spinal cord. These processes may be part of the reason that the pain associated with deafferentation is so resistant to treatment by procedures that produce further deafferentation (45). For example, the pain of postherpetic neuralgia, which is associated with deafferentation of one dermatome, can be relieved transiently by cutting the nerve or the dorsal root innervating the painful segment; however, more often than not the pain returns. The failure of deafferenting procedures to permanently relieve the pain supports the notion that there is some process by which aberrant inputs from an area within or adjacent to a denervated region can produce excessive excitation of central pain transmission neurons.

Another relevant manifestation of the plasticity of somatosensory pathways is that, in the presence of deafferentation and chronic nociceptive input, central neurons whose activity normally does not produce pain become capable of producing it. This is suggested by the observation that, whereas surgical interruption of the spinothalamic and spinoreticular pathways (anterolateral cordotomy) produces profound hypalgesia with immediate relief of severe clinical pain, the pain usually returns within 1 to 2 years (66). There is no evidence that regeneration occurs in the CNS, so the return of the pain must represent a functional change in undamaged neurons. Somehow, over a period of months, these undamaged neurons acquire the capacity to provide a bypass route for the nociceptive message.

There seem to be two critical requirements for this process. First, there must be a sustained noxious input. Second, there must be deafferentation of a central pain transmission neuron. Provided these conditions are met, the pain message can detour or bypass a lesion of the normal somatosensory conduction pathway.

Clinical studies using electrical stimulation in the CNS of patients with neuropathic pain also support the concept that plasticity of somatosensory pathways plays an important role in neuropathic pain (59). In those patients with an intact nervous system and pain from a long-term peripheral tissue–damaging process such as cancer, electrical stimulation at the midbrain level produces reports of pain, but only when the electrode is in the vicinity of the spinothalamic tract. Stimulation of midbrain sites medial to the spinothalamic tract rarely produces pain in these patients. In contrast, in patients with chronic neuropathic pain, stimulation of these same medial sites characteristically produces burning pain. Furthermore, in the patients with neuropathic pain, such stimulation actually reproduces the quality and location of the patient's pain, something that does not occur in patients whose pain is not due to a neuropathic process. It is interesting in this regard that stimulation of the somatosensory cortex in humans rarely produces pain, except in cases of chronic neuropathic pain (28), in which the stimulation is reported to reproduce the patient's clinical pain. These observations raise the possibility that chronic neuropathic pain is associated with functional changes in central somatosensory pathways such that neurons that are not normally part of the pain transmission pathway contribute to sustaining chronic neuropathic pains. Lesion data are also consistent with the idea that alternate pathways for nociception develop concomitantly with chronic neuropathic pain. Thus, although lesions of the spinothalamic tract at the midbrain level relieve patients with non-neuropathic pain, such lesions do not help patients with neuropathic pains (59).

Figure 6.9 illustrates one possible explanation for these clinical observations. Normally, a noxious input will activate both spinothalamic and spinoreticular tracts. The spinothalamic input is relayed via the contralateral spinal cord and brainstem to the thalamus and cortex. Noxious inputs also activate both ipsilateral and contralateral spinoreticular pathways, but the input ascending over these medial pathways may be inhibited under normal conditions. According to this proposal, when the contralateral anterolateral quadrant is cut, noxious input would be relayed via the ipsilateral spinoreticular pathway. With time, this ipsilateral pathway becomes increasingly effective. Under these conditions medial brainstem stimulation would produce pain, and lesions of the spinothalamic tract in the lateral brainstem will not give pain relief.

Whether or not this proposal is valid, it seems likely that, in certain patients, neural pathways not normally involved in pain perception can develop the capacity to signal it. It is not surprising that patients with such pains are rarely helped by surgical interruption of the classical pain transmission pathways.

Pain From Lesions of the CNS

Lesions of the CNS rarely produce pain in previously pain-free individuals. Although pain and dysesthesias are not unusual following surgical procedures performed for pain relief, these cases are complicated by the likelihood that the original cause of the pain is still present and may contribute to the postsurgical problem (see above). This section will focus on pathological lesions that produce pain in previously pain-free individuals.

Lesions of the CNS that result in pain are typically traumatic or vascular and are located in or very near the pain transmission pathways (6, 51). The most common pain-producing lesion of the CNS is a stroke involving the ventral posterolateral thalamus. In most, but not all, thalamic cases there is impairment of pain and temperature sensation. The distal limbs are usually the sites of most intense pain, although it may involve the entire contralateral body. The essential features are similar to those of the pains resulting from lesions of the peripheral

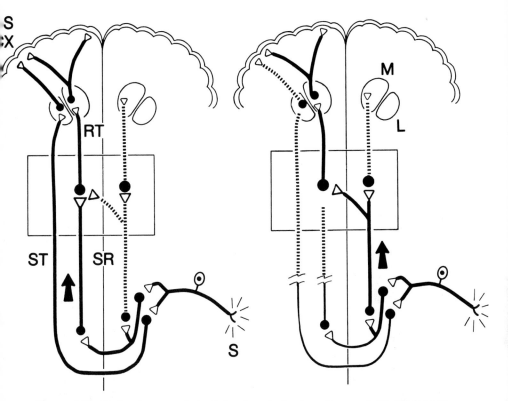

Figure 6.9 Redundancy and plasticity of central pain pathways. **Left:** Under normal circumstances, noxious stimuli (*S*) activate the contralateral spinothalamic (*ST*) and the spinoreticular (*SR*) pathways (*arrow*). ST projects directly to the lateral thalamus, which projects to somatosensory cortex (*SSCX*). The reticulothalamic (*RT*) projection terminates in the medial thalamus, which projects to wide areas of cortex, including SSCX. Noxious stimuli also activate the ipsilateral spinoreticulothalamic pathway (*dashed line*); however, the profound analgesic effect of contralateral cordotomy indicates that ipsilateral SR pathways normally contribute little to nociception. **Right:** A possible mechanism for the progressive recovery of nociceptive function after cordotomy. Because the ipsilateral SR pathway projects bilaterally to RT neurons, it can provide a "bypass" (*arrow*) for the pain message to the contralateral thalamus and cortex. *M,* medial thalamus; *L,* lateral thalamus.

nervous system: spontaneous pain and an exaggerated response to noxious stimuli. In some cases, the severe pain and hyperalgesia coexist with a significant impairment of cutaneous sensation. In these cases the hyperalgesia can be demonstrated by pressure over deep structures. The spontaneous pain may be steady, but usually there are spasms of severe pain superimposed. These bouts of severe pain may be triggered by light stroking of the skin, loud noises, bright lights, or other mild irritants.

The pain due to thalamic lesions was originally described by Dejerine and Roussy in 1906 (7). This description has not been improved upon, and is excerpted below [as translated by Wilkins and Brody (67)].

Case 6.2

"In our analytical study of the symptoms of the thalamic syndrome, we shall examine the signs as they appear a few months, or even better a year, after the onset of the hemiplegia.

"It is, in fact, in this period that the syndrome appears in all its purity, and then it is easiest to affirm its existence.

"The disorders of sensation take on major importance in the clinical picture we are studying by virtue of their intensity, their constancy, their character, and their modality. They dominate the symptomatology of the thalamic syndrome.

"*Superficial sensation* is affected by the thalamic lesions in its three modalities: touch, pain, and temperature. There is not a complete abolition of peripheral sensations but modification of sensory impressions as they occur in the cerebral anesthesias with all their classical characteristics. We will only enumerate them rapidly: The anesthesia is never absolute as in hysterical hemianesthesia; it predominates in the distal portion of the limb and diminishes from the periphery proximally; and finally, on the trunk and the face this anesthesia goes slightly over the midline of the body, 1 to 2 cm. on the healthy side.

"*Deep sensation* is affected much more, and in its various components: articular, muscular, tendinous, osseous."

The presence of pains on the hemiplegic side are important to note.

"They appear early, dating from the onset of the hemiplegia, or a few months later. They reside not only in the paralyzed limbs, but also in the face and trunk. It is very hard to obtain from the patients an exact idea of the localization of these pains concerning whether they are superficial or deep. Most of the patients, though, insist that they are rather superficial and that it is the skin and the subjacent adipose tissue which are painful.

"In any case, these pains are continuous with paroxysmal exacerbations, sometimes bringing cries from the patients and keeping them from sleep or awakening them rudely.

"One of our patients keeps telling us that what prevents her from moving her left hand, or walking, are the intense pains in her arm and leg. Here is a true *painful impotence*.

"Moreover, the pain is not exclusively spontaneous. In some cases it may be provoked by simply touching the skin with the finger. Pinprick, contact with cold and heat, and pressure are very painful. The patients are sometimes very hyperesthetic.

"The patients sometimes compare their pains to superficial or deep burns, sometimes to twinges, to violent and painful pressure placed on the skin, sometimes to the stabbing of a dagger. These phenomena have a paroxysmal character. Between crises, there are formications, numbness in the tips of the limbs and sometimes around the face.

"Finally we note another important characteristic. These pains are not suppressed by any internal or external analgesic treatment. Nothing gives relief to the patient, whose suffering is sometimes intolerable."[2]

Subsequent reports have established that lesions of other sites in the CNS can give rise to a pain syndrome that is qualitatively identical to that resulting from thalamic lesions. Such sites include the spinal cord, medulla, pons, and cortex. A careful review of the cord, medulla, and pons in previously pain-free individuals who develop central pain syndromes has clearly shown that pain-producing lesions usually include or are adjacent to the spinothalamic tract (6). The distribution of the pain in these cases is topographically related to the body region served by the damaged spinothalamic tract at that level, that is, it usually overlaps the area of impairment of pain and temperature sensation.

Lesions of the cerebral cortex can produce a pain syndrome that is indistinguishable from that produced by thalamic lesions. Although this condition, called pseudothalamic syndrome, is exceptionally rare, there are a few well-documented cases in the published literature (13).

The attempt to understand the mechanism or mechanisms underlying the pain that results from lesions of the CNS is complicated not only by the rarity of the clinical cases but, more importantly, by the fact that in the majority of patients apparently identical lesions are painless. What does seem clear, however, is that lesions must be in or near the pain pathway at some point between the spinal cord and cortex and that an exaggerated response to noxious stimuli is often present.

Several authors have suggested that the lateral neospinothalamic tract exerts a damping action on the medial paleospinothalamic and spinoreticulothalamic pathways (6). According to this idea, damage to the neospinothalamic tract that spares the medial pathways would release the latter from inhibition, resulting in summation and hyperalgesia. This is analogous to what happens when dorsal horn nociceptors excited by unmyelinated primary afferents are released from the inhibitory influence of myelinated afferents.

Despite the plausibility of theories that emphasize loss of central inhibition in the etiology of these painful conditions, it is likely that other factors also play an important role. One important possibility is that efferent sympathetic activity contributes to the pain. This concept is suggested by the clinical observation that peripheral sympathetic blockade can sometimes relieve the pain associated with CNS lesions (30).

Laboratory research into the mechanism of pain due to CNS lesions is hampered by the lack of an animal model. The reader is referred to other authors for a more detailed discussion of possible pathophysiological mechanisms (6).

[2]Reprinted by permission from Wilkins, R. H., and Brody, I. A.: The thalamic syndrome. *Arch. Neurol.* **20:**559–562, 1969.

Pain Due to Epileptic Discharge

In addition to the pathophysiological mechanisms discussed above, pain can be produced by focal epileptic discharge. Focal epilepsy is a feature of the damaged cerebral cortex characterized by hypersynchronous discharge of neighboring cortical cells. The abnormal discharge has the characteristic property of spreading to involve adjacent undamaged cortical regions. Unless a patient is actually injured by the motor manifestations of the seizure (falls and tongue biting are common), seizures are typically painless. However, approximately 2 percent of patients with focal epilepsy report pain either prior to or concomitant with other, more typical seizure manifestations. Gowers (15) divided patients with painful seizures into three groups: unilateral body pain, head pain, or abdominal pain.

The following case, quoted from Young and Blume (69), is typical of the unilateral body pain type:

Case 6.3

A 14-year-old girl with a congenital left hemiparesis developed seizures when aged 10 years. The seizures began with a "burning, tingling pain" in the left forearm which progressed to a "shooting pain" to the left shoulder. This sometimes proceeded to macropsia and then a generalized tonic-clonic seizure. On examination her paresis was most marked in her left arm and hand. The small left hand was analgesic and anaesthetic distal to the wrist, with pin prick sensation reduced but still perceived in the remainder of the left upper limb, left upper thorax, left side of the neck and left lower face. Position sense was impaired in the left wrist. A seizure recorded on the EEG showed reduction in voltage in the right central region just prior to the onset of left arm pain. Quasi-periodic right central sharp waves followed this flattening.

At operation, an area of shrunken gliotic cortex was present in the post central gyrus and superior temporal area on the right. This shrunken area probably included the "hand area" as stimulation just above this area produced a sensation of tingling in the left forearm. Cortical epileptiform activity was present superior and posterior to the gliotic area on the post central gyrus. Resection of the atrophic area and immediately adjacent cortex relieved her of her seizures.

Electroencephalographic recording has established that for patients with unilateral body pain the sensation is perceived during epileptiform discharge in the contralateral parietal (somatosensory) cortex. There are several reports, such as the one quoted above, of patients in whom surgical excision of the cortical region containing the seizure focus relieved the pain and the other manifestations of the seizure. The pain often has a tingly, abnormal quality similar to the dysesthesias produced by peripheral nerve injury. In these cases it seems likely that the pain is a projected sensation due to electrical activation of cortical cells that are normally involved in pain sensation. Whether the pain is due directly to the discharge of the somatosensory cortical cells or to other cells to which they project is not clear. These clinical findings do, however, support the idea that the somatosensory cortex plays a role in pain sensation.

In some cases abdominal pain is a major manifestation of the seizure. Another case of Young and Blume's is typical:

Case 6.4

> This 21-year-old man had hemiconvulsions in childhood. His seizures subsequently began with a "sharp" abdominal pain, "like someone hitting me with an axe", followed by loss of consciousness with automatisms. Apart from dull normal intelligence, there was no neurological deficit. His EEG showed multiple independent spikes, maximal in the right anterior temporal and superior frontal regions. A recorded clinical and electrographic seizure began in the right anterior-midtemporal region.

In these abdominal cases the pain is associated with a seizure focus in the temporal lobe. In the cases of head pain due to epilepsy, it is not certain that the pain results directly from the epileptiform discharge. The pain is usually described in terms similar to common headache. Furthermore, the pain is often ipsilateral to the seizure focus, occasionally directly over it, raising the possibility that the headache is due to local factors related to increased blood flow or focal brain swelling.

Summary

In this chapter I have discussed several clinical neuropathic pain syndromes and a variety of potential mechanisms. The mechanisms that may contribute to neuropathic pain are listed in Table 6.4. At the present time only two processes have definitely been associated with clinical pain syndromes: cortical epileptiform discharge, which is actually a rare cause of pain, and sympathetic efferent facilitation (or sensitization) of the peripheral terminals of primary afferents. It is not clear whether sympathetically maintained pains depend on increased or abnormal discharge in sympathetic efferents, increased sensitivity of primary afferents, a change in the central actions of afferents sensitive to sympathetic efferents (52), or some combination of these factors.

The contribution to clinical pain of the other mechanisms discussed in this chapter is not known with any certainty. There are psychophysical, neurophysiological, and clinical data to support the concept that loss of myelinated afferent inhibition of spinal pain transmission cells contributes to clinical pain. Thus, in normal subjects, with selective blockade of peripheral nerve myelinated axons, cutaneous stimuli result in exaggerated, summating sensations that have a burning, dysesthetic quality similar to what is reported by many patients with painful injuries to peripheral nerve. On the other hand, since most patients with nerve injuries do not have spontaneous pain, it is likely that the pain of nerve injury is due to a combination of factors. For example, in causalgia, the pain may result from a combination of loss of myelinated afferent inhibition, ectopic impulse generation at the site of nerve injury, and sympathetic activation of primary afferents (52). In tic douloureux, and the lancinating pains associated with demyelinating disease, the sympathetic nervous system does not contribute to the pain, and ectopic impulse generation from a demyelinated patch of axon is a more likely cause of the distinctive pain pattern. With brachial plexus avulsion, the pain may be primarily due to hyperactivity of deafferented spinal pain transmission cells. Because there is presently no satisfactory animal model of neuropathic pain, the investigation of these problems will require physiological studies of patients. Until the results of such studies are available, postulated mechanisms of most neuropathic pains will remain speculative.

References

1 Blumberg, H., and Janig, W.: Changes of reflexes in vasoconstrictor neurons supplying the cat's hindlimb following chronic nerve lesions: A model for studying mechanisms of reflex sympathetic dystrophy. *J. Autonomic Nerv. Syst.* **7**:399–411, 1983.

2 Blumcke, S., and Niedorf, H. R.: Electronenoptische untersuchungen und wachstumsendkolben regenierender peipherer nervenfasern. *Virchows Arch.* **340**:93, 1965.

3 Bonelli, S., Conoscente, F., Movilia, P. G., Restelli, L., Francucci, B., and Grossi, E.: Regional intravenous guanethidine vs. stellate ganglion block in reflex sympathetic dystrophies: A randomized trail. *Pain* **16**:297–307, 1983.

4 Burchiel, K. J.: Abnormal impulse generation in focally demyelinated trigeminal roots. *J. Neurosurg.* **53**:674–683, 1980.

5 Calvin, W. H., Loeser, J. D., and Howe, J. F.: A neurophysiological theory for the mechanism of tic douloureux. *Pain* **3**:147–154, 1977.

6 Cassinari, V., and Pagni, C. A.: *Central Pain, a Neurosurgical Survey.* Harvard University Press, Cambridge, MA, 1969.

7 Dejerine, J., and Roussy, G.: Le syndrome thalamique. *Rev. Neurol.* **14**:521–532, 1906.

8 De Takats, G.: Reflex dystrophy of the extremities. *Arch. Surg.* **34**:939–956, 1937.

9   Devor, M.: The pathophysiology and anatomy of damaged nerve. In P. D. Wall and R. Melzack (eds.), *Textbook of Pain*. Churchill-Livingstone, Edinburgh, 1984, pp. 49–64.

10 Devor, M., and Janig, W.: Activation of myelinated afferents ending in a neuroma by stimulation of the sympathetic supply in the rat. *Neurosci. Lett.* **24:**43–47, 1981.

11 Devor, M., and Wall, P. D.: Plasticity in the spinal cord sensory map following peripheral nerve injury in rats. *J. Neurosci.* **1:**679–684, 1981.

12 Doupe, J., Cullen, C. H., and Chance, G. Q.: Post-traumatic pain and the causalgic syndrome. *J. Neurol. Psychiatry* **7:**33–48, 1944.

13 Fields, H. L., and Adams, J. E.: Pain after cortical injury relieved by electrical stimulation of the internal capsule. *Brain* **97:**169–178, 1974.

14 Fowler, T. J., and Ochoa, J.: Unmyelinated fibres in normal and compressed peripheral nerves of the baboon: A quantitative electron microscopic study. *Neuropathol. Appl. Neurobiol.* **1:**247–265, 1975.

15 Gowers, W. R.: *Epilepsy and other Chronic Convulsive Diseases: Their Causes, Symptoms and Treatment*. Churchill, London, 1901.

16 Granit, R., and Skoglund, C. R.: Facilitation, inhibition and depression at the 'artificial synapse' formed by the cut end of a mammalian nerve. *J. Physiol. (Lond.)* **103:**435–448, 1945.

17 Hannington-Kiff, J. G.: Intravenous regional sympathetic block with guanethidine. *Lancet* **1:**1019–1020, 1974.

18 Head, H., and Holmes, G.: Sensory disturbances from cerebral lesions. *Brain* **34:**102–254, 1911.

19 Hongo, T., Jankowska, E., and Lundberg, A.: Postsynaptic excitation and inhibition from primary afferents in neurones of the spinocervical tract. *J. Physiol. (Lond.)* **199:**569–592, 1968.

20 Howe, J. F., Loeser, J. D., and Calvin, W. H.: Mechanosensitivity of dorsal root ganglia and chronically injured axons: A physiological basis for the radicular pain of nerve root compression. *Pain* **3:**25–41, 1977.

21 Janig, W.: Causalgia and reflex sympathetic dystrophy: In which way is the sympathetic nervous system involved? *TINS* **8:**471–477, 1985.

22 Jefferson, D., and Eames, R. A.: Subclinical entrapment of the lateral femoral cutaneous nerve: An autopsy study. *Muscle Nerve* **2:**145–154, 1979.

23 Kerr, F. W. L.: Pathology of trigeminal neuralgia: Light and electronmicroscopic observations. *J. Neurosurg.* **26:**151–156, 1967.

24 Kibler, R. F., and Nathan, P. W.: Relief of pain and paraesthesiae by nerve block distal to a lesion. *J. Neurol. Neurosurg. Psychiatry* **23:**91, 1960.

25 Kirk, E. J., and Denny-Brown, D.: Functional variation in dermatomes in macaque monkey following dorsal root lesions. *J. Comp. Neurol.* **139:**307–320, 1970.

26 Kozin, F., McCarty, D. J., Sims, J., and Genant, H.: The reflex sympathetic dystrophy syndrome. 1. Clinical and histologic studies: Evidence for bilaterality, response to corticosteroids and articular involvement. *Am. J. Med.* **60:**321–331, 1976.

27 Levine, J. D., Dardick, S. J., Basbaum, A. I., and Scipio, E.: Reflex neurogenic inflammation. 1. Contribution of the peripheral nervous system to spatially remote inflammatory responses that follow injury. *J. Neurosci.* **5:**1380–1386, 1985.

28 Lewin, W., and Phillips, C. G.: Observations on partial removal of the post-central gyrus for pain. *J. Neurol. Neurosurg. Psychiatry* **15:**143, 1952.

29 Livingston, W. K.: *Pain Mechanisms.* Macmillan, New York, 1943.

30 Loh, L. Nathan, P. W., and Schott, G. D.: Pain due to lesions of central nervous system removed by sympathetic block. *Bri. Med. J.* **282:**1026–1028, 1981.

31 Lombard, M. C., and Larabi, Y.: Electrophysiological study of cervical dorsal horn cells in partially deafferented rats. *Adv. Pain Res. Ther.* **5:**147–154, 1983.

32 Markus, H., Pomeranz, B., and Krushelnycky, D.: Spread of saphenous somatotopic projection map in spinal cord and hypersensitivity of the foot after chronic sciatic denervation in adult rat. *Brain Res.* **296:**27–39, 1984.

33 Matthews, W. B., Acheson, E. D., Batchelor, J. R., and Weller, R. O.: *McAlpine's Multiple Sclerosis.* Churchill-Livingstone, London, 1985.

34 Melzack, R., and Wall, P. D.: Pain mechanisms: A new theory. *Science* **150:**971–978, 1965.

35 Melzack, R., and Wall, P. D.: *The Challenge of Pain.* Basic Books, New York, 1982.

36 Mendell, L. M., Sassoon, E. M., and Wall, P. D.: Properties of synaptic linkage from long ranging afferents onto dorsal horn neurons in normal and deafferented cats. *J. Physiol. (Lond.)* **285:**299–310, 1978.

37 Merzenich, M. M., Nelson, R. J., Stryker, M. P., Cynader, M. S., Schoppmann, A., and Zook, J. M.: Somatosensory cortical map changes following digit amputation in adult monkeys. *J. Comp. Neurol.* **224:**591–605, 1984.

38 Meyer, G. A., and Fields, H. L.: Causalgia treated by selective large fibre stimulation of peripheral nerve. *Brain* **95**:163–168, 1972.

39 Meyer, R. A., Campbell, J. N., and Raja, S.: Peripheral neural mechanisms of cutaneous hyperalgesia. *Adv. Pain Res. Ther.* **9**:53–71, 1985.

40 Mitchell, S. W.: *Injuries of Nerves and Their Consequences.* Dover, New York, 1965.

41 Nashold, B. S., and Ostdahl, R. H.: Dorsal root entry zone lesions for pain relief. *J. Neurosurg.* **51**:59–69, 1979.

42 Nathan, P. W., and Wall, P. D.: Treatment of post-herpetic neuralgia by prolonged electric stimulation. *Br. Med. J.* **3**:645–647, 1974.

43 Nixon, B. J., Doucette, R., Jackson, P. C., and Diamond, J.: Impulse activity evokes precocious sprouting of nociceptive nerves into denervated skin. *Somatosensory Res.* **2**:97–126, 1984.

44 Noordenbos, W.: *Pain.* Elsevier, Amsterdam, 1959.

45 Noordenbos, W., and Wall, P. D.: Implications of the failure of nerve resection and graft to cure chronic pain produced by nerve lesions. *J. Neurol. Neurosurg. Psychiatry* **44**:1068–1073, 1981.

46 Nystrom, B., and Hagbarth, K. E.: Microelectrode recordings from transected nerves in amputees with phantom limb pain. *Neurosci. Lett.* **27**:211–216, 1981.

47 Ochoa, J.: Pain in local nerve lesions. In W. J. Culp and J. Ochoa (eds.), *Abnormal Nerves and Muscles as Impulse Generators.* Oxford University Press, New York, 1982.

48 Ochoa, J., and Noordenbos, W.: Pathology and disordered sensation in local nerve lesions: An attempt at correlation. *Adv. Pain Res. Ther.* **3**:67–90, 1979.

49 Pak, T. J., Martin, G. M., Magness, J. L., and Kavanaugh, M. D.: Reflex sympathetic dystrophy. *Minn. Med.* **53**:507–512, 1970.

50 Patman, R. D., Thompson, J. E., and Persson, A. V.: Management of post-traumatic pain syndromes: Report of 113 cases. *Ann. Surg.* **177**:780–787, 1973.

51 Riddoch, G.: The clinical features of central pain. *Lancet* Volume 1:1093–1209, 1938.

52 Roberts, W. J.: An hypothesis on the physiological basis for causalgia and related pains. *Pain* **24**:297–311, 1986.

53   Roberts, W. J., and Elardo, S. M.: Sympathetic activation of A-delta nociceptors. *Somatosensory Res.* **3**:33–44, 1985.

54   Roberts, W. J., Elardo, S. M., and King, K. A.: Sympathetically induced changes in the responses of slowly adapting type I receptors in cat skin. *Somatosensory Res.* **2**:223–236, 1985.

55   Scadding, J. W.: Development of ongoing activity, mechanosensitivity and adrenaline sensitivity in severed peripheral nerve axons. *Exp. Neurol.* **73**:345–364, 1981.

56   Seltzer, Z., and Devor, M.: Ephaptic transmission in chronically damaged peripheral nerves. *Neurology* 29:1061–1064, 1979.

57   Shibasaki, H., and Yoshigoro, H.: Painful tonic seizure in multiple sclerosis. *Arch. Neurol.* **30**:47, 1974.

58   Stewart, J. D., and Aguayo, A. H.: Compression and entrapment neuropathies. In P. J. Dyck, P. K. Thomas, E. H. Lambert, and R. Bunge (eds.), *Peripheral Neuropathy* (2nd ed.). Saunders, Philadelphia, 1984.

59   Tasker, R. R., Tsuda, T., and Hawrylyshyn, P.: Clinical neurophysiological investigation of deafferentation pain. *Adv. Pain Res. Ther.* **5**:713–738, 1983.

60   Thomas, P. K.: The anatomical substratum of pain, evidence derived from morphometric studies on peripheral nerve. *Can. J. Neurol. Sci.* **1**:92–97, 1974.

61   Walker, A. E., and Nulson, F.: Electrical stimulation of the upper thoracic portion of the sympathetic chain in man. *Arch. Neurol. Psychiatry* **59**:559, 1948.

62   Wall, P. D., and Devor. M.: Sensory afferent impulses originate from dorsal root ganglia as well as from the periphery in normal and nerve injured rats. *Pain* **17**:321–339, 1983.

63   Wall, P. D., and Gutnick, M.: Properties of afferent nerve impulses originating from a neuroma. *Nature* **248**:740–743, 1974.

64   Wall, P. D., and Sweet, W. H.: Temporary abolition of pain in man. *Science* **155**:108–109, 1967.

65   Wallin, G., Torebjörk, E., Hallin, R. Preliminary observations on the pathophysiology of hyperalgesia in the causalgic pain syndrome. In Y. Zotterman (ed.), *Sensory Functions of the Skin in Primates.* Pergamon Press, Oxford, England, 1976.

66   White, J. C., and Sweet, W. H.: *Pain and the Neurosurgeon. A Forty-Year Experience.* Charles C. Thomas, Springfield, IL, 1969.

67 Wilkins, R. H., and Brody, I. A.: The thalamic syndrome. *Arch. Neurol.* **20:**559–562, 1969.

68 Wynn-Parry, C. B.: Pain in avulsion lesions of the brachial plexus. *Pain* **9:**41–53, 1980.

69 Young, G. B., and Blume, W. T.: Painful epileptic seizures. *Brain* 106:537–554, 1983.

70 Zimmermann, M., and Sanders, K.: Responses of nerve axons and receptor endings to heat, ischemia, and algesic substances. Abnormal excitability of regenerating nerve ending. In W. J. Culp and J. Ochoa (eds.), *Abnormal Nerves and Muscles as Impulse Generators.* Oxford University Press, New York, 1982.

Chapter 7

The Psychology of Pain

I have reviewed the anatomy, physiology, and pharmacology of pain and attempted to relate what is known about neural mechanisms to clinical problems. Although there are major gaps in our knowledge of these basic pain mechanisms, there is general agreement about the body of knowledge presented. In the present chapter I outline some of the current ideas about the psychology of pain. This is an area of great importance and active research, but one where there are few definitive observations. Because our understanding of the psychology of pain is so primitive, there are many different approaches to its study, and many plausible but unproven theories have been proposed. What we do know of the psychology of pain is derived primarily from uncontrolled clinical observations and from studies of experimental pain in human subjects. The reproducibility of the findings in different experimental and clinical studies is limited, and the literature is rife with controversy (39). Despite this problem, there has been progress and some areas of general agreement are beginning to emerge. I will try to stay as close as possible to areas of agreement while presenting several different approaches to the analysis of the psychological aspects of pain.

In Chapter 3, I contrasted the sensory and affective (emotional) aspects of pain and discussed the evidence that these two aspects have at least partially separate neuroanatomic substrates. Knowledge of the sensory aspect of pain is much more extensive and certain than that of the affective aspect. However, from the patient's point of view, only the affective aspect, i.e., the unpleasantness of pain is significant. Pain becomes a problem when, for whatever reason, it can no longer be ignored. At that point, pain has significant effects on behavior and on the emotional life of the person experiencing it.

People experience pain frequently. This point was documented dramatically by a recent telephone survey of adults in the United States (40). This study revealed, for example, that nearly 15 percent of the population had at least 30 days of backache in the preceding year. In addition, headaches or joint pains lasting 30 days or more were each reported by more than 10 percent of the population. Most people accept these common pains as a normal, if unpleasant, part of life. They ignore the pain or treat themselves with over-the-counter drugs or home remedies, and go about their lives. Although there are no systematic studies of the psychological impact of these common pains on the individuals who suffer from them, it is likely that mild frustration, irritability, and impatience are the normal responses. Obviously, the psychological reaction will be greater when the pain is sufficient to interfere with normal activities. The telephone survey referred to above also found that functional impairment resulting from pain is very common in the general population. For example, back pain alone causes over 5 percent of adults to lose 7 or more days of work per year, and about the same number have at least 7 sleepless nights each year for the same reason.

It is not clear why pain produces a functional impairment in some people, whereas most are able to carry on with their lives despite it. Intensity is obviously a major factor. A second important factor is the *meaning* of the pain to the individual. This is closely tied to location and quality. For example, chest pain in a person who has previously suffered myocardial infarction may be particularly disabling because it is interpreted as life threatening. In addition, clinical observations suggest that differences in personality traits between individuals contribute to the variation in their responses to pain. Finally, there is evidence that psychosocial factors in the home or at work can help perpetuate pain complaints and functional impairment.

Affective responses to painful injury or disease range from annoyance to agony and desperation. These affective responses, which are the major determinant of impairment, can be produced by problems other than somatic pain, for example, personal loss or endogenous depression. If a painful injury or disease occurs in a person who has such problems, the degree of suffering is likely to be out of proportion to the severity of the somatic pain. Thus a major task for the clinician dealing with pain patients, especially those with chronic pain, is to assess the relative contribution of psychological and somatic factors. Unfortunately, there is always a degree of uncertainty about such assessments because there is no way to objectively measure how intense a person's pain actually is.

The problem of assessment is also compounded by the fact that patients are often unaware of or reluctant to discuss the most relevant psychological issues. A mild somatic pain may be emphasized by a depressed or anxious patient because it is more socially acceptable to seek medical than psychiatric help (15–17). Thus, the type of help sought by the patient is often inappropriate to his or her most significant problem (16, 17). Individuals complaining of chronic pain frequently deny that they have any problems unrelated to their pain (3) and resist psychiatric evaluation (10). Unfortunately, for many such patients approaches that ignore the psychological factors are not likely to produce any long-term benefit. Clearly, the adequate assessment and treatment of patients with persistent pain demands attention to both somatic and psychological factors.

In this chapter, I will focus on three issues. One is the psychological effects produced in the individual by somatic pain. The second is how a person's preexisting psychological traits affect his or her response to noxious stimuli. The third is how environmental factors can perpetuate pain-induced behaviors through psychological mechanisms.

Psychological Consequences of Pain

ACUTE AND EXPERIMENTAL PAIN

At the present time the psychological effects of pain are most effectively assessed by questioning patients and evaluating their verbal reports. By definition, pain is associated with negative affect. If the pain is of sufficient duration, the negative affect develops into a distinctly unpleasant mood or emotion. The contribution of affect to the overall experience of pain is verified by the frequency with which patients use emotionally charged words such as "unbearable" or "excruciating" to describe their pain.

One of the first systematic approaches to evaluating the affective aspect of pain in humans was to record the words people use to describe their experience. Melzack and Torgerson (21, 22) pioneered this approach by obtaining lists of the most common words used by people to describe their pain. They attempted to come to a consensus among patients, students, and physicians about the meaning of the words and their relative magnitudes. They came up with 20 lists of words (Table 7.1), which fall into two broad categories—sensory and affective. Some of the sensory words communicate a definite somatic sensation (e.g., itchy, tingling, aching), whereas others describe the sensation in terms of an objective stimulus that might produce it (e.g., burning, pinching, tugging, cutting). Both types of sensory words clearly refer to phenomena that are localized to a specific part of the body. In contrast, the affective words (e.g., fearful, dreadful) describe negative feelings that usually do not have a specific location in the body. They refer to feelings that can also occur in emotionally charged situations where there is no somatic pain. Thus the words that people commonly use to describe their subjective experience of pain support the idea that affective responses, similar to those produced by other unpleasant life events, are an integral part of "normal" pain perception.

Because of the close tie of pain with fear and anxiety one might expect individuals who tend to be fearful or anxious to experience more pain. As dis-

Table 7.1   Words Commonly Used by People to Describe Pain

1	2	3	4
1 Flickering	1 Jumping	1 Pricking	1 Sharp
2 Quivering	2 Flashing	2 Boring	2 Cutting
3 Pulsing	3 Shooting	3 Drilling	3 Lacerating
4 Throbbing		4 Stabbing	
5 Beating		5 Lancinating	
6 Pounding			

5	6	7	8
1 Pinching	1 Tugging	1 Hot	1 Tingling
2 Pressing	2 Pulling	2 Burning	2 Itchy
3 Gnawing	3 Wrenching	3 Scalding	3 Smarting
4 Cramping		4 Searing	4 Stinging
5 Crushing			

9	10	11	12
1 Dull	1 Tender	1 Tiring	1 Sickening
2 Sore	2 Taut	2 Exhausting	2 Suffocating
3 Hurting	3 Rasping		
4 Aching	4 Splitting		
5 Heavy			

13	14	15	16
1 Fearful	1 Punishing	1 Wretched	1 Annoying
2 Frightful	2 Gruelling	2 Blinding	2 Troublesome
3 Terrifying	3 Cruel		3 Miserable
	4 Vicious		4 Intense
	5 Killing		5 Unbearable

17	18	19	20
1 Spreading	1 Tight	1 Cool	1 Nagging
2 Radiating	2 Numb	2 Cold	2 Nauseating
3 Penetrating	3 Drawing	3 Freezing	3 Agonizing
4 Piercing	4 Squeezing		4 Dreadful
	5 Tearing		5 Torturing

Reprinted by permission from Melzack, R.: The McGill Pain Questionnaire: Major properties and scoring methods. *Pain* **1:**277–299, 1975.

cussed in Chapter 1, some people with low pain tolerance have exaggerated expectations of harm (42). In fact, individuals in whom anxiety is a prominent personality trait report more pain and require more analgesic medication following surgery (39), and there is evidence that people tolerate more severe pain if they feel they have some control over it [see Thompson (41) for review]. The control may simply consist of a belief that the noxious stimulus can be reduced or terminated by some action of the subject. Another means of control is for a person to have a strategy for distraction, for example, listening to music or imagining that the painful area is numb (2). In clinical situations, control may be sought by attributing the pain to a cause that implies personal responsibility (e.g., I wouldn't have sprained my ankle if I had been more careful) (41). The common element in these approaches is that they give the subject a feeling that he or she can do something to reduce the intensity or the occurrence of pain. They would therefore be expected to reduce anxiety.

Understanding the effect of individual differences in psychological makeup on responses to pain can be of great practical help in treatment. Relief of anxiety by reassurance, instilling a sense of control, or the short-term use of anxiolytic drugs can be of immense help for some patients, especially those with acute pain of somatic origin.

CHRONIC PAIN

It is likely that the same personality traits that predispose certain individuals with acute pain to more suffering would have an even greater effect on those with persistent pain. However, direct evidence on this question is not available. Although many patients with chronic pain have characteristic psychological abnormalities (26, 36), it is not clear which of the abnormalities were caused by the pain and which predisposed the patients to it. A major problem is that most studies of the psychological attributes of chronic pain have been carried out in the setting of a pain clinic. The patients who are referred to pain specialists represent a highly selected population whose characteristics differ from other populations of chronic pain patients, for example, those treated by primary care physicians (7). Furthermore, those individuals with chronic pain who do not seek medical attention and continue to function despite their pain constitute an important group rarely subject to psychological studies. It is likely that the psychological profile of chronic pain patients seen in a pain clinic is shaped not only by the fact of chronic pain but by the selection process that channeled them to the pain clinic. The psychological effect of chronic pain and the role of predisposing personality factors in its genesis can only be accurately determined by studies of patients that begin before their pain becomes chronic. Since only a small percentage of patients with acute pains go on to have chronic pain, such prospective studies would require large numbers of patients. It is obviously very

Table 7.2   Some Common Symptoms in Patients with Persistent Pain

Depressed mood

Sleep disturbance

Somatic preoccupation

Reduced activity

Reduced libido

Fatigue

important that methods be developed to identify those patients who are at high risk for chronicity.

Setting aside for the moment the problem of patient selection, there is agreement among experienced clinicians about some of the psychological features that are common in patients with chronic pain (Table 7.2) (3, 5, 26, 36). It is well established that many chronic pain patients are depressed. For example, using a standardized scale to evaluate depression, one recent study found clinically significant depression in 79 percent of chronic low back pain patients (8). Vegetative signs typical of depression, including early morning awakening, weight loss, and decreased libido, were common in this patient group.

In addition to changes in mood there are disturbances in thinking and behavior. Pain tends to capture and dominate a person's attention. Patients become preoccupied with it and they can often describe its location and qualities in exquisite detail. They seem to notice little else. They will tell you that the persistent unpleasant sensation has taken the joy out of their lives. They tend to withdraw from social contact and from other activities, including sports, hobbies, and housework. Sexual activity is reduced and, because ambulation often makes them feel worse, many retreat to a bed or a chair and become increasingly dependent on family and friends. If they cannot work, financial problems ensue with additional worry and loss of independence and self-esteem.

A common complaint of patients with persistent pain is that it interferes with their sleep (3, 8). This problem not only leads to chronic fatigue, it presents the patient with lonely, sleepless nights. The absence of nighttime distraction intensifies the misery. The pain is difficult enough to ignore during the day; at night it becomes impossible. It is obvious that chronic pain is demoralizing and potentially devastating.

In addition to the analysis of individual case studies, the psychology of chronic pain patients has been studied by administering standardized questionnaires. The one most commonly used is the Minnesota Multiphasic Personality Inventory (MMPI). Although the interpretation of the MMPI is somewhat confounded by the fact that many of the questions relate to somatic symptoms that could be due to either emotional disturbance or somatic disease (e.g., palpitations, light-headedness), it is of value as a way to compare the work of different investigators (35). Patients with chronic pain score very high on the hysteria, depression, and hypochondriasis scales (6, 36).

In an attempt to approach the question of the impact of chronicity, Sternbach et al. (38) compared patients with low back pain of less than 6 months' duration (acute pain) to patients who had had the same type of pain for more than 6 months (chronic pain). Although the "acute" low back pain patients did have elevations in the MMPI hysteria, depression, and hypochondriasis scales, the elevations were significantly greater in the chronic low back pain patients. A similar relationship between acute and chronic pain was found (6). These studies are consistent with the idea that the MMPI abnormalities resulted from the persistent painful condition. This conclusion is also supported by the observations of Sternbach and Timmermans (37). They studied 113 patients with low back pain of at least 6 months' duration. Twenty-nine underwent surgery followed by a rehabilitation program, and the other 84 received rehabilitation only. Both groups were evaluated before and 6 weeks after treatment. Following treatment, both groups showed reduced pain and both were significantly less abnormal on the MMPI hysteria and hypochondriasis scales. The surgical group had a greater posttreatment reduction in pain and a greater reduction in MMPI abnormalities. These results are consistent with the idea that the chronic pain contributed to the psychological abnormalities.

In an interesting extension of these studies Naliboff and his colleagues (23) compared a group of patients with chronic pain to a group with chronic *nonpainful* illnesses that included diabetes and hypertension. The patients were studied using the MMPI and a standardized scale that assessed the patients' ability to carry out their normal daily activities (work, household, social, sexual, recreational). They found that, within each patient group, abnormalities on the MMPI correlated significantly with the self-assessed functional impairment. Although this study does not tell us whether the functional impairment or the MMPI abnormality was primary, it raises the possibility that at least part of the psychological abnormality associated with chronic pain is related to the functional impairment and thus only **indirectly** related to the pain.

In summary, extensive clinical experience and some systematic studies using standard psychological tests agree that pain is associated with significant emotional disturbances. Acutely, anxiety and fear predominate; chronically, depression develops along with persistent anxiety and a somatic preoccupation.

Psychological Processes and Syndromes That Predispose Patients to Chronic Pain

There is a broad range of individual responses to chronic pain. At one extreme there are those who are able to ignore the pain, who do not seek medical attention and continue their work and their personal lives. Since these individuals have little contact with the medical profession, little is known about how they cope successfully with chronic pain. At the other extreme are those patients whose lives are literally destroyed by pain. In some cases, for example, in patients with cancer, there is an obvious somatic cause for severe persistent pain; more puzzling are those individuals who have little in the way of objective evidence to explain their pain. There is convincing evidence that some of the latter group have psychological abnormalities that predispose them to the development of chronic pain. Many experienced clinicians believe that these patients suffer from a condition that is best understood as a mental rather than somatic illness (3, 10).

To examine this possibility, Blumer and Heilbronn (3) compared two different groups of patients with chronic pain. One group consisted of 36 patients with advanced rheumatoid arthritis, an easily diagnosed condition with a clearly identifiable somatic source of pain. The other group consisted of patients with pains of undiagnosed cause in a variety of locations, including the face, abdomen, and low back. Patients in the rheumatoid arthritis group tended to be older and to have had their pain for a longer period of time, but the groups were otherwise demographically similar and had approximately the same level of functional impairment. Although both groups had significant depressive symptoms and impairments in social, sexual, and recreational activity, a significantly higher percentage of patients in the undiagnosed pain group were depressed and had insomnia. Furthermore, a strikingly high percentage of patients in the undiagnosed pain group had close relatives with mental illness (42 percent) and/or a physically abusive spouse (23 percent). The authors concluded that the group with undiagnosed chronic pain included individuals with predominantly psychological abnormalities.

There are a variety of emotional disorders that are associated with increased susceptibility or decreased tolerance for pain. These include Major Depression, Dysthymic Disorder, Somatization Disorder, Conversion Disorder, and Hypochondriasis.[1] In the absence of objective biological markers for diagnosis, these terms refer to descriptive entities or syndromes as defined in the third edition of the American Psychiatric Association's *Diagnostic and Statistical Manual of Mental Disorders* (Referred to as the DSM-III). The differentiation between these entities is often difficult. This is particularly true for patients with chronic pain, in whom symptoms of depression, somatization, and hypochondriasis may all be present. Nonetheless, it is useful to outline the features of each of the

[1]In the following discussion, I will use terms such as *somatization, depression,* and *hypochondriasis* in two ways: as symptoms and as diagnostic entities. When referring to one of them as a symptom or process, I will use lower case first letters. When referring to a specific diagnostic entity as outlined in the American Psychiatric Association's *Diagnostic and Statistical Manual of Mental Disorders* (3rd ed., 1980; DSM-III), I will capitalize the first letter of each word.

conditions separately in order to clarify the different psychological mechanisms that influence the behavior of pain patients.

DEPRESSION AND PAIN

Accumulated clinical experience clearly associates persistent pain with symptoms of depression. There is evidence that chronic pain causes depression and, conversely, that patients whose major problem is depression frequently complain of pain.

One source of confusion in the literature concerning this subject is the frequent failure to adequately define depression (13, 28). The term *depression* has been used to refer to a sad mood or emotion that all of us have had at one time or another as a normal response to an important unhappy life event such as a failure, illness, or personal loss. In a clinical context, depression refers to the symptom of persistent sadness occurring as part of a somatic or mental illness. Many patients with chronic pain have the symptom of depression. The question in any given patient is whether the depression is a normal reaction to the painful illness or represents psychopathology and is therefore a problem distinct from whatever it is that caused the somatic pain. It is obviously difficult to know how much depression is "normal" since the pain intensity cannot be directly measured.

In its most restricted and specific sense, depression refers to a group of several psychiatric syndromes characterized primarily by long periods of persistent, deep, and pervasive sad mood. The most common of these syndromes is Major Depression. Major Depression is the DSM-III term for what used to be called endogenous depression (1). (For a complete list of the diagnostic criteria for Major Depression see Appendix A at the end of this chapter.) In addition to an unpleasant (dysphoric) mood, usually sadness, patients with Major Depression feel hopeless, worthless, and guilty and often have suicidal thoughts. They may have delusions that some part of their body is being destroyed by a disease. So-called vegetative symptoms such as early morning awakening, poor appetite, constipation, slowed thinking, fatigue, inactivity, and loss of libido are prominent. The dysphoric mood change is profound in Major Depression, and both it and the other signs are persistent and usually recurrent.

Dysthymic Disorder is the DSM-III term for what used to be called neurotic or reactive depression (1) (see Appendix B for diagnostic criteria). In patients with Dysthymic Disorder the depressed mood is chronic, but is neither as profound or as pervasive as in Major Depression, vegetative signs are not prominent, and, although the patients are often pessimistic, tearful, and socially withdrawn, they are not delusional (31).

As discussed above, it is common for chronic pain patients to have depression as a symptom. Major Depression occurs in a significant number of chronic pain patients, although the incidence varies greatly depending on the patient population (8, 11, 13, 26, 28). Dysthymic Disorder also occurs in a significant number of chronic pain patients (11). Although the association between pain and depression is well established, it is not clear whether the pain or the depressive syndrome is primary.

It seems logical that chronic pain would cause depression; however, the task of determining the incidence, severity, and quality of the depressive symptoms caused by chronic pain is complicated by the fact that primary depressive illness is so common. For example, there is a lifetime risk of over 15 percent for Major Depression (31). This means that chronic pain patients are at significant risk for Major Depression *independent* of their pain problem. Looking at this issue the other way, it is likely that a subset of patients complain of persistent pain because they have Major Depression (3, 13, 16). In fact, pain complaints are very common in patients referred to psychiatrists for the treatment of Major Depression (13, 16). Furthermore, a high percentage of patients who contact primary care physicians with a variety of somatic complaints have clinically significant depression (33). In a recent study using standardized scales to assess depressive symptoms in patients attending a primary care clinic, 44 percent were found to be at least mildly depressed and 6 percent had Major Depression (15). Pain complaints were common in this patient population, and there was a positive correlation between the severity of depression and the frequency of office visits and telephone calls.

Although there is little doubt that complaints of somatic pain are common in patients whose major problem is depression, the reason for this is not obvious. One possibility is that the pain that depressed patients complain of is somatic in origin but is mild and would not be bothersome if the patient were not depressed. Since pain complaints are so common in the general population (20, 40), the effect of depression might simply be to lower pain tolerance so that "normal" day-to-day aches and pains become unbearable. This could occur at a neuro-chemical level if depressed patients had lower levels of pain-inhibiting neurotransmitters such as serotonin, norepinephrine, or endogenous opioid peptides. It could also occur at a cognitive level if the depressed patient interprets a mild pain as evidence of a serious organic illness (i.e., hypochondriasis).

Another potentially important set of contributing factors results from learning and selective attention. Katon and his colleagues (16, 17) proposed that some people actually experience depression as a feeling of ill health and somatic discomfort. They ascribe this somatization of depression to a developmental process in which individuals learn from others how to describe and communicate the subjective experience of depression. When patients become depressed they have mood changes, somatic discomfort, a lowering of pain tolerance, and a tendency to interpret daily events in a negative way. Some of these changes are easier to communicate than others. Compared to headache, for example, the symptoms of self-deprecation, guilt, and hopelessness are rather subtle judgments that are, in part, culturally determined. Some cultures—indeed, some families in our own culture—ignore or discourage complaints of emotional disturbance but attend to and express sympathy for somatic complaints. This would encourage people to focus on and express the somatic rather than the psychological manifestations of depression.

Whatever the explanation, it is quite clear that a small but significant proportion of patients with Major Depression present to physicians with multiple somatic symptoms including pain. Because these patients do not volunteer the information that they are depressed, the physician may miss the diagnosis (24). This is a particular tragedy because Major Depression is both a treatable and a potentially fatal illness. The value of rapid depression screening in patients with persistent unexplained somatic complaints is obvious (24, 32).

In summary, there is an intimate link between depression and pain. Both are characterized by negative affect, and when both are present in the same individual they are reciprocally linked. Pain produces depressive symptoms directly and, as a signal of real or feared disease, provides a reason for worry and pessimism. The presence of depression impairs a patient's ability to cope with pain. Chronic pain patients who are depressed are more preoccupied with their bodily pain and more certain that they have a serious somatic illness (28). The pain and depression feed on each other, the pain serving to deepen the sadness and pessimism and the depression lowering the tolerance for pain. The optimal management of pain patients requires an active search for depression and specific efforts to treat it. Frequently, successful treatment of depression will allow a patient to cope with his or her pain and return to a relatively normal life.

SOMATIZATION AND HYPOCHONDRIASIS

In addition to Major Depression, there is a group of psychiatric diseases that are characterized by multiple, persistent, unexplained somatic symptoms and excessive demand for medical attention. These are now classified generically as Somatoform Disorders and include Somatization Disorder, Conversion Disorder, Hypochondriasis, and Psychogenic Pain Disorder (1). Psychogenic Pain Disorder will be considered separately.

Appendix C gives the DSM-III diagnostic criteria for Somatization Disorder. This is a severely disabling, chronic syndrome that usually begins in adolescence or early adulthood and always before age 30. The patients must have at least 12 different somatic symptoms (14 for women). At different times the symptoms are referable to different organ systems. The patients are convinced that they are chronically ill with a serious somatic disease. They are usually not reassured by normal tests or examinations, and, if their physician does not take their complaint seriously, they will shop around for another one who will. Their relentless pursuit of medical attention for their imagined or feared illness results in tremendous utilization of health care resources (30, 34), often including multiple surgical procedures. Pain complaints are very common in this group of patients. For example, the diagnosis of lumbar disc disease is frequently made

(34). Once the existence of Somatization Disorder is appreciated it is usually not difficult to recognize. The diagnosis can be made on the basis of the history and the absence of a somatic explanation of their symptoms. Case 7.1. is a typical example of a patient with Somatization Disorder (30).

Case 7.1[2]

A 74-year-old woman was referred by her gastroenterologist for primary care. Her chief complaints were severe headache and weakness that persisted for more than six months. Her recent evaluation by a neurologist had included two computed tomographic scans of the head, two electroencephalograms, nerve conduction studies, and a muscle biopsy, none of which was definitive. She spontaneously offered that she was not depressed and that there must be a physical reason for her distress. She warned that other doctors had falsely believed that she had psychological problems, only to be proved wrong when the proper tests had been obtained or the proper surgery undertaken.

In the past year she had been evaluated by a cardiologist for chest pain, a gastroenterologist for abdominal pain, and a pulmonologist for shortness of breath. The evaluations included an echocardiogram, two avionics, a stress-thallium test, a cardiac catheterization, an upper gastro-intestinal tract series, a barium enema examination, two endoscopies, two colonoscopies, pulmonary function tests, and two ventilation-perfusion scans. Each physician believed her to be a diagnostic puzzle, but they gave tentative diagnoses of coronary artery spasm, inflammatory bowel disease, and microscopic pulmonary emboli.

Her more remote history showed over 30 operations, often for vague indications, beginning at the age of 24 years with a cesarean section. She carried over 50 separate medical diagnoses but no psychiatric diagnoses. The specific data on which her diagnoses were based were vague and conflicting. She was taking six prescription medications regularly (nifedipine, nitrates, furosemide, indomethacin, antacids, and a mixture of chlordiazepoxide hydrochloride and clidinium bromide [Librax]), as well as narcotic analgesics for pain. She was allergic to many antibiotics and analgesics.

She described having had a "hard life," including two siblings who had died violent deaths, a mother who had died painfully of bowel carcinoma, and a long marriage to an alcoholic husband who had physically abused her. She had worked hard since childhood, the only respite being periods when she was ill.

Her physical examination showed a thin, downcast woman, who seemed remarkably well despite her medical ailments. With the exception of the numerous surgical scars all over her body, her examination results were within normal limits. . . . Results of screening laboratory tests, including complete blood cell count, sedimentation rate, electrolyte levels, liver function tests, stool guaiacs, total serum thyroxine, Papanicolaou smear, and mammmograms, were normal.

[2]Reprinted by permission from Quill, T. E.: Somatization disorder: one of medicine's blind spots. *JAMA* **254**:3075–3079, 1985.

Conversion Disorder (see Appendix D), previously known as hysterical neurosis, conversion type, has much in common with Somatization Disorder (cf. Appendix C), including age of onset, predominance in women, and multiple recurrent symptoms and signs that are not explained by somatic disease. In Conversion Disorder, the most common symptoms and signs superficially resemble alterations in nervous system function, for example, paralysis, sensory loss, blindness, and seizures. Despite the gravity of the apparent loss of function, patients characteristically appear untroubled by their symptoms (9). In this disorder, clinical findings occur in relation to a precipitating emotional event, and the patient obtains a psychological benefit from either the impairment or the attention. The role of the precipitating event is central to the diagnosis. Conversion Disorder may be monosymptomatic or oligosymptomatic. The particular form and location of the symptom often has symbolic meaning to the patient, and the disability is thought to help the patient resolve an emotional conflict (9, 29).

Hypochondriasis is a pervasive preoccupation with somatic symptoms and a conviction that the symptoms indicate actual or impending serious bodily disease, despite repeated assurances from physicians (see Appendix E). Hypochondriasis may occur as a symptom of depression; however, many hypochondriacs have no other psychopathology (27). In fact, the current DSM-III criteria for diagnosis of Hypochondriasis require that the patient have no other psychiatric illness.

As with Somatization Disorder, Hypochondriasis is a chronic condition that persists for years and results in repeated medical consultations, unwarranted diagnostic tests, and unsuccessful treatments. In contrast to persons with Somatization Disorder, hypochondriacs usually focus their concern on a specific organ system or fear of a specific disease (29, 30). Hypochondriacs are quite vigilant with respect to their bodies, and they pay inordinate attention to a variety of bodily sensations such as heartbeat, itch, bowel sounds, fatigue, dizziness, and minor musculoskeletal aches, which they interpret as indicative of serious illness. It is important to remember that the symptoms commonly reported by hypochondriacs are widespread in populations of healthy subjects who do not seek medical care (20). Some of the symptoms, such as palpitations, tingling in the extremities, and shortness of breath, may be signs of anxiety. In contrast to patients with Conversion Disorder, hypochondriacs are excessively worried about their symptoms, but the condition produces no loss or impairment of bodily function (1).

Although hypochondriasis is an important element of the chronic pain syndrome, it is not clear in any given patient whether it is a primary problem or develops in response to the pain. As with depression, hypochondriasis and pain interact because the attentiveness to the pain and the fear of what it means reduce a patient's ability to tolerate it. In pain clinic patients, the symptom of hypochondriasis is positively correlated with depressive symptoms (27) and is more severe if the pain has been present for more than 6 months (38).

When persistent pain is the patient's most prominent problem, there is no identifiable tissue injury or somatic disease to explain it, and no other psychiatric diagnosis can be made, the patient may be diagnosed as having Psychogenic Pain Disorder (see DSM-III criteria in Appendix F). This syndrome will be discussed in the next section.

In summary, the Somatoform Disorders are a group of psychiatric syndromes characterized by chronic preoccupation with bodily symptoms, fear of disease, and intensive utilization of health care resources. The symptoms cannot be accounted for by objective evidence of injury or disease. In these disorders the assumption is that the severity and significance of a symptom are greatly exaggerated because of an emotional disturbance. In other words, most individuals with the same level of somatic sensation either would not notice or would not be concerned. The complaint of pain is often a prominent feature of Somatization Disorder and Hypochondriasis. Patients with these conditions are important to identify, if only to protect them from invasive tests and unnecessary surgery.

There is a range of severity in the manifestations of the mental processes that underly hypochondriasis and somatization. When isolated and severe, they constitute distinct disabling psychiatric syndromes. When less severe and pervasive they represent mental processes that operate in most patients with chronic pain, adding to but not completely accounting for the patient's impairment.

Psychogenic Pain

The term psychogenic pain refers to a pain that is not elicited by noxious stimuli, nor due to gross dysfunction of pain transmission or modulation neurons. If it does exist, this sort of pain would, mechanistically, more closely resemble a dream, hallucination, or memory than a receptor-elicited sensation (4, 10).

Perceptual experiences originating in the brain are accepted in other sensory spheres. Dreams are an almost universal example of such a phenomenon. In dreams and certain drug intoxications, vivid visual experiences occur that are generated within the central nervous system. The eyes are closed, yet there is a completely formed, colorful visual image. Without getting into the issue of whether dreams are real, it is easy to confirm (or deny) that a visual experience reported by a person is due to visible objects in the outside world. Dreams and hallucinations are images that require no sensory input. They are "constructed" using material stored in memory. Such constructed experiences also occur in the auditory sphere. For example, the self-accusatory thoughts of certain schizophrenics are commonly projected into the outer world and experienced by them as other people's voices. These examples show that there can be perceptions originating in the brain that are very similar to those elicited by sensory stimuli. By analogy, one could argue that pain can also originate within the brain.

On the other hand, that pain can be generated by mental mechanisms similar to those underlying dreams and hallucinations (10) is a very difficult assertion to confirm. First of all, in contrast to vision and hearing (or for that matter olfaction or temperature sensation), pain is a subjective interpretation of a bodily feeling and not a description of an externally verifiable object. That another person has a fractured bone can be confirmed, but not that they feel pain. Furthermore, memories of previous painful experiences are often vague and dreams of somatic pain are unusual, at least in patients who are not in pain while awake. This indicates that, if psychogenic pain does occur, the mechanism that generates it may differ from those that underlie dreams and hallucinations. At the present time, the existence of purely psychogenic pain can be accepted as an unproven but reasonable idea, supported by evidence that is circumstantial and arguments that are indirect.

Although the idea of *purely* psychogenic pain is of theoretical importance, from a practical standpoint it is not crucial. Pains are so common in everyday life that it is not necessary to invoke a purely psychogenic mechanism when there are no objective signs to confirm the pain or proximate cause to account for it. For example, at one time or another, most people suffer from transient headache, heartburn, sore muscles, and joint or back pain. Occasionally, these common minor pains persist for days, even weeks, without an obvious explanation. In certain patients, psychological mechanisms could amplify and perpetuate these otherwise mild pains. Technically speaking, this pain would not be purely psychogenic. It is likely that many of the cases of chronic pain that are referred to in the literature as psychogenic actually represent a psychologically amplified pain of somatic origin. These are pains that would be ignored by a patient were it not for a significant psychological disturbance. Whatever the actual mechanism, it is clear that, for some patients, it is most helpful to think of their pain as representating a primarily psychological disturbance.

As discussed above, pain may appear in several psychiatric syndromes, including Major Depression, Somatization Disorder, Conversion Disorder, and, possibly, Hypochondriasis. In addition, there are many patients whose symptom complex does not conform to any of the above syndromes, although it may incorporate some features of each. I believe that most of these patients have a condition that is a type of somatoform disorder; however, the DSM-III criteria for Psychogenic Pain Disorder (see Appendix F), do not quite catch the flavor of most of these patients. It is likely that, with further clinical studies, a syndrome (or syndromes) will become more clearly defined and the diagnostic criteria will be refined.

One of the most thorough and persuasive descriptions of psychogenic pain was that presented by George Engel (10). Building on the classic observations of Breuer and Freud (4), Engel described a series of patients with chronic pain and significant behavioral disturbance, discussed the clinical evidence indicating that their pain was of psychological origin, and gave a detailed, plausible hypothesis to explain how psychological mechanisms can produce and sustain pain. For Engel, pain is a subjective experience that can be vividly recalled, and there-

Table 7.3   Historical Features Suggesting a Significant Psychogenic Component to Chronic Pain

Multiple locations of pains at different times

Pain problems dating from adolescence

Pain without obvious somatic cause, especially in the perineal or face region

Physically abusive parents or spouse

Multiple surgical procedures of an elective nature

Alcohol or drug abuse (patient and/or spouse)

Frequent failure in job and social life

fore purely psychogenic pain is possible. The key assumption underlying Engel's formulation is that there are circumstances in which the experience of pain can ameliorate feelings that are even more unpleasant, such as guilt, anxiety, and depression. In this way it could reduce the overall level of suffering and even be pleasant, at least in a relative sense. If one accepts the possibility of this paradoxical effect of pain, the arguments he presents are reasonable.

In what way could pain possibly be pleasurable? Engel points out that, in a young child, a painful experience such as a fall is often followed by extra attention and signs of parental affection. In this way, mild pains could contain a pleasurable element of anticipation of affectionate parental behavior. Another contributing factor emerges from the relationship of pain to punishment. Engel pointed out, and others have confirmed (3), the high frequency with which chronic pain patients report physically abusive parents. The patient identifies with the punishing parent and comes to view having pain as a legitimate way either to control unacceptable aggressive or sexual thoughts and behaviors or to deal with the guilt and anxiety engendered by them (e.g., Case 7.3, below). A third situation conducive to psychogenic pain occurs when a patient loses a loved one who suffered (or is imagined by the patient to have suffered) a painful illness or injury. Through the psychological process of identification the patient experiences what he or she imagines to be a similar pain, and this identification assuages the psychic "pain" of the loss. This process seems more likely to occur when patients have ambivalent feelings about the loved one or feel guilt about the circumstances of the loss (e.g., Case 7.2, below).

According to Engel, there are certain individuals who are susceptible to a life of chronic pain by virtue of their psychological makeup. Although these patients include some who could be diagnosed as having Conversion Disorder or Hypochondriasis, their characteristics set them apart (Table 7.3). Engel's patients had no objective somatic pathology to explain their pain, which was often in the head or face. The pain complaint was part of what was usually presented by the patients as a hard life, with problems starting in childhood. In addition to the frequent occurrence of painful injury and illness, the patients seemed to be attracted to situations that would cause them to be exploited, injured, or defeated. Their need to suffer is indicated by the fact that their pain is usually exacerbated when their life situation improves. This is illustrated by the following vignette from Engel's classic paper.

Case 7.2[3]

> A forty-one year old unmarried woman, a teacher, lived with and took care of her ailing mother for many years until her death one month before the beginning of the patient's face pain. She slept in the same bed as her mother. On the night of her mother's death she had awakened to find that the right side of her mother's face was drawn and a short time later it became blue. She was breathing heavily and the patient *believed* her to be suffering great pain. She called for help but when unable to secure any climbed back into bed only to realize that her mother was dead.
>
> She had been engaged to a man for many years but had not married because she could not leave her mother. However, upon her mother's death, she first felt emancipated, and bought a house, but then pain developed in the right side of her face and because of it she gave up both her home and fiancé. She expressed remorse at her feelings of emancipation after her mother's death and consciously considered the pain as punishment, a sign that she was being inconsiderate of her mother's memory.

This case illustrates several important common features of patients with psychogenic pain: the patient's self-denial, her sacrificing her personal life in order to care for her mother; the location of the pain in a site apparently determined by where the patient thought the mother had pain; her guilt surrounding the mother's death (because the patient felt relieved); and the exacerbation of the pain when her life was materially improved.

According to Engel's formulation, guilt is the unifying theme in patients with psychogenic pain. The self-denial and inability to extricate themselves from unpleasant situations can be seen not as hard luck but as "deliberate" masochistic behavior that would serve the same self-punitive purpose as the pain, that is, to assuage excessive feelings of guilt. The guilt and consequent pain may also appear in the setting of aggressive or sexual acts or fantasies that are unacceptable to the patient, as illustrated by the following case.

[3]Reprinted by permission from Engel, G. L.: "Psychogenic" pain and the pain-prone patient. *Am. J. Med.* **26:**899–918, 1959.

Case 7.3[4]

A twenty-six year old woman with a variety of hysterical manifestations had several episodes of pain and burning at the end of urination. The urine examination was always negative but she referred to it as "my cystitis." One episode occurred during her first year of marriage. Her husband proved less capable sexually than she hoped for and she felt both frustrated and angry. As a child the bathroom was the scene of many sexual fantasies of masturbation, which included poking things in and around the urethra. These symptoms recurred briefly during the course of psychoanalysis when her husband had a severe case of flu and was sexually inattentive for several weeks. She developed fleeting sexual fantasies about the analyst and then her "cystitis" recurred. The painful dysuria promptly disappeared when these transference sexual feelings were brought up during the analytic hour and connected with the childhood fantasies and masturbatory activities.

This case is particularly instructive because the location of the pain relates to the forbidden fantasies and because of the relief that occurred when the unconscious mechanisms were revealed to the patient. It is quite similar to the cases described in great detail by Breuer and Freud (4).

In summary, Engel believes that pain-prone patients are people afflicted by excessive guilt feelings that are ameliorated by their pain. They have a long history of suffering both "physical" and emotional pain and a behavioral pattern suggesting that they seek, rather than avoid, situations that will have negative consequences for them. The location of the pain often has symbolic meaning. The severity of their pain increases when things are otherwise going well, or if they indulge themselves in aggressive or sexually gratifying behavior.

The psychoanalytic approach, as exemplified by the writings of Engel, is valuable because it provides an explanation for the disturbed thinking and behavior of many chronic pain patients and suggests treatment strategies. For some patients, for example, the woman in Case 7.3, pain relief occurs when the unconscious factors producing it are brought to light. Unfortunately, this is usually a slow, expensive, and highly individual process. Even with the help of experienced and talented professionals, many people are not helped. Even when these patients improve, it is difficult to prove that the analytic approach was responsible. Nonetheless, for some patients, this approach appears to be dramatically effective.

Pain Behavior and Learning

Responses to noxious stimuli fall into two distinct categories: one is the subjective experience of pain, and the other is a complex set of observable behaviors.

[4]Reprinted by permission from Engel, G. L.: "Psychogenic" pain and the pain-prone patient. *Am. J. Med.* **26:**899–918, 1959.

I will use the word *pain* to refer to the unpleasant subjective experience. I will use the term *pain behavior* to refer to observable behaviors that are usually indicative of subjective pain or are attributed by a patient to his or her pain. In medical practice, the usual focus is on the subjective experience as described by the patient. Physicians ask patients about the quality of the pain, its location, duration, and severity. This information is used both to establish a diagnosis and as a guide to the efficacy of therapy.

Pain behaviors include withdrawal, grimacing, moaning, limping, rubbing the painful part, splinting, guarding, and other forms of immobilization. There are also more "organized" behaviors such as seeking medical care, taking analgesics, avoiding sex, and staying home from work. In a class by itself is the patient's verbal communication of pain. This is an observable behavior that describes the pain but is quite distinct from the actual sensation. Language is obviously a very complex, learned, and culturally determined behavior.

When we see a patient exhibit pain behaviors we assume that he or she hurts because the behaviors are characteristically associated with noxious stimuli, and because of how *we* feel when we act that way. In general, health professionals pay little attention to nonverbal pain behaviors except as a way of corroborating that a patient has severe pain or to judge its severity. They are considered to be epiphenomena.

The tacit assumption in medicine is that pain is completely explainable by processes within somatic tissues or the nervous system. Either nociceptors are activated, or neural dysfunction activates central pain pathways or a psychological abnormality gives rise to pain memories or hallucinations. According to this assumption, pain, whatever its cause, is the subjective experience that results from somatic, neural, or mental pathology within the individual. This is the disease or medical model of pain.

Learning theorists take a fundamentally different view (12). Although they accept that processes within the individual can cause subjective pain, they are more concerned with pain behaviors, which are objective and can be influenced by environmental factors *outside the individual.* It is critical to understand that, in contrast to subjective pain, which is by definition unpleasant, pain behaviors are inherently neutral. It is the consequences of the pain behavior that are meaningful. Depending on environmental factors, pain behaviors can lead to either reward or punishment. The major advance provided by the behavioral or learning model of pain is the idea that, under certain circumstances, reinforcement of pain behaviors will be sufficiently strong to sustain them in the absence of the noxious somatic stimulus that initially elicited them (12).

Pain behaviors fall into two categories, innate (or reflex) and learned. Withdrawal, groans, autonomic changes, and perhaps certain facial expressions are genetically determined reflexes that can be elicited directly by noxious stimuli. Other pain behaviors require learning. We learn the nuances of pain behavior in childhood (12), partly by mimicking older individuals and partly by having them reward our pain behavior when it is appropriate (e.g., when we fall down the stairs and cut our lip, particularly if we need stitches). The reward may consist of attention, cuddling, and not having to wash the dishes. On the other hand, if the crying is excessive or inappropriate (e.g., in response to a light shove from a brother who doesn't want you to play with his toy), the parent may ignore or even reprimand the sufferer. By this process the individual learns which behaviors are appropriate in a given situation. The point is that the behavior is obvious and susceptible to change by reinforcement or punishment.

The learning theorist is concerned primarily with reinforcement, not pain and pleasure. According to the behavioral model, the chronic pain patient is a person who acts like a chronic pain patient, and it is immaterial whether the pain is somatogenic, neurogenic, or psychogenic (or for that matter, whether there "really" is any subjectively experienced pain). If the patient is reinforced in some way when he or she takes analgesics, stays in bed, or complains of pain, he or she will continue to do so. If these pain behaviors are not rewarded, or if not performing them is rewarded, the chronic pain patient will cease acting like a chronic pain patient. The power of the learning model is that, in its approach to the pain problem, it goes beyond the individual to include a search for the interpersonal factors in the family, workplace, and physician's office that reinforce pain behaviors or discourage "well" behaviors.

According to Fordyce (12), a given pain behavior, for example, a grimace or moan, can result either from nociceptive input or because it has been reinforced (Figure 7.1). In fact, at any given time, *both* nociceptor activity and reinforcement can contribute to the occurrence of a given pain behavior. For example, whether a person stays home with a headache is determined partly by nociceptive input (pain intensity) and partly by the interpersonal consequences of staying home. Similarly, the decision to take an analgesic drug will be determined by the severity of the pain and by the rewarding or aversive effects of the drug, such as euphoria, sedation, or nausea. It is important to point out that drug-taking behavior can be reinforced either because it relieves pain (negative reinforcement) or because it has a euphoriant action (positive reinforcement) or both.

From the learning model perspective, the first step in evaluating a patient is to determine the relative contributions of nociception and reinforcement in producing his or her pain behavior. Part of this process is to identify the environmental factors that reinforce pain behaviors or that punish well behaviors.

Table 7.4 lists some typical pain behaviors, common reinforcers, and examples of possible predisposing factors. Each of these factors has been described in detail by Fordyce, whose book on this subject (12) I highly recommend. I shall just briefly mention each.

Vocalizations and Verbal Complaints Moans and groans, exclamations such as "ouch," and detailed descriptions of pain are usually indicative of subjective pain. They are communications and are thus more likely to have positive consequences when someone is around to hear them. These behaviors can be-

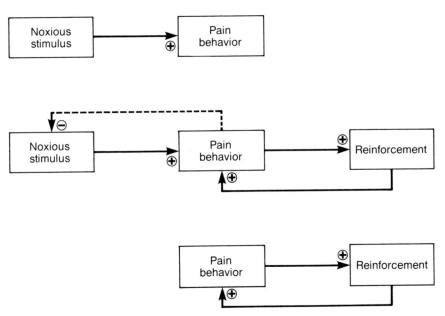

Figure 7.1   Reinforcement of pain behavior. **Top:** Noxious stimulus elicits a pain behavior (e.g., rest). **Middle:** Noxious stimulus elicits a pain behavior that is reinforced in two ways: first, it reduces the pain, and second, in the case of rest, it permits the patient to avoid unpleasant jobs or situations. To the extent that it occurs because of reinforcement rather than the continued presence of a noxious stimulus, rest is a learned pain behavior. **Bottom:** No noxious stimulus. The pain behavior is sustained solely by avoidance of unpleasant jobs or situations.

come operant if the attention or nurturance they elicit from others is rewarding. This could be the case if, for example, a neglectful, hostile, or cruel spouse becomes gentle, kind, and attentive when the person communicates that he or she is in pain.

Medical Consultation   People usually have a fairly high threshold for seeking medical attention. It is time consuming, often uncomfortable, and can be expensive. As with all pain behaviors, it is initiated because there is hope of obtaining relief. There may also be other, less obvious reinforcers, especially in the chronic pain setting. For example, in addition to pain relief, the physician offers validation of the pain behavior; medications, which can be reinforcers in their own right; and a social interaction, which for some patients seems to be very rewarding. For some, particularly elderly patients living alone, the health care professional may be their major social contact (16, 17).

Medication Intake   If a drug is effective it will be reinforcing because it relieves pain. It can act in this way only as long as the pain is present. If, in

Table 7.4 Reinforcements and Environmental Factors Involved in Pain Behavior

Pain behavior	Mode of reinforcement	Possible risk factors
Complaint of pain, moans, tears	attention, nurturing	hostile or inattentive spouse
Medical consultation	pain relief, psychoactive drugs, attention, nurturing, validate sick role	depression, hypochondriasis, loneliness, drug abuse
Drug intake or alcohol	euphoria, analgesia, relief of anxiety	trait anxiety, previous drug or alcohol abuse
Compensation, disability	money	low pay, poverty
Rest, inactivity	pain relief, avoid unpleasant job or interpersonal responsibilities	low self-esteem, low job satisfaction

addition, it has pleasant psychological effects it will have a double reinforcing action. For example, opiates can produce an elevation of mood or have an anti-anxiety effect that is independent of their analgesic action. Such drugs, as well as many of the minor tranquilizers, are reinforcing. Because of this, patients, particularly those who are depressed or anxious, are at risk for continued drug intake even after the somatic cause of their pain has subsided. A small percentage of chronic pain patients are at least psychologically dependent on opiates or anxiolytic drugs, not because they have pain but because the drugs are reinforcing by themselves. Alcohol is another "drug" that is used by many chronic pain patients, who claim that it relieves their pain. It has an action very similar to anxiolytic drugs, inducing a pleasant state of relaxation. As with opiates and minor tranquilizers, patients who use alcohol are at risk for becoming dependent.

In any given pain patient it is possible that the major reason for many of his or her pain behaviors is the reinforcing effect of the drug or drugs he or she is taking. This is particularly difficult to sort out (or to change) when the patients insist that the drugs are the only thing that helps alleviate the pain. Because of this, many behaviorally oriented pain treatment programs make withdrawal of all psychoactive and analgesic drugs a high priority. Once this is done, it may be somewhat easier to evaluate and deal with other environmental reinforcers.

Disability Payments This is powerful positive reinforcement for staying away from work. The ratio between the patient's wages and the amount of the disability payment is the critical factor. As disability or workmen's compensation payments rise relative to wages, an increasing proportion of workers apply for benefits (18). For a certain percentage of people, disability payments are greater than their wages from full-time work (18). In addition, these payments can be indirectly reinforcing if they permit the patient to avoid an unpleasant work situation (see below).

Rest and Inactivity   These terms refer to the avoidance of movement. Initially, the movements avoided are those that cause pain. Pain patients frequently report that their pain worsens with fatigue and that rest ameliorates it. In this situation activity is punished by the pain. Pain also provides negative reinforcement for rest (i.e., rest is rewarded by the *removal* of pain). When the somatic cause of the pain subsides, activity is no longer painful and rest is no longer reinforcing for most people; they return to their normal activity level. However, if rest is reinforcing for reasons other than pain relief, patients will continue to rest even after the somatic cause of the pain has subsided. For example, rest may enable a patient to avoid unpleasant or threatening conditions at work, onerous household chores, social responsibilities, or situations that expose real or imagined personal inadequacies.

The major contribution of learning theory to the understanding of chronic pain is its recognition that environmental factors, especially interpersonal relationships, play a major role in producing and perpetuating pain behavior. Many pain behaviors are learned in childhood and plastic in adulthood. Pain behaviors are reinforced when they provide pain relief. They can be reinforced in the absence of somatic pain if they have consequences that meet the patient's emotional or material needs.

It is important to emphasize that it is not only the *patient's* behavior that is subject to reinforcement. Application of the learning model makes it obvious that the people with whom the patient comes in contact can also be rewarded for their caretaking behavior. Family members who have the patient's best interest at heart can unwittingly perpetuate his or her impairment (12, 25). These well-intentioned people derive emotional and financial rewards from tending to the chronic pain patient. There is evidence that treatment programs directed toward correcting family interactions that sustain disability can be effective in returning patients to a more normal life (14).

Physicians may also inadvertently contribute to the perpetuation of pain behaviors. Because the possibility of somatic disease is so threatening, the patient with somatic pain is treated solicitously. The physician can contribute to the problem by focusing exclusively on the somatic aspects of a patient's problem. Afraid of missing something "organic" (and possibly being sued), no stone is left unturned. The patient's pain behaviors are validated by expensive tests and occasionally by exploratory surgery. It is only after the physician has exhausted all approaches to finding a somatic source for the pain that psychological factors are seriously considered.

Behaviorally oriented pain treatment programs provide a way out of this

Table 7.5   Psychosocial Factors Contributing to "Unexplained" Chronic Pain

Problem	Somatic stimulus	Cause of pain (complaint)
Malingering	0	conscious benefit
Conversion	0	unacceptable sexual or aggressive conflict, desire for attention
Somatization	±	somatic preoccupation, environmental reinforcers, anxiety
Depression	±	reduced pain tolerance, poor coping ability
Hypochondriasis	±	disease conviction, anxiety, somatic preoccupation
Operant pain behavior	+/0	environmental reinforcers
Psychogenic pain (Engel)	0	amelioration of guilt

situation by recognizing and eliminating the reinforcers that perpetuate pain behavior. Many such programs have reported returning a high percentage of patients to a productive life and reducing their intake of analgesics (19); however, randomized, controlled prospective studies are not yet available.

Summary

In this chapter I have outlined some of the psychiatric syndromes and psychological abnormalities that predispose patients to chronic pain or pain behavior. The major problem confronting the clinician is how to deal with a patient who complains of somatic pain but has no obvious somatic cause for it. It is likely that many such patients actually do have a somatic cause for their pain but physicians lack the tools to demonstrate it. On the other hand, a variety of psychiatric syndromes and psychological mechanisms may also contribute to the problem. Table 7.5 lists some of the possibilities to be considered in the "differential diagnosis" of unexplained chronic pain. These possibilities are by no means mutually exclusive. In a given patient, several could be at work.

It is clear that there are distinctly different approaches to the study and analysis of the psychology of chronic pain patients. Although there is some overlap, each approach deals with somewhat different issues and uses different terminology. There are at least three schools: the biological or descriptive, the psychodynamic, and the behavioral. Each of the approaches has contributed in a different way to our understanding of pain patients. The descriptive-biological approach focuses on psychiatric disease. It seeks to classify emotional disorders and assign patients to diagnostic categories. This approach is of value for those patients whose chronic pain is caused by or associated with a distinct psychiatric disorder. Of particular importance is the recognition of Major Depression, because there are specific treatments for it. Somatization Disorder, Hypochondriasis, and Conversion Disorder are also distinct syndromes that are often manifested by the complaint of pain. Although it is less clear how to treat them, they are important to recognize in order to prevent unnecessary, expensive, and potentially harmful utilization of health care resources. The psychodynamic or psychoanalytic approach, as exemplified by Engel's analysis of pain-prone patients, has provided an exposition of the role of guilt in the creation of psychogenic pain. The major advance provided by the behavioral or learning model approach is the recognition of the important role played by environmental factors in the development and perpetuation of pain behaviors.

Each of these approaches has something different to offer. Under ideal circumstances, a patient should be evaluated using each of these approaches and the decision about treatment should be based on the type of problem that the individual has. For some, antidepressant medication will clearly be the best treatment. For others, recovery is unlikely if environmental reinforcers are not removed. Unfortunately, in current practice the diagnostic and treatment approach suggested for a given patient depends to a large extent on the professional to whom the patient happens to be referred. Psychologists and psychiatrists presently use a combination of cognitive, behavioral, and pharmacologic methods, the therapy being tailored to both the background of the clinician and the needs of the individual patient. It is to be hoped that this somewhat haphazard approach will be replaced in the future by a more comprehensive, systematic, and uniform method of evaluation and treatment.

References

1   American Psychiatric Association Committee on Nomenclature and Statistics: *Diagnostic and Statistical Manual of Mental Disorders,* 3rd ed. American Psychiatric Association, Washington, D.C., 1980.

2   Blitz, B., and Dinnerstein, A. J.: Role of attentional focus in pain perception: Manipulation of response to noxious stimulation by instructions. *J. Abnorm. Psychol.* **77:**42–45, 1971.

3   Blumer, D., and Heilbronn, M.: Chronic pain as a variant of depressive disease— the pain-prone disorder. *J. Nerv. Ment. Dis.* **170:**381–406, 1982.

4 Breuer, J., and Freud, S.: *Studies in Hysteria*. Beacon Press, Boston, 1961.

5 Chapman, C. R., and Bonica, J. J.: Chronic pain. *Curr. Concepts*, August, pp. 1–68, 1985.

6 Cox, G. B., Chapman, C. R., and Black, R. G.: The MMPI and chronic pain: The diagnosis of psychogenic pain. *J. Behav. Med.* **1**:437–443, 1978.

7 Crook, J., and Tunks, E.: Defining the "Chronic Pain Syndrome": An Epidemiological Method. In Fields, H. et al. (ed.) *Adv. Pain Res. Ther.* **9**:871–877, 1985.

8 Davidson, J., Krishnan, R., France, R., and Pelton, S.: Neurovegetative symptoms in chronic pain and depression. *J. Affective Disord.* **9**:213–218, 1985.

9 Engel, G. L.: Conversion symptoms. In Blacklow, R. S. (ed.), *MacBryde's Signs and Symptoms*, 6th ed. Lippincott, Philadelphia, 1983, pp. 623–646.

10 Engel, G. L.: "Psychogenic" pain and the pain-prone patient. *Am. J. Med.* **26**:899–918, 1959.

11 Fishbain, D. A., Goldberg, M., Meagher, B. R., Steele, R., and Rosomoff, H.: Male and female chronic pain patients categorized by DSM-III psychiatric diagnostic criteria. *Pain* **26**:181–197, 1986.

12 Fordyce, W.: *Behavioral Methods for Chronic Pain and Illness*. Mosby, St. Louis, 1976.

13 Gupta, M. A.: Is chronic pain a variant of depressive illness? *Can. J. Psychiatry* **31**:241–248, 1986.

14 Hudgens, A. J.: Family-oriented treatment of chronic pain. *J. Marital Fam. Ther.* **5**:67–78, 1979.

15 Katon, W., Berg, A. O., Robins, A. J., and Risse, S.: Depression—medical utilization and somatization. *West. J. Med.* **144**:564–568, 1986.

16 Katon, W., Kleinman, A., and Rosen, G.: Depression and somatization: A review—Part I. *Am. J. Med.* **72**:127–135, 1982.

17 Katon, W., Kleinman, A., and Rosen, G.: Depression and somatization: A review—Part II. *Am. J. Med.* **72**:241–247, 1982.

18 Lando, M. E., Coate, M. B., and Kraus, R.: Disability benefit applications and the economy. *Social Security Bull.* **42**(10):3–10, 1979.

19 Linton, S. J.: Behavioral remediation of chronic pain: A status report. *Pain* **24**:125–141, 1986.

20 Mechanic, D.: Social psychologic factors affecting the presentation of bodily com-
    plaints. *N. Engl. J. Med.* **286:**1132–1139, 1972.

21 Melzack, R.: The McGill Pain Questionnaire: Major properties and scoring methods.
    Pain **1:**277–299, 1975.

22 Melzack, R., and Torgerson, W. S.: On the language of pain. *Anesthesiology* **34:**50–
    59, 1971.

23 Naliboff, B. D., Cohen, M. J., and Yellen, A. N.: Does the MMPI differentiate
    chronic illness from chronic pain? *Pain* **13:**333–341, 1982.

24 Nielson, A. C., and Williams, T. A.: Depression in ambulatory medical patients.
    Arch. Gen. Psychiatry **37:**999–1004, 1980.

25 Payne, B., and Norfleet, M. A.: Chronic pain and the family: A review. *Pain* **26:**1–
    22, 1986.

26 Pelz, M., and Merskey, H.: A description of the psychological effects of chronic
    painful lesions. *Pain* **14:**293–301, 1982.

27 Pilowsky, I.: Primary and secondary hypochondriasis. *Acta Psychiatr. Scand.*
    46:273–285, 1970.

28 Pilowsky, I., Chapman, C. R., and Bonica, J. J.: Pain, depression, and illness be-
    havior in a pain clinic population. *Pain* **4:**183–192, 1977.

29 Purcell, S. D.: Somatoform disorders. In Goldman, H. H. (ed.), *Review of General
    Psychiatry.* Lange Medical Pub., Los Altos, CA, 1984, pp. 376–384.

30 Quill, T. E.: Somatization disorder, one of medicine's blind spots. *JAMA* **254:**3075–
    3079, 1985.

31 Reus, V. I.: Affective disorders. In Goldman, H. H. (ed.), *Review of General Psy-
    chiatry.* Lange Medical Pub., Los Altos, CA, 1984, pp. 346–361.

32 Rucker, L., Frye, E. B., and Cygan, R. W.: Feasibility and usefulness of depression
    screening in medical outpatients. *Arch. Intern. Med.* **146:**729–731, 1986.

33 Schurman, R. A., Kramer, P. D., and Mitchel, J. B.: The hidden health network:
    Treatment of mental illness by non-psychiatrist physicians. *Arch. Gen. Psychiatry*
    42:89–94, 1985.

34 Smith, G. R., Jr., Monson, R. A., and Ray, D. C.: Patients with multiple unex-
    plained symptoms. *Arch. Intern. Med.* **146:**69–72, 1986.

35 Southwick, S. M., and White, A. A.: The use of psychological tests in the evaluation
    of low-back pain. *J. Bone Joint Surg.* **65-A:**560–565, 1983.

36 Sternbach, R. A.: *Pain Patients: Traits and Treatment*. Academic Press, New York, 1974.

37 Sternbach, R. A., and Timmermans, G.: Personality changes associated with reduction of pain. *Pain* **1**:177–181, 1975.

38 Sternbach, R. A., Wolf, S. R., Murphy, R. W., and Akeson, W. H.: Traits of pain patients: The low-back "loser". *Psychosomatics* **14**:226–229, 1973.

39 Taenzer, P., Melzack, R., and Jeans, M. E.: Influence of psychological factors on postoperative pain, mood and analgesic requirements. *Pain* **24**:331–342, 1986.

40 Taylor, H., and Curran, N. M.: *The Nuprin Pain Report*. Louis Harris & Assoc., New York, 1985.

41 Thompson, S. C.: Will it hurt less if I can control it? A complex answer to a simple question. *Psychol. Bull.* **90**:89–101, 1981.

42 Turk, D. C., and Kerns, R. D.: Conceptual issues in the assessment of clinical pain. *Int. J. Psychiatry Med.* **13**:1983–1984, 1983.

Appendixes[5]

APPENDIX A: A MAJOR DEPRESSION

Diagnostic criteria for Major Depression
A. One or more major depressive episodes. [see below]
B. Has never had a manic episode . . . or hypomanic episode. [see DSM-III, pp. 208 and 209, respectively]

Diagnostic criteria for major depressive episode [in adults]
A. Dysphoric mood or loss of interest or pleasure in all or almost all usual activities and pastimes. The dysphoric mood is characterized by symptoms such as the following: depressed, sad, blue, hopeless, low, down in the dumps, irritable. The mood disturbance must be prominent and relatively persistent, but not necessarily the most dominant symptom, and does not include momentary shifts from one dysphoric mood to another dysphoric mood, e.g., anxiety to depression to anger, such as are seen in states of acute psychotic turmoil.

B. At least four of the following symptoms have each been present nearly every day for a period of at least two weeks.

[5]Reprinted by permission from American Psychiatric Association Committee on Nomenclature and Statistics: *Diagnostic and Statistical Manual of Mental Disorders*, 3rd ed. American Psychiatric Association, Washington, D.C., 1980.

(1)   poor appetite or significant weight loss (when not dieting) or increased appetite or significant weight gain
(2)   insomnia or hypersomnia
(3)   psychomotor agitation or retardation (but not merely subjective feelings of restlessness or being slowed down)
(4)   loss of interest or pleasure in usual activities, or decrease in sexual drive not limited to a period when delusional or hallucinating
(5)   loss of energy; fatigue
(6)   feelings of worthlessness, self-reproach, or excessive or inappropriate guilt (either may be delusional)
(7)   complaints or evidence of diminished ability to think or concentrate, such as slowed thinking, or indecisiveness not associated with marked loosening of associations or incoherence
(8)   recurrent thoughts of death, suicidal ideation, wishes to be dead, or suicide attempt

C.   Neither of the following dominate the clinical picture when an affective syndrome (i.e., criteria A and B above) is not present, that is, before it developed or after it has remitted:

(1)   preoccupation with a mood-incongruent delusion or hallucination (see definition below)
(2)   bizarre behavior

D.   Not superimposed on either Schizophrenia, Schizophreniform Disorder, or a Paranoid Disorder.

E.   Not due to any Organic Mental Disorder or Uncomplicated Bereavement.

Fifth-digit code numbers and criteria for subclassification of major depressive epidose
(When psychotic features and Melancholia are present the coding system requires that the clinician record the single most clinically significant characteristic.)

6— In Remission.   This fifth-digit category should be used when in the past the individual met the full criteria for a major depressive episode but now is essentially free of depressive symptoms or has some signs of the disorder but does not meet the full criteria.

4— With Psychotic Features.   This fifth-digit category should be used when there apparently is gross impairment in reality testing, as when there are delusions or hallucinations, or depressive stupor (the individual is mute and unresponsive). When possible, specify whether the psychotic features are mood-congruent or mood-incongruent. (The non-ICD-9-CM fifth-digit 7 may be used instead to indicate that the psychotic features are mood-incongruent; otherwise, mood-congruence may be assumed.)

Mood-congruent Psychotic Features. Delusions or hallucinations whose content is entirely consistent with the themes of either personal inadequacy, guilt, disease, death, nihilism, or deserved punishment; depressive stupor (the individual is mute and unresponsive).

Mood-incongruent Psychotic Features. Delusions or hallucinations whose content does not involve themes of either personal inadequacy, guilt, disease, death, nihilism, or deserved punishment. Included here are such symptoms as persecutory delusions, thought insertion, thought broadcasting, and delusions of control, whose content has no apparent relationship to any of the themes noted above.

3— With Melancholia
A. Loss of pleasure in all or almost all activities
B. Lack of reactivity to usually pleasurable stimuli (doesn't feel much better, even temporarily, when something good happens).
C. At least three of the following:

(a) distinct quality of depressed mood, i.e., the depressed mood is perceived as distinctly different from the kind of feeling experienced following the death of a loved one
(b) the depression is regularly worse in the morning
(c) early morning awakening (at least two hours before usual time of awakening)
(d) marked psychomotor retardation or agitation
(e) significant anorexia or weight loss
(f) excessive or inappropriate guilt

2— Without Melancholia

APPENDIX B: DYSTHYMIC DISORDER

Diagnostic criteria for Dysthymic Disorder
A. During the past two years (or one year for children and adolescents) the individual has been bothered most or all of the time by symptoms characteristic of the depressive syndrome but that are not of sufficient severity and duration to meet the criteria for a major depressive episode (although a major depressive episode may be superimposed on Dysthymic Disorder).

B. The manifestations of the depressive syndrome may be relatively persistent or separated by periods of normal mood lasting a few days to a few weeks, but no more than a few months at a time.

C. During the depressive periods there is either prominent depressed mood (e.g., sad, blue, down in the dumps, low) or marked loss of interest or pleasure in all, or almost all, usual activities and pastimes.

D.   During the depressive periods at least three of the following symptoms are present:

(1)   insomnia or hypersomnia
(2)   low energy level or chronic tiredness
(3)   feelings of inadequacy, loss of self-esteem, or self-deprecation
(4)   decreased attention, concentration, or ability to think clearly
(6)   social withdrawal
(7)   loss of interest in or enjoyment of pleasurable activities
(8)   irritability or excessive anger (in children, expressed toward parents or caretakers)
(9)   inability to respond with apparent pleasure to praise or rewards
(10)   less active or talkative than usual, or feels slowed down or restless
(11)   pessimistic attitude toward the future, brooding about past events, or feeling sorry for self
(12)   tearfulness or crying
(13)   recurrent thoughts of death or suicide

E.   Absence of psychotic features, such as delusions, hallucinations, or incoherence, or loosening of associations.

F.   If the disturbance is superimposed on a preexisting mental disorder, such as Obsessive Compulsive Disorder or Alcohol Dependence, the depressed mood, by virtue of its intensity or effect on functioning, can be clearly distinguished from the individual's usual mood.

APPENDIX C: SOMATIZATION DISORDER

Diagnostic criteria for Somatization Disorder
A.   A history of physical symptoms of several years' duration beginning before the age of 30.

B.   Complaints of at least 14 symptoms for women and 12 for men, from the 37 symptoms listed below. To count a symptom as present the individual must report that the symptom caused him or her to take medicine (other than aspirin), alter his or her life pattern, or see a physician. The symptoms, in the judgment of the clinician, are not adequately explained by physical disorder or physical injury, and are not side effects of medication, drugs or alcohol. The clinician need not be convinced that the symptom was actually present, e.g., that the individual actually vomited throughout her entire pregnancy; report of the symptom by the individual is sufficient.

Sickly: Believes that he or she has been sickly for a good part of his or her life.

Conversion or pseudoneurological symptoms: Difficulty swallowing, loss of voice, deafness, double vision, blurred vision, blindness, fainting or loss of consciousness, memory loss, seizures or convulsions, trouble walking, paralysis or muscle weakness, urinary retention or difficulty urinating.

Gastrointestinal symptoms: Abdominal pain, nausea, vomiting spells (other than during pregnancy), bloating (gassy), intolerance (e.g., gets sick) of a variety of foods, diarrhea.

Female reproductive symptoms: Judged by the individual as occurring more frequently or severely than in most women: painful menstruation, menstrual irregularly, excessive bleeding, severe vomiting throughout pregnancy or causing hospitalization during pregnancy.

Psychosexual symptoms: For the major part of the individual's life after opportunities for sexual activity: sexual indifference, lack of pleasure during intercourse, pain during intercourse.

Pain: Pain in back, joints, extremities, genital area (other than during intercourse); pain on urination; other pain (other than headaches).

Cardiopulmonary symptoms: Shortness of breath, palpitations, chest pain, dizziness.

APPENDIX D: CONVERSION DISORDER

Diagnostic criteria for Conversion Disorder
A.   The predominant disturbance is a loss of or alteration in physical functioning suggesting a physical disorder.

B.   Psychological factors are judged to be etiologically involved in the symptom, as evidenced by one of the following:

(1)   there is a temporal relationship between an environmental stimulus that is apparently related to a psychological conflict or need and the initiation or exacerbation of the symptom
(2)   the symptom enables the individual to avoid some activity that is noxious to him or her
(3)   the symptom enables the individual to get support from the environment that otherwise might not be forthcoming

C.   It has been determined that the symptom is *not* under voluntary control.

D.   The symptom cannot, after appropriate investigation, be explained by a known physical disorder or pathophysiological mechanism.

E.   The symptom is not limited to pain or to a disturbance in sexual functioning.

F.   Not due to Somatization Disorder or Schizophrenia.

APPENDIX E: HYPOCHONDRIASIS

Diagnostic criteria for Hypochondriasis
A.   The predominant disturbance is an unrealistic interpretation of physical signs or sensations as abnormal, leading to preoccupation with the fear or belief of having a serious disease.

B.   Thorough physical evaluation does not support the diagnosis of any physical disorder that can account for the physical signs or sensations or for the individual's unrealistic interpretation of them.

C.   The unrealistic fear or belief of having a disease persists despite medical reassurance and causes impairment in social or occupational functioning.

D.   Not due to any other mental disorder such as Schizophrenia, Affective Disorder, or Somatization Disorder.

APPENDIX F: PSYCHOGENIC PAIN DISORDER

Diagnostic criteria for Psychogenic Pain Disorder
A.   Severe and prolonged pain is the predominant disturbance.

B.   The pain presented as a symptom is inconsistent with the anatomic distribution of the nervous system; after extensive evaluation, no organic pathology or pathophysiological mechanism can be found to account for the pain; or, when there is some related organic pathology, the complaint of pain is grossly in excess of what would be expected from the physical findings.

C.   Psychological factors are judged to be etiologically involved in the pain, as evidenced by at least one of the following:

(1)   a temporal relationship between an environmental stimulus that is apparently related to a psychological conflict or need and the initiation or exacerbation of the pain
(2)   the pain's enabling the individual to avoid some activity that is noxious to him or her
(3)   the pain's enabling the individual to get support from the environment that otherwise might not be forthcoming

D.   Not due to another mental disorder.

Chapter 8

Evaluation of Patients with Persistent Pain

A patient's report of pain is influenced by a variety of neural and psychological factors that cannot be explained as a direct consequence of a tissue-damaging process. These factors often play a major role in determining the suffering and disability of the patient, and optimal patient care demands that they be evaluated. Ideally, such factors should be evaluated as soon as the patient's pain becomes a major persistent problem. At present, however, this is rarely done. The major problem is that current medical training does not equip any single physician to evaluate the full range of problems that could be producing or perpetuating pain in any given patient. For example, a patient with persistent back pain might have an inflammatory disease (ankylosing spondylitis), a structural lesion (herniated disc, cyst, tumor), nerve damage with deafferentation, a somatoform disorder, a myofascial syndrome, or reflex sympathetic dystrophy. The diagnosis and treatment plan pursued will depend on the window through which the clinician views the patient. For example, an orthopedic surgeon might focus on surgically treatable musculoskeletal problems. An anesthesiologist would look for a problem that can be treated by blocking sympathetic or somatic nerves or by myofacial trigger point injection. The clinical psychologist will investigate stressful environmental factors and interpersonal relationships that may be perpetuating the pain. Specialists consider primarily those conditions with which they are most familiar and treat the one most likely to be causing the problem. In some cases, the patient's major problem is not under consideration, and nothing happens that is of benefit to the patient.

This is not meant to imply that any one of these different approaches is inherently wrong for pain patients. Obviously, each specialty does help certain patients. The problem is getting the patient to the appropriate specialist (or specialists). The current fragmentation of diagnosis and care, wherein each health care professional works within his or her expertise for a while and then, if that fails to provide lasting benefit, refers the patient on to the next specialist, results both in unnecessary treatments and delays in appropriate therapy.

In this chapter I will outline a general comprehensive approach to the initial evaluation of patients in whom persistent pain is a major diagnostic or treatment problem. Five distinct areas will be covered: possible tissue-damaging diseases, functional somatic perpetuating factors, pain associated with nerve damage, psychiatric factors, and interpersonal and behavioral perpetuating factors. Investigation of all five areas is necessary for optimal patient care.

Tissue-Damaging Diseases

This part of the evaluation needs no emphasis in medical circles. Physicians are trained to diagnose somatic diseases and are good at it. Medical students are taught how to interview and examine patients, order appropriate diagnostic studies, evaluate the information, arrive at a diagnosis, and, finally, develop and carry out a plan for treatment.

The symptom of pain and the sign of tenderness, although most important for the patient, are just two among the many clinical findings that are evaluated in the process of diagnosis. For each disease or syndrome the pain has a characteristic pattern, consisting of location, quality, intensity, time course, and exacerbating and relieving factors. Knowledge of the specific pain pattern for a disease is extremely useful in clinical practice. However, it is not my purpose to comprehensively review the characteristics of the pain in each of the medical conditions that can produce it. That information is found in textbooks that describe the various disease entities. In fact, it is inappropriate to discuss the pain of a given disease in isolation from its other diagnostic features because for most patients, the disease, not the pain, is the meaningful entity. Although the focus may shift when pain becomes a chronic problem, initially it is the diagnosis that determines therapy, not the characteristics of the pain. Furthermore, for each type of pain that presents a diagnostic or management problem, there is a medical specialty specifically trained to evaluate it. Examples are: for headaches, neurologists; for abdominal pains, gastoenterologists and general surgeons; and for musculoskeletal problems, rheumatologists and orthopedic surgeons. Each specialty is familiar with the differential diagnosis of particular types of pains and with the spectrum of therapeutic approaches to the different diagnostic entities.

Most of the time, the location, quality, and time course of the pain fit with the constellation of other signs and symptoms that lead to a diagnosis and to the initiation of appropriate therapy. With cure of the disease, the symptoms subside. In the vast majority of patients, this is the ideal way to deal with their pain. On the other hand, it is appropriate under certain circumstances to single out the symptom of pain and to treat it. For example, it is appropriate to treat pain in patients whose underlying disease is known but in whom appropriate treatment does not give complete relief (e.g., rheumatoid arthritis, pneumococcal pneumonia), or if effective treatment of the disease is not available (e.g., terminal cancer). A similar situation arises when pain is the expected sequela of a recent surgical procedure or obvious accidental injury. In still other cases, the cause of the pain is unknown but the syndrome is characteristic enough for a diagnosis to be made and treatment instituted for alleviation of the pain (e.g., trigeminal neuralgia or migraine headache). The decision to treat pain symptomatically in these cases has to be based on sound clinical judgment; the major guiding principal is that the clinician must know the diagnosis (or at least the diagnostic possibilities) before instituting palliative treatment.

Beyond the Somatic Diagnosis

Despite the appropriate application of medical knowledge and clinical judgment, there are patients who do not respond to curative or palliative therapies based on a probable medical diagnosis. Either the pain does not respond despite what should be appropriate therapy or it persists despite objective evidence that the disease or injury that originally caused it has healed. Such patients puzzle, worry, and occasionally torment the treating physician. Physicians usually have two major concerns about such patients: that their patient has a potentially diagnosable somatic disease that was missed; or that, although the diagnosis is correct and the treatment of the disease is appropriate, the patient does not respond because he or she has a particularly severe or intractable case. Some patients with migraine headache, rheumatoid arthritis or degenerative spine disease seem to fall into this latter category; they just don't do as well as other patients with the same disease.

The tendency to focus exclusively on these two possibilities (i.e., that the patient has an undiagnosed somatic disease or that they have a severe form of a correctly diagnosed disease that has not responded to conventional therapy) is not totally misplaced, but it does represent a bias that is common in current medical practice. That bias is to view persistent pain exclusively as a symptom of an objectively verifiable somatic injury or disease. This bias leads to extensive diagnostic studies aimed at finding a somatic source of the pain. In the extreme, this approach can culminate in exploratory surgery. The therapeutic approaches to such patients reflect a desperation and somatic preoccupation that is communicated by the patient and accepted by the treating physician. The treatments include high-dose narcotics and tranquilizers and repeated surgical procedures aimed at either removing the cause of the pain (e.g., multiple tooth extractions, spine fusions, lysing of adhesions) or blocking the pain transmission pathways (cutting the nerves, dorsal roots, or central pain pathways). Although such 'heroic' measures are occasionally appropriate and effective, more often they do not help. Accumulated clinical experience indicates that such extensive workups and drastic treatments often fail because the patient's major problem, which could be an emotional disturbance or a regional pattern of muscle spasm, is overlooked. Few physicians are trained to look beyond the well-established somatic diseases for alternate explanations of persistent pain. Improved management of patients with chronic pain requires broadening the conceptual framework of their evaluation to include assessment of a range of somatic and psychological factors that may intensify or perpetuate their pain.

Table 8.1 lists some of the causative and perpetuating factors that should be considered in evaluating patients with persistent pain. Pain may persist indefinitely because of functional somatic perpetuating factors such as sympathetic hyperfunction, myofascial trigger points, and nerve damage. The pain complaints may also persist because of major psychological problems, reinforcement by analgesic drugs or disability payments or because they help the patient avoid unpleasant situations. These will be discussed in the section on interviewing patients with persistent pain.

Functional Somatic Factors Perpetuating Pain

SYMPATHETICALLY MAINTAINED PAINS

In Chapter 6 I discussed the mechanisms by which activity of the sympathetic nervous system can sustain pain. In questioning patients, certain historical features should raise the index of suspicion that the sympathetic nervous system is contributing to the pain. In such cases, the pain often begins after a delay from the time of the inciting trauma or the onset of the precipitating disease. In some cases, the pain begins weeks or months later, long after the primary injury has healed. The pain characteristically builds in intensity with a time course of weeks. Patients note that their skin is hypersensitive and cold in or near the perceived location of their pain. Very often, the pain is exacerbated by cold weather.

Table 8.1 Factors Contributing to Persistent or Recurrent Pain Complaints

Factor	Example
Sympathetic nerve activity	Reflex sympathetic dystrophy, causalgia
Myofascial trigger points	Myofascial pain syndrome
Damage to sensory nerves	Brachial plexus avulsion, postherpetic neuralgia
Psychiatric illness	Major depression, somatization disorder
Environmental reinforcers	Disability payments, litigation
Habitual drug use	Alcoholism, analgesic abuse

On physical examination, patients with sympathetically maintained pain may have mild edema, mottling of the skin, loss of hair, and ridging of the nails in the affected area. The skin is objectively cold and often sweaty. When these objective findings are present, the diagnosis of reflex sympathetic dystrophy is straightforward and can be confirmed by radiographic evidence of patchy osteo-porosis and a bone scan consistent with increased bone resorption in the affected region (10). There are some patients who do not have the full-blown syndrome but in whom sympathetic activity contributes in a major way to perpetuation of their pain. Thermography may be useful in such patients since it is sensitive to small changes in skin temperature (17, 18). Thermography can also be used to document a topographical relationship between the pain and a disturbance of sympathetic function. Dramatic relief of pain by sympathetic block is diagnostic and should be carried out in all patients with persistent pain complaints who have cutaneous hypersensitivity and signs of sympathetic dysfunction, or unex-plained focal osteoporosis with active bone resorption in the painful region.

MYOFASCIAL PAIN

The most common persistent and disabling pains are of musculoskeletal origin. The potential sources of musculoskeletal pain include the joints and muscles and their connective tissue attachments. When the pain is localized to one or more joints, the diagnosis of arthritis is usually straightforward. It can be confirmed by such objective signs as local swelling and tenderness as well as X-ray changes. Another large group of patients with musculoskeletal pain have persis-tent, deep aching pains that are not localized to joints. In these patients the origin of the pain is not as obvious as in arthritis patients. However, most have pain that can be shown to originate in specific muscles that have well-delineated, highly sensitive tender spots. These patients have myofascial pain syndrome (MPS).

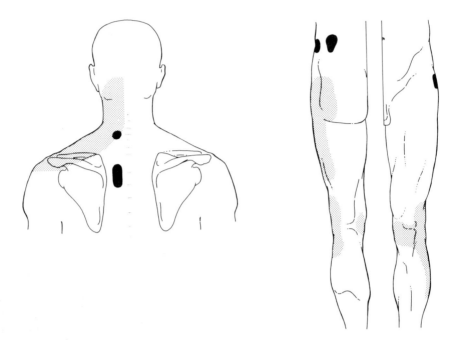

Figure 8.1   Left (Case 8.1): Solid black regions were trigger areas; pressure on them elicited pain distributed over the region indicated by the stipple. **Right** (case 8.2): Solid and stipple same as at left.

Clinical Features of MPS

Although MPS can occasionally be traced to a twisting or straining movement or to an obvious injury, often there is no precipitating event and the patient is vague about the exact date of onset of the pain. The pain is characteristically deep and aching, but nonarticular. It usually has a regional rather than a spinal segmental or peripheral nerve distribution. Frequently, the tender spots in the muscles are present over palpable firm nodules or stringlike bands (7, 8, 15, 16). Pressure on these tender spots, called myofascial trigger points, reproduces the patient's pain. It is important to point out that although the trigger points are small, highly localized, and usually restricted to a small number of muscles, the pain they generate is typically referred to a much more extensive area that may or may not include the muscle containing the trigger points (Figure 8.1) (8, 16). The diagnosis of MPS is confirmed if inactivation of the small trigger point area relieves the larger area of pain. This can be done by one of several methods, including stretching the muscle or injecting local anesthetic into the trigger points (16).

Although MPS is common and not difficult to diagnose, many physicians are unaware of its existence. There are several reasons for this, including its varying severity, duration, and location and the fact that its cause is unknown. Furthermore, in contrast to arthritis, in which the pain is centered in and around the affected joint, in MPS the pain is typically experienced at a site that is near to but distinct from the location of the offending trigger points. The paucity of objective signs, the normal radiographs, and the lack of a diagnostic laboratory test all add to the confusion. These factors have led to a profusion of names for the syndrome, including fibrositis, muscular rheumatism, and fibromyalgia (16).

Our knowledge of MPS owes much to the pioneering work of Kellgren (8, 9, 11). As discussed in Chapter 4, he demonstrated that the injection of a particular muscle with a noxious irritant generates a consistent pattern of pain over a region that is much larger than the muscle injected. Armed with this knowledge, he subsequently described a group of patients with spatially extensive and persistent pain, the origin of which could be traced to one or two muscles that contained small, excruciatingly tender spots (8). Because local anesthetic injection of these small spots relieved pain over the much larger region of ongoing pain, Kellgren postulated that the pain in the larger region represented reflex-induced contraction in segmentally related muscles. The reflex contraction in these muscles was presumed to be caused by nociceptors in the muscle with the trigger points. His original descriptions of what we now call myofascial pain syndrome were confirmed and extended by subsequent studies (see ref. 16 for review). The following illustrative cases are quoted from Kellgren's original series (8).

Case 8.1

A builder, aged 41, who had suffered for six months from pain in the left side of his neck. This came on gradually while he was doing overhead work to which he was unaccustomed. The pain was a continuous ache felt over the left side of the neck from the shoulder-tip to the occiput. The pain was aggravated by any use of the left arm; his neck felt stiff, and he had sudden exacerbations of pain on attempting to move his head. For the two weeks before he was seen the pain had been worse and had kept him awake at night.

He was a muscular man who appeared in fair general health. He held his head flexed to the right, and all neck movements were greatly limited by pain. He had a full range of passive movement in the left shoulder, but active movements were painful. Two tender spots were found—one in the erector spinae at the root of the neck, and the other by the vertebral border of the scapula (trapezius or rhomboids). The tender spots were infiltrated with 16 c.cm. novocain. This abolished the pain and he could move his head and neck painlessly through an almost normal range. One week later he was quite free from symptoms and had a full range of movements in the neck, though he had had some pain for two days after the injection.

Case 8.2

A baker of 36, who for seven months had suffered on and off from pain in both hips and legs. For the last week he had had a continuous aching pain in the left knee and in the outside of the left thigh and calf.

He was a muscular man who appeared in good general health and had a normal posture. He had limitation of abduction and rotation in both hips, but only the left was painful; there was full and painless movement in both knees and back. Straight knee leg-raising to 75 degrees on both sides. His knee- and ankle-jerks were present, and there were no sensory changes in the skin. Radiographs showed bilateral coxa vara, with very slight osteo-arthritic changes. Tender spots were found in the left gluteus medius and tensor fasciae femoris. These spots were infiltrated with 70 c.cm. novocain. During injection there was a momentary increase of pain in the knee. When the infiltration was complete the pain in the knee was abolished, but there was still slight pain in the hip. There was no change in the range of movement. One week later he had been free from pain for six days, though the night after the injection he had had much pain. The movements of both hips were still limited, though painless.

These two cases are typical. The subacute time course, the aching quality of the pain, the restricted range of movement in the affected muscles, and the presence of points in the muscle where moderate pressure reproduces the patient's pain are all characteristic features of MPS patients. These cases are also typical in that the distribution of the spontaneous pain is not coextensive with the location of the trigger areas producing it (Figure 8.1). The lasting benefit of trigger point injection is diagnostic.

Table 8.2 lists some of the most important features of MPS. Since Kellgren's description, other common features have been described that are helpful in confirming the diagnosis. As mentioned above, the trigger points are frequently located in areas of the muscle that are palpably firmer than the rest of the muscle (7). Patients often give a startled jump when even slight pressure is applied to the trigger area (jump sign). With pressure or needling of the trigger point, a local twitch is often elicited that is palpable and sometimes visible (16). This twitch does not involve the entire muscle; only those muscle fibers in the immediate vicinity of the trigger point contract. The local occurrence of the twitch raises the possibility that the muscle fibers in that area are hyperexcitable to direct mechanical stimulation.

It must be stressed that the presence of trigger points is necessary but not sufficient for the diagnosis of MPS. There is good evidence that a high percentage of asymptomatic people have tender spots in certain muscles. For example, in 200 randomly selected military personnel (males and females, ages 17–35), Sola et al. (14) examined the posterior shoulder muscles for the occurrence of tender points. Although none of the subjects had any ongoing pain problem, half had at least one tender area indistinguishable from a myofascial trigger point.

Table 8.2 Clinical Features of Myofascial Pain

Continuous, dull, deep aching pain

Pressure on tender spots or bands (trigger areas) in muscles reproduces pain

Pain relief by inactivating trigger area

Restricted range of movement in affected muscle

Local muscle twitch produced by trigger point stimulation

Patient startle or jump sign with trigger point pressure

Trigger points in patients with no pain are said to be latent. Since trigger points occur so often in normal people, their diagnostic significance is limited. The point to remember is that a trigger point can only be implicated if pressure on it reproduces the patient's spontaneous pain.

Mechanism of MPS

The mechanism of myofascial pain syndrome is uncertain. Travell and Simons (16) believed that MPS occurs when latent trigger points are activated. We do know that a noxious input from any source can, by reflex action, induce muscle contraction (11), and experimentally induced muscle pain has been shown to be correlated with active muscle contraction (2). Furthermore, muscle contraction will produce a more severe and sustained secondary pain if the contracting muscle contains a latent trigger point. These observations suggest that injury or disease (at a primary site) can give rise to pain through reflex-induced contractions of muscles at secondary sites (see Chapter 4).

If the original source of noxious input is necessary to sustain the myofascial pain, MPS should fade when the input from the original site has stopped. This is probably what happens in most people. However, in some patients, myofascial pain continues long after the original injury has healed. Input from the primary site that initiated the reflex muscle contraction is no longer required. In such patients, the secondary nociceptive input from the contracting muscle is sufficient to sustain its own contraction. That the process generating the pain and muscle contraction is self-sustaining is supported by the clinical observation that temporary inactivation with local anesthetic often leads to long-lasting, frequently permanent relief—like a fire or a spinning top, MPS requires an outside process to start but not to continue. The contraction could be generated by activity arising in the motor nerve or the muscle fibers or it may require a neural reflex loop through the spinal cord.

These observations indicate that MPS is a functional (i.e., rapidly and completely reversible) problem that depends on active muscle contraction with consequent activation of muscle nociceptors. This process involves restricted zones (trigger points) within the contracting muscles where there are sensitive muscle nociceptors. The muscle nociceptor input from these trigger points then feeds back to the spinal cord to cause further muscle contraction and sustain the pain.

Primary and Secondary Myofascial Pain Syndrome

If this hypothesis for the genesis of MPS is correct, it is clear that the problem can either be primary or secondary. In primary MPS, the initiating process occurs within the muscle that contains the trigger points. This may be abnormal strain or mild trauma. In some cases there may be no obvious precipitating event. In secondary MPS, the initiating stimulus is outside the trigger point muscle and could be any process that activates nociceptors and produces secondary muscle contraction. It is important to consider the possibility of secondary MPS, even in patients with another likely cause of pain. MPS can be a complicating factor in patients with such persistent problems as cancer, nerve injury, or arthritis. In patients with these and other painful diseases, MPS may add to the severity of pain and to its resistance to therapy.

On the other hand, patients with what appears to be primary MPS may actually have an underlying primary problem. These patients may obtain significant relief when their trigger points are inactivated, but the pain invariably returns. In cases where repeated trigger point inactivation fails to provide more than transient relief, the possibility of occult underlying diseases or perpetuating factors must be investigated (16).

Summary: The Myofascial Contribution to Persistent Pain

Although MPS is usually benign and self-limited, there are a very large number of patients in whom the condition does not resolve spontaneously. It should be considered in all cases of unexplained pain not only because it is treatable, but because, when unrecognized, it is a major cause of confusion and of delay in effective treatment. Although common, most physicians miss the diagnosis of MPS because its clinical presentation is protean and they do not examine their patients for trigger points. This is a serious problem because the diagnosis can only be made by physical examination; there are no imaging, electrodiagnostic, or laboratory tests diagnostic of MPS. The frustration and suffering of the patient with undiagnosed MPS can be compounded in situations in which MPS mimics a cardiac, gastrointestinal or neurological disease (9). In such cases there is not only prolonged pain but excessive fear and expensive, uncomfortable, and occasionally dangerous diagnostic workups.

PAIN ASSOCIATED WITH NERVE DAMAGE

Nerve injury or dysfunction is another important cause of persistent pain. Although injuries of the nervous system are typically not painful, when they are, the pain can be particularly bothersome because the sensations have a peculiar quality and analgesic medications are often ineffective. Because static nerve injury can produce persistent pain in the absence of noxious stimuli, the possibility of a neuropathic cause comes up in pain patients who have no "objective" evidence of ongoing tissue damage.

The possibility of neuropathic pain should always be considered whenever there is persistent pain plus evidence of injury to the nervous system. Establishing that neural injury is the cause of a patient's pain depends on the history, the description of the pain, and the findings on neurological examination. Damage to the nervous system is manifested by weakness or sensory loss and can be documented by imaging or electrodiagnostic tests.

Pain is much more likely to occur with peripheral than with central nervous system (CNS) damage. Accidental trauma, tumors, cervical or lumbar spine disease, and surgical procedures are common causes of painful nerve injury. These injuries usually involve one or two peripheral nerves or nerve roots, and the pain is felt in the body region normally innervated by the damaged nerves. There are also toxic, metabolic, and hereditary causes of painful polyneuropathies (e.g., alcohol abuse, diabetes mellitus). These polyneuropathies tend to be symmetrical and are most severe on the distal limbs. The pain follows the distribution of the sensory loss and weakness.

Table 6.1 (p. 134) lists some of the prominent clinical features of neuropathic pain. Typically, there is a latent period between the neural injury and the onset of the pain. This delay is more prominent in patients with pain due to CNS injury. The intensity of the pain gradually builds over weeks or months to a stable plateau. Very often, pain due to nerve injury is significantly worse in the evening and much better in the morning, so that some patients report that they wake up in the morning relatively pain free.

Neuropathic pain is often reported to have a burning and/or tingling quality. It is characteristically reported as an unfamiliar or strange sensation. Whereas visceral pain is commonly sharp and cramping, headaches throbbing or pulsing, and musculoskeletal pain deep and aching, the pain associated with neural injury often has a shooting or shocking, electrical quality. Patients report annoying, if not frankly painful sensations like insects crawling under the skin or deep ripping or tearing sensations. Another feature of neuropathic pain is the presence of hypersensitive skin. Patients complain that a slight breeze or the touch of their clothes in certain skin areas produces a brief burst of sharp pain (allodynia; see Chapter 6).

Although neuropathic pain is due in part to the activation of nociceptive neurons, its strange quality probably results from the disruption of the sensory apparatus so that a normal pattern of neural activity is no longer transmitted to the perceptual centers. Although the message that reaches these centers is clearly unpleasant, patients recognize that the sensations are not "normal" pain sensations.

Interviewing Patients with Persistent Pain

The form of the history and physical examination of chronic pain patients differs somewhat from that for patients with other medical problems. This is because the type of information needed is different. Occasionally such patients have a somatic disease that was simply missed by their physicians. In other cases, the diagnosis was correct but not all the potentially effective treatment modalities were tried. Common sense dictates that these possibilities be the first consideration, and often there is a gratifying response to treatment. More commonly, the patients have a significant undiagnosed psychiatric disease, a maladaptive social situation, or a functional somatic process such as sympathetic hyperfunction or MPS. Such problems can produce pain directly or significantly complicate the treatment of an otherwise manageable somatic pain.

The evaluation process has several goals. The first is to determine if there is a structural lesion causing the pain. The second is to determine whether there are somatic and psychosocial factors that are perpetuating the pain or are reducing the patient's tolerance for it. The third is to determine the impact of the pain on the patient's life. The final goal is to develop a treatment plan that will relieve or ease the intensity of the pain and lessen its impact on the patient. Thus the physician seeks information that will help to determine both the underlying somatic (or psychological) cause of the pain and the level and nature of the disability produced by it.

The adequate evaluation of patients with chronic pain usually requires a great deal of clinical information. Some of it is straightforward and will come out in the history. However, unless the physician has taken the time to establish some degree of trust, patients will occasionally deny and usually will not volunteer facts about significant marital or family problems or drug dependence. Forming a therapeutic alliance can be difficult in patients with chronic pain, who are often angry, impatient, and mistrustful. However, forming this alliance is essential in order to gain crucial facts about the patient and his or her situation. It is also essential in gaining patient compliance with a treatment plan. The physician is aided in this endeavor by the fact that the patient has decided to seek help and, at some level, wants to get better.

A very important practical problem is that history taking in chronic pain patients is extremely time consuming. Their hospital records are thick, their interpersonal relationships complicated, and, because they are usually preoccupied with their bodies, they often provide extremely detailed descriptions of different somatic sensations that either worry them or that they believe are important to tell the physician. Because of this wealth of information, it is very helpful, at least initially, to be directive in asking questions. Furthermore, a systematic approach is required to ensure that certain basic information is obtained from all patients. I have found that using a questionnaire is very helpful as a guide for interviewing patients. The questionnaire that I use is included as Appendix A. By having the patient fill out a questionnaire, much essential information can be obtained prior to the interview. This allows the physician to expand the interview in the most relevant areas.

DESCRIPTION OF PRESENT PAIN (Sections D through G, Patient Questionnaire)

Determine the location of the pain or pains. The best way to do this is to have the patient indicate the location of their pain (or pains) on a body diagram (questionnaire, section F). Ask whether the pain is superficial or deep and whether there are tender places in muscle or hypersensitive patches of skin (these can also be shown on the body diagram).

Have the patient briefly describe the quality of the pain in his or her own words. If, for some reason, a standardized approach is desirable, a list of descriptive words (questionnaire, section E) can also be presented. Ask whether there is more than one type of pain.

Have the patient list the maneuvers that make the pain worse and, if any, the things (other than pain medications) that help. Are there particular movements or positions that are painful or give relief? A list of some typical exacerbating and relieving factors is given on the questionnaire (section E).

Although the intensity of the pain cannot really be compared in different patients, it is helpful to know whether the pain has a diurnal variation. Here again, a diagram is useful (questionnaire, section E) so the patient can give a graphic presentation of the typical daily changes.

HISTORY

Trace the onset and course of the pain beginning with any injury or disease that the patient feels might be related to it (see Physician Interview Guide, Appendix B). If the pain was precipitated by an injury, what were the circumstances of the injury? What was the patient doing at the time? Why? For example, if it was an automobile accident, who was driving and what was the destination and purpose of the trip? Who else was in the car? If the patient attributes the pain to a work-related injury, did the patient have a history of disability or extensive use of sick leave prior to the injury?

Has the pain changed in quality, location, or intensity over the course of time? Were there ever any remissions or exacerbations for several days or more? If so, what were the circumstances (include surgical procedures or other treatments here only if they had some effect on the pain)?

CONSEQUENCES OF THE PAIN (Sections H through J, Patient Questionnaire)

An important part of the assessment of a patient's pain problem is the determination of its behavioral impact. As opposed to the subjective (i.e., intensity, suffering) aspect, which cannot be directly assessed, it is possible to determine the impact of pain on the patient's daily activities (behavior). The behavioral impact of pain is a complex function of its location, the movements that exacerbate it, its response to analgesics, its diurnal variation, and the patient's pain tolerance. Although complicated to interpret, it is helpful to determine because it is an objective measure of just how "sick" the patient is.

Behavioral impact is determined by making specific inquiries about such things as exercise tolerance, work, household chores, driving, sitting, hobbies, sports, shopping, and social activities. Other important areas include interpersonal relations, sexual activity, and sleep. These inquiries can be done in a quantitative and reproducible way by using the Sickness Impact Profile, a questionnaire that takes about 30 minutes to complete and has been shown to be valid for pain patients (1, 5). A simple way to determine the impact of pain is to have the patient describe a typical day and contrast this to a typical day before the pain problem began. It is also useful to ask the patient specifically what they would like to do that they presently cannot do because of their pain.

MEDICATION (Section K, Patient Questionnaire)

Detailed information about medication is extremely important. A complete list should be made of all medications that were tried, the dose taken, the duration of use, and the effect. Was the medication stopped because it was not effective or because the patient could not tolerate the drug? If the patient is currently taking medications, are they used on a regular basis or only when there is pain? If the patient is taking tranquilizers, barbiturates, or opiates, do the drugs actually relieve the pain or are they mainly taken because they relax the patient, permit sleep, or elevate his or her mood? Finally, it is important to know who is prescribing the medications.

It is useful to inquire about alcohol, tobacco, and other recreational drugs. Patients should be pushed a little on this and reassured that the information is considered confidential. The patient should be asked if he or she has ever had a drug or alcohol problem. The presence of pain may exacerbate such problems and vice versa. Information about medication, "self-medication," and potential for drug abuse is essential for the overall evaluation of pain patients.

PREVIOUS PAIN PROBLEMS AND PAST MEDICAL HISTORY (Sections L and M, Patient Questionnaire)

The purpose of inquiring about painful illnesses other than the present problem is to determine whether the patient is pain prone. Is the current problem just the most recent in a lifelong pattern of pain problems involving different regions of the body? Inquire about all hospitalizations and surgical procedures, including tonsillectomy and appendectomy. For women, ask about menstrual cycle pain. Do not stop with the diagnosis; have the patient tell about his or her symptoms.

The general medical history and review of systems has two aims: to assess the patient's general health, and to look for evidence of somatization and hypochondriasis (see Chapter 7). It is important to determine whether the patient has sought treatment for a variety of vague complaints, including pain, which appear to involve multiple body regions and organ systems. A checklist and questionnaire is particularly useful for this purpose, which can otherwise be extremely time consuming. A history of persistent contact with physicians and other health care professionals for treatment of multiple apparently unrelated somatic problems is characteristic of somatization.

In summary, the purpose of this part of the patient evaluation is to examine whether the current pain problem is a singular event or the continuation of a long-standing pattern of multiple, distinct somatic complaints, including pain, which involve different regions of the body.

PSYCHOSOCIAL ASSESSMENT

As discussed in Chapter 7, there are a variety of psychological factors that influence pain. For some patients, the psychosocial factors complicate a problem that is primarily somatic. In others, the major problem is a psychiatric disorder or a reinforced maladaptive behavior. In either case, a psychosocial assessment will be rewarding because a very high proportion of patients with chronic pain have a significant and diagnosable psychiatric disorder (4).

Although this type of assessment is optimally performed by a psychiatrist or clinical psychologist experienced with pain patients, it is possible for the nonpsychiatrist to uncover significant psychological abnormalities by focusing on specific problem areas (see Physician Interview Guide, Appendix B). In fact, because pain patients are usually convinced that their major problem is a somatic illness, they are less threatened and therefore more open to "psychological" questions from medical doctors. Since the information is taken along with questions about somatic problems, the stigma attached to a psychiatric evaluation is removed. Furthermore, if the patient believes that his or her somatic complaint is being taken seriously and the initial evaluation includes a thorough physical examination looking for possible somatic problems, the patient will be more compliant with referral for more extensive psychological evaluation.

Depression

Questions designed to elicit evidence of substance abuse, and somatization disorder were discussed above. It is also important to look for major depression, which is probably the most common psychological problem in pain patients (4). Patients should be asked if there has been a recent personal loss such as the death of a spouse, parent, or child. Divorce and financial problems are also common causes of depression. Depressed patients usually look sad, are frequently tearful, and may have difficulty concentrating. In addition to signs of current depression it is important to determine if the patient has a personal or family history of depressive illness. Specific inquiry should be made about suicidal ideation or attempts, and psychiatric hospitalization or outpatient care (see Patient Questionnaire, section N, and Physician Interview Guide for other points).

Psychogenic Pain

Although this entity is not universally accepted, there are patients whose pain problem seems to be best understood in terms of a psychodynamic model (see Chapter 7). That a patient falls into this category is supported by the following findings: the patient has a physically or sexually abusive spouse (or had an abusive parent), the patient has a "model" for the pain (a loved one with pain in a similar location), and the patient's life is characterized by excessive or inappropriate guilt feelings (3). In the absence of objective evidence of somatic disease, the presence of these findings is presumptive evidence of psychogenic pain.

Behavioral Reinforcers

The role of learning in the maintenance of pain complaints and disability was discussed at length in Chapter 7. At first glance, most of these behaviors, such as rest, taking pain medication, seeking medical attention, and avoidance of work and social situations seem appropriate because they lessen the pain. The central question is whether the patient derives any significant reward other than pain relief from these behaviors. One obvious example is the reinforcing potential of psychoactive drugs. Other rewards may derive from relief from unpleasant work or social situations.

A simple aid for uncovering potential behavioral problems is to have the patient fill out a pain diary (see Appendix C) for a couple of weeks. For each period during the day the patient records the time spent doing various activities (e.g., watch TV, sleep, eat dinner, drive, play cards), the amount of each medication taken, and the relative level of pain experienced. The diary will provide a guide for further questioning about the behavioral impact of the pain as well as a baseline for the assessment of therapy.

The pain and disability may yield financial rewards, and to this end it is important to determine if the patient is receiving disability payments, a pension, or workmen's compensation. It is also useful to know if there is any litigation pending that involves a potential payment based on pain or disability (Patient Questionnaire, Section J).

Marriage and family interactions are powerful determinants of behavior. For a woman with an abusive or uncaring spouse, the pain may be a way for the patient to protect herself or obtain nurturance from the spouse (or from other family members and physicians). On the other hand, an overprotective spouse who will not let the patient do anything may be a strong factor in perpetuating pain complaints. It is crucial to interview the spouse and the patient separately about their marital and sexual adjustment and about the impact of the *patient's* pain on the spouse (see Physician Interview Guide, Appendix B). For many patients, successful treatment requires that the spouse be actively involved.

The evaluation of behavioral reinforcers is obviously a complex task (6). It involves extensive questioning of patients and family members. The physician often can do little more than ask a few probing questions to determine whether a more extensive workup is needed. If it is indicated, further workup is best carried out in the setting of a behaviorally oriented pain treatment program.

Physical Examination

The physical examination of patients with persistent pain will depend on several factors, including the location of the pain and the diagnoses that are being entertained. Good medical practice demands that the examination be tailored to the complaint (i.e., the differential diagnosis). For example, a patient with face pain should have a careful neurological examination that focuses on the cranial nerves. In a patient with low back pain, the examiner will concentrate on local tenderness, weakness of the leg, and abnormalities of sensation and reflexes. It is obviously not feasible to describe how to examine patients for all the different possible causes of persistent pain. However, there are elements of the physical examination that can provide information of potential importance for all pain patients. It is these aspects of the exam that have general relevance to pain patients that I will describe here.

Before starting the formal examination note the facial expression and listen carefully to the patient's voice. Is the patient obviously sad (tearful)? Does his or her voice indicate anxiety? If the patient is with a spouse or significant other, who does the talking? Does the spouse appear to be a major caretaker?

Try to observe the patient's gait and posture as they come into the examining room, before they know they are being examined. Is there a limp? Grimacing with changes of position? Guarding? Does the patient appear to sit comfortably during the interview? When examining the patient, note whether any muscles are painful when stretched and whether there is a restricted range of movement around particular joints. How does this compare with the patient's movements before the formal examination started?

Look for evidence of inflammation and sympathetic nervous system dysfunction. Note whether there is any swelling, mottling, dampness, or other unusual appearance of the skin in the painful area. Feel the skin temperature (use the palmar surface of the wrist) and compare it with an unaffected area of skin, preferably the mirror image area.

EXAMINING PATIENTS WITH SUSPECTED NEUROPATHIC PAIN

A neurological examination should be carried out in all patients with suspected neuropathic pain. Muscle tone, bulk and strength, and reflexes should be examined. The greatest emphasis, however, should be on the sensory exam because there are certain sensory abnormalities that indicate the presence of neuropathic pain.

Attention should be focused on the skin area that the patient indicates is nearest the location of his or her pain. Stimuli to be used include innocuous heat (a test tube with warm water), cold (a tuning fork at room temperature), pinprick, and light touch using a few strands of cotton. Brush the cotton strands lightly against the skin, instructing the patient to report if any sensation at all is detected. If there is an area of deficit, map out its boundaries by moving the stimulus from the area of greatest deficit outward toward the boundary with normally innervated skin. Once this is done, repeat the mapping process with the thermal stimuli, asking the patient to report if the stimulus is felt as distinctly cool or warm. Finally, using a pin, stimulate with a force that is felt by the patient as sharp (and/or painful) in normal skin. Then, stimulating in the affected area, ask the patient to report whether the sensation is sharp or dull. Alternate stimulation with the point and the head of the pin as a control.

Once any areas of deficit are mapped out, the presence of allodynia and hyperalgesia should be documented. First, using a few strands of cotton fiber, rapidly and lightly stroke the skin in the painful area and in normal areas (preferably the contralateral mirror-image region). The patient should be asked whether the sensation in the two areas is the same. Note whether the patient jumps or winces when this stimulation is being carried out. If this stimulation produces a sensation of greater intensity in the painful (i.e., abnormal) region, the patient is said to have hyperesthesia. If the sensation is unpleasant it is a dysesthesia and, if painful, the patient is said to have allodynia. Next, apply the warm (or cold) stimulus for 15–30 seconds alternately to the affected area and to normal skin and ask the patient to compare the sensations. Then have the patient compare the effect of pinprick in normal and painful areas. If the pinprick is more painful in the affected area, the patient is said to have hyperalgesia.

In the sensory examination of patients with pain pay particularly close attention to the border zone between the affected areas and the adjacent normally innervated skin. These areas are most likely to manifest allodynia and hyperalgesia. Figure 8.2 illustrates this in two patients with painful nerve injuries.

Summation and Spatial Spread

It is important to examine the patient for summation and spatial spread of sensation because these two findings are highly correlated with neuropathic pain (12, 13). If a zone of hyperesthesia is present, summation and spread should be sought there; if not, examine the region close to the boundary of normal and abnormal sensation. Use the point of a pin, and stimulate with a force that is felt as sharp in normally innervated skin. Stimulate the same spot repeatedly (about two to three times per second) for at least 30 seconds and ask the patient whether the perceived intensity grows with successive stimuli (summation), whether there is any spread of the sensation beyond the area being stimulated (spatial spread), and whether the unpleasant sensation persists after the stimulation has stopped (after discharge).

EXAMINATION FOR MYOFASCIAL PAIN

All patients with persistent aching pain should be examined for MPS. The examination consists of passively stretching the muscles in the painful area looking for painful restriction of the range of movement. The muscles that might be generating the pain are then carefully palpated for trigger points using the thumb or index finger. Figures 8.3, 8.4, and 8.5 illustrate some of the common referral patterns for MPS generated by trigger points in muscles of the head, shoulder, and hip. For more complete charts see Travell and Simons (15, 16). Occurrence of the local twitch and jump sign are helpful but not required for diagnosis. It is most critical that the patient's original pain complaint be mimicked by pressure on the trigger point and/or that inactivation of the trigger points gives significant relief.

In my experience, the best way to inactivate trigger points is by injection

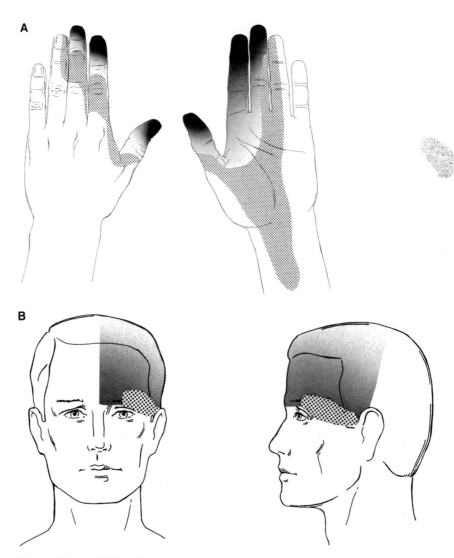

Figure 8.2   A: Thirty-eight-year-old man with complete transection of the left median nerve. This resulted in a burning, throbbing hand pain that, when severe, spread up into the forearm. In the stippled region, very light stimuli and pinprick were exquisitely painful. In the shaded region, all modalities of sensation were diminished; the darkness of the shading indicates the degree of sensory impairment. (Adapted from Denny-Brown, D.: The release of deep pain by nerve injury. *Brain* **88:**725–738, 1965.) **B:** A man with pain following herpes zoster of the first division of the left trigeminal nerve. The pain was described as a continual burning headache with intermittent jolts of severe electric shock-like pain above the left eye. He was particularly bothered by an area of skin (*stipple*) where very light touch triggered the jolts of pain. Stippling and shading as in **A.**

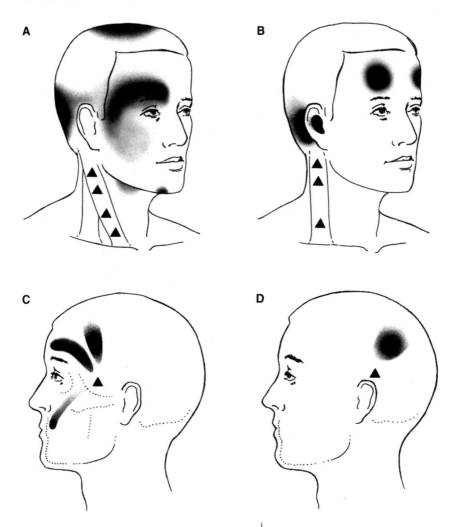

Figure 8.3   Representative myofascial pain syndromes of the head. Examples of the topography of trigger points in muscles (*triangles*) and the distribution of the referred pain that they can produce (darker *shading* indicates regions more likely to be the locus of referred pain). **A:** Sternocleidomastoid (sternal division). **B:** Sternocleidomastoid (clavicular division). **C:** Temporalis (anterior). **D:** Temporalis (posterior). (Adapted from Travell, J. G., and Simons, D. G.: *Myofascial Pain and Dysfunction: The Trigger Point Manual.* Williams & Wilkins, Baltimore, 1983.)

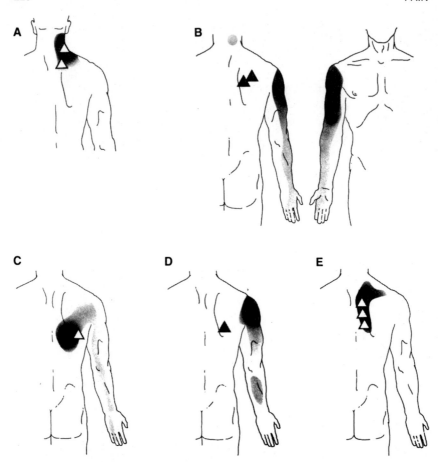

Figure 8.4 Representative myofascial pain syndromes of the neck and shoulder (symbols and shading as in Figure 8.2). **A:** Levator scapulae. **B:** Infraspinatus. **C:** Latissimus dorsi. **D:** Teres major. **E:** Rhomboids. (Adapted from Travell, J. G., and Simons, D. G.: *Myofascial Pain and Dysfunction: The Trigger Point Manual.* Williams & Wilkins, Baltimore, 1983.)

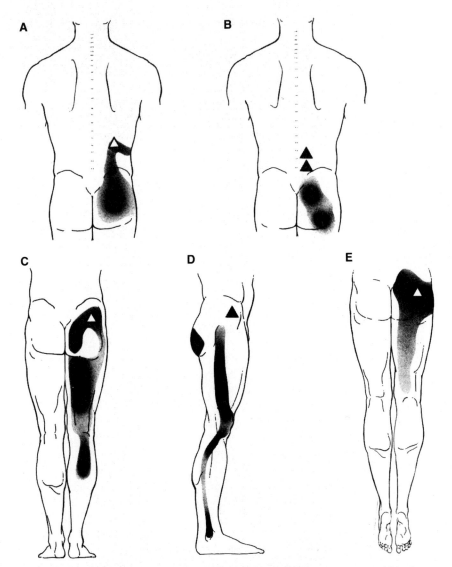

Figure 8.5 Representative myofascial pain syndromes of the hip and leg (symbols and shading as in Figure 8.2). **A:** Iliocostalis lumborum. **B:** Quadratus lumborum. **C:** Gluteus minimus (posterior). **D:** Gluteus minimus (anterior). **E:** Piriformis. (Adapted from Simons, D. G., and Travell, J. G.: Myofascial origins of low back pain. *Postgrad. Med.* **73:**66–108, 1983.)

of local anesthetic. After marking the location of the trigger points with an ink mark, I prep the skin with alcohol. It typically takes about 5–15 ml of a 0.5% solution of procaine or lidocaine for each muscle. A wheal is raised in the skin above the trigger point. With the first and second finger exerting slight pressure on either side of it, the needle is slowly advanced directly toward the trigger point. The muscle will often twitch when the needle hits the trigger point and the patient may experience a sharp pain radiating into the region of spontaneous pain. Inject 3–4 ml at that point. Withdraw the needle almost to the surface and then advance it again to the same depth but about 0.5–1 inch to the side of the original injection. In this way two to four more injections are made around the target site to assure complete inactivation of the trigger point. The patient should be warned that the pain may return, but the physician should avoid being specifically optimistic or pessimistic about what will happen. Trigger points can also be inactivated by "dry needling," injection of sterile saline, or stretching the trigger muscle while the skin is cooled with a vapocoolant spray. These methods are thoroughly and meticulously described by Travell and Simons in their recent book, which also covers the patterns of referred pain for most of the muscles in the upper body (16).

Diagnostic Tests

By the time the extensive evaluation described above has been carried out, you should have a good idea about the probable causative and perpetuating factors for the patient's pain. In some cases it will be helpful to carry out further diagnostic tests and procedures either to confirm the suspected problem or to differentiate between alternative explanations. Nerve damage can be confirmed using electromyography and nerve conduction studies. These tests are particularly useful for determining whether a lesion involves a spinal root or a peripheral nerve. Thermography, which gives a picture of the topography of skin temperature, is useful for documenting the presence of excess sympathetic activity (cool areas), inflammation (warm areas), and root lesions. Radioisotope bone scans are useful for picking up unsuspected areas of active bone resorption (10) and inflammation. They can also be used to detect tumors affecting bone.

In addition to standard imaging tests like radiography, computed tomography, and myelography, there are several procedures for confirming functional somatic problems. I have already described the use of trigger point injections to confirm and treat myofascial pain syndrome. Another useful procedure is sympathetic block. For pains in the head, shoulder, and arm the stellate ganglion is blocked. The sympathetic chain can be blocked anywhere along its length, depending on the location of the pain. If the pain is relieved by sympathetic block and there is no evidence that the anesthetic has spread to involve somatic nerves it is likely that the patient has a sympathetically maintained pain. The relief produced by the block should outlast the duration of action of the local anesthetic. Such pains are often relieved by a series of four or five sympathetic blocks.

Summary

In this chapter I have outlined a general approach to the evaluation of pain patients. This approach has evolved gradually, shaped by my experience with certain types of pain patients. I have presented it as an example of a method to obtain the sort of information that I believe is crucial for understanding and treating pain patients. I am sure there are many other approaches that are just as good; the major requirement for effectiveness is that the approach be comprehensive and systematic.

References

1 Bergner, M., Bobbitt, R. A., Carter, W. B., and Gilson, B. S.: The Sickness Impact Profile: Development and final revision of a health status measure. *Med. Care* **19:**787–805, 1981.

2 Cobb, C. R., DeVries, H. A., Urban, R. T., Luekens, C. A., and Bagg, R. J.: Electrical activity in muscle pain. *Am. J. Physical Med.* **54:**80–87, 1975.

3 Eisendrath, S. J., Way, L. W., Ostroff, J. W., and Johanson, C. A.: Identification of psychogenic abdominal pain. *Psychosomatics* **27:**705–712, 1986.

4 Fishbain, D. A., Goldberg, M., Meagher, B. R., Steele, R., and Rosomoff, H.: Male and female chronic pain patients categorized by DSM-III psychiatric diagnostic criteria. *Pain* **26:**181–197, 1986.

5 Follick, M. J., Smith, T. W., and Ahern, D. K.: The Sickness Impact Profile: A global measure of disability in chronic low back pain. *Pain* **21:**67–76, 1985.

6 Fordyce, W. E.: *Behavioral Methods for Chronic Pain and Illness*. C.V. Mosby, St. Louis, 1976.

7 Gutstein, M.: Diagnosis and treatment of muscular rheumatism. *Br. Med. J.* **1:**302–321, 1938.

8 Kellgren, J. H.: A preliminary account of referred pains arising from muscle. *Br. Med. J.* **1:**325–327, 1938.

9 Kellgren, J. H.: Somatic simulating visceral pain. *Clin. Sci.* **4:**303–309, 1940.

10   Kozin, F., Ryan, L. M., Carerra, G. F., Soin, J. S., and Wortmann, R. L.: The reflex sympathetic dystrophy syndrome (RSDS). III. Scintigraphic studies, further evidence for the therapeutic efficacy of systemic corticosteroids, and proposed diagnostic criteria. *Am. J. Med.* **70:**23–30, 1981.

11   Lewis, T., and Kellgren, J. H.: Observations relating to referred pain, visceromotor reflexes and other associated phenomena. *Clin. Sci.* **4:**47–71, 1939–42.

12   Lindblom, V.: Sensory abnormalities in neuralgia. In J. J. Bonica et al. (eds.), *Advances in Pain Research and Therapy*, Vol. 3. Raven Press, New York, 1979.

13   Noordenbos, W.: *Pain*. Elsevier, Amsterdam, 1959.

14   Sola, A. E., Rodenberger, M. L., and Gettys, B. B.: Incidence of hypersensitive areas in posterior shoulder muscle. *Am. J. Physical Med.* **34:**585–590, 1955.

15   Simons, D. G., and Travell, J. G.: Myofascial origins of low back pain. *Postgrad. Med.* **73:**66–108, 1983.

16   Travell, J. G., and Simons, D. G.: *Myofascial Pain and Dysfunction: The Trigger Point Manual*. Williams & Wilkins, Baltimore, 1983.

17   Uematsu, S.: Thermagraphic imaging of cutaneous sensory segment in patients with peripheral nerve injury. *J. Neurosurg.* **62:**716–720, 1985.

18   Uematsu, S., Hendler, N., Hungerford, D., Long, D., and Ono, N.: Thermography and electromyography in the differential diagnosis of chronic pain syndromes and reflex sympathetic dystrophy. *Electromyogr. Clin. Neurophysiol.* **21:**165–182, 1981.

APPENDIX A: UCSF PAIN SERVICE
PATIENT QUESTIONNAIRE

INSTRUCTIONS: This questionnaire is designed to provide information that will help us to understand your particular pain problem. Please read each question carefully. Please print your answers clearly so they are easy to read. If you feel you would like to clarify or add to a particular answer, please feel free to use additional pages. Because this is an account of your personal experience, please complete it by yourself, without assistance from anyone else.

A   *Identification Data*

    1   Name _____

    2   Address _____

    3   Telephone # Work _____ # Home _____

4 Social Security # _____ Date of Birth _____

5 Age _____ Sex _____ Race _____

6 Weight _____ Height _____

B *Referral Information*

   1 Who referred you to the UCSF Pain Program?

     _____ Doctor   _____ Attorney   _____ Insurance Company

     _____ Self   _____ Other

     Their name and telephone number: _____

   2 Who do you regard as your primary doctor? _____

     Telephone number _____

   3 What is his or her specialty? _____

C *Personal Information*

   1 Marital Status: ( ) Married   ( ) Remarried   ( ) Single

                               ( ) Divorced   ( ) Separated   ( ) Widowed

   2 With whom do you live?

     Name(s): _____   Relationship: _____

            _____   _____

            _____   _____

            _____   _____

            _____   _____

            _____   _____

   3 Check the highest grade of schooling you have completed?

     ( ) less than high school   ( ) high school

     ( ) vocational technical   ( ) vocational business

     ( ) college   ( ) graduate or professional

     ( ) other (describe) _____

   4 Please list the *name, sex* and *age* of each of your children:

     _____

     _____

D *Information About Your Pain*

   1 What is the problem you would like us to help you with?

   _____

   _____

   2 Is this your major problem?   YES / NO

     If not, what is? _____

   _____

   3 What event or events lead to your present pain:

     _____ accident   _____ cancer

     _____ other injury   _____ no obvious cause

     _____   _____ other disease _____

                             _____ following an operation

                             _____ other _____

   4 Indicate what *you* think is the cause of your pain

   _____

   _____

   _____

E *Temporal Pattern and Exacerbating Factors*

   1 How often does your pain occur?

     _____ continuously (nonstop)

     _____ several times a day

     _____ once or twice a day

     _____ several times a week

     _____ less than 3–4 times per month

     _____ once or twice a month

     _____ less than once a month

   2 How has the *intensity* of the pain changed throughout the time you have had it?

     _____ increased   _____ decreased   _____ stayed the same

3 If you have pain-free periods, how long do they last?

_____ minutes _____ hours _____ days

_____ weeks _____ months

4 Describe the circumstances of your last pain-free period of 3 or more days if you had one? _____

_____

5 Which of the following affect your pain? (Mark "B" for better, "W" for worse, and leave blank for "no effect")

_____ heat   _____ cold   _____ massage or rubbing

_____ sitting   _____ standing   _____ lying down

_____ walking   _____ running   _____ getting out of bed

_____ coughing   _____ fatigue   _____ straining

_____ vibration   _____ anxiety   _____ sudden movements

_____ wet climate   _____ hot climate   _____ cold climate

_____ alcoholic drinks   _____ noise

_____ caffeinated drinks (coffee, tea, colas)

_____ strong emotion (anger, excitement, surprise, etc.)

_____ other _____

_____ particular movements (explain) _____

_____

6 Which, if any, of the preceding activities bring on the pain when you are pain free? _____

7 Which posture or body position causes you the least pain? _____

_____

8 Do you have any points or areas of your body that, when touched or rubbed, produce or worsen pain?   YES / NO

9 Does light touching or rubbing in the affected area produce unpleasant sensations?   YES / NO

10 If yes, please describe the sensation and location:

_____

_____

_____

11 Please show us how your pain changes during the course of an average day by making a graph like the one in this example (10 indicates the worst pain you can imagine). It would also be helpful to indicate your usual hours of sleep.

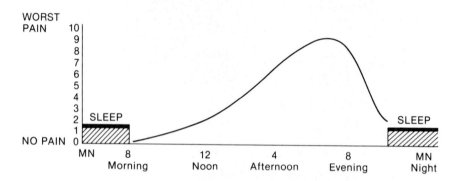

As you can see, the person who drew the example graph showed us that his pain is least severe in the morning, and that it gradually increases during the day until the late afternoon, when it is worst, and then it gradually improves until sometime after he goes to bed. The person went to bed at 10 P.M. and woke up at 8 A.M.

Please draw a line on the graph below to show us how *YOUR* pain changes through the day. If it does not change, draw a straight line at the approximate pain level:

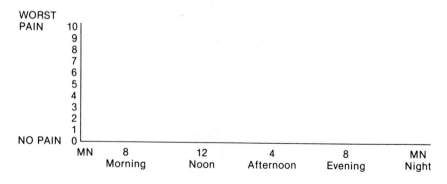

12 Please make another graph on the form below to show us generally how your pain has progressed in severity over the entire period of time since it began.

```
WORST
PAIN    10│
         9│
         8│
         7│
         6│
         5│
         4│
         3│
         2│
         1│
NO PAIN  0└_____
                                TIME
         Onset of                                        Now
         Pain (Date_____)
```

13 If your pain is due to an injury, a short illness, or a surgical procedure give the date of that problem:

_____

If you can't give an exact date, please give the time period over which

the problem began: _____

14 How much time went by between your injury and the beginning of your pain?

_____ immediate _____ hours _____ days _____ weeks

_____ months _____ not applicable

15 How much time went by between the start of your pain and your first visit to a health care professional?

_____ immediate _____ hours _____ days _____ weeks

_____ months _____ years _____ not applicable

16 How much time went by between first onset of pain and when pain became its worst?

_____ immediate _____ hours _____ days _____ weeks

_____ months _____ years _____ not applicable

F   *Location of Your Pain*

Using these pictures and the ones on the next page, indicate which parts of your body are affected by pain by shading them with a pen or pencil.

If you have more than one type of pain, you may use a different color for each.

If you have any particularly sensitive areas or trigger points, label them with an "X."

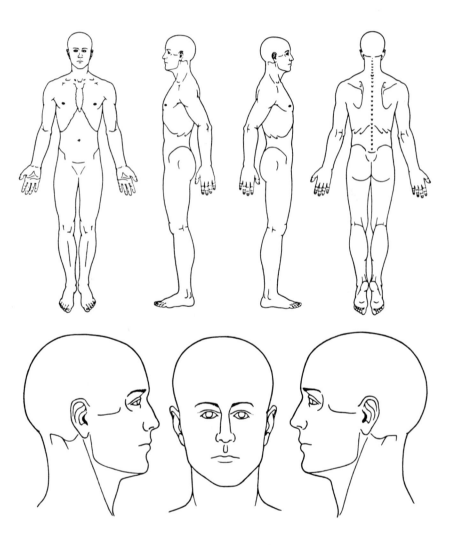

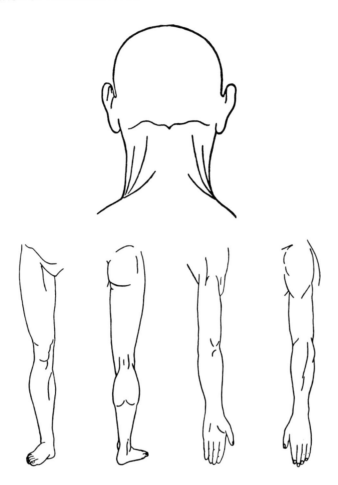

G *Quality of the Pain*

    1 Describe the *quality* of your current pain (i.e., what it feels like?) *in your own words*. If there is more than one type of pain, describe each separately.

_____

_____

_____

_____

2 Some of the words below may describe your *present* pain. Circle only
one in each of the 20 groups *if* the group contains a word that describes
your pain. Leave out any group that is not suitable.

1	2	3	4
Flickering	Jumping	Pricking	Sharp
Quivering	Flashing	Boring	Cutting
Pulsing	Shooting	Drilling	Lacerating
Throbbing	Shocking	Stabbing	
Beating		Lancinating	
Pounding			

5	6	7	8
Pinching	Tugging	Hot	Tingling
Pressing	Pulling	Burning	Itchy
Gnawing	Wrenching	Scalding	Smarting
Cramping		Searing	Stinging
Crushing			

9	10	11	12
Dull	Tender	Tiring	Sickening
Sore	Taut	Exhausting	Suffocating
Hurting	Rasping		
Aching	Splitting		
Heavy			

13	14	15	16
Fearful	Punishing	Wretched	Annoying
Frightful	Grueling	Blinding	Troublesome
Terrifying	Cruel		Miserable
	Viscious		Intense
	Killing		Unbearable

17	18	19	20
Spreading	Tight	Cool	Nagging
Radiating	Numb	Cold	Nauseating
Penetrating	Drawing	Freezing	Agonizing
Piercing	Squeezing	Icy	Dreadful
	Tearing		Torturing

H   *Effect of Pain on Activity*

1   Please tell us how your pain interferes with your activities by writing the number of the descriptive term in the blank next to the type of activity:

_____ Work

_____ Family activities

_____ Chores

_____ Play/Recreation

_____ Exercise

1. Continuously
2. Several times a day
3. Once a day
4. Several times a week
5. Several times a month
6. Once a month
7. Less than once a month
8. Never

2   List your usual daily activities before your pain problem started:

Type of Activity	*Hours per Day*
_____	_____
_____	_____
_____	_____
_____	_____

3   List your *current* activities on a typical day:

_____	_____
_____	_____
_____	_____
_____	_____

4 Before you had any pain problems, how far could you walk?

_____ miles _____ blocks _____ less than a block

5 How far now? _____

6 What time do you usually go to bed? _____

7 How long after you close your eyes before you fall asleep?

_____

8 What time do you usually wake up in the morning? _____

9 Number of times you wake up at night due to pain: _____

10 Could you drive a car before your pain problems? _____

If yes, how long? _____ (hours) How long now? _____ (hours)

11 If your pain was reduced to an acceptable level, list the activities you would engage in that your current pain level prevents you from doing. Be specific.

a. _____

b. _____

c. _____

I *Employment Information*

1 What is your current employment status?

( ) employed full time   ( ) employed part time

( ) retired   ( ) homemaker

( ) unemployed due to pain   ( ) self-employed

( ) unemployed for other reasons

2 How many hours per week do you presently work? _____

3 Present or most recent occupation? _____

4 If employed, has your pain forced you to limit your work

activities?   YES / NO   (circle one, if applicable)

5 If unemployed, when did you last work? _____

6 Spouse's occupation? _____

J   *Financial Information*

   1   What are your present sources of financial support?

      (　) personal earnings   (　) workmen's compensation

      (　) disability payment   (　) insurance _____

      (　) spouse's earnings   (　) other _____

      (　) pension/retirement   (　) none

   2   Are you hoping to receive other income or compensation:

      (　) disability payment   (　) workmen's compensation

      (　) legal settlement   (　) other _____

   3   Who is the source of payment or reimbursement for your medical

      care? _____

      _____

   4   Do you have any legal action pending related to this pain or any

      other pain or present health problem?   YES / NO   (Circle one)

K   *Pain Medication and Other Treatments*

   1   Please list *all* the medications you are *now* taking specifically for
      pain (prescription or not):

	Drug	*Strength*	*# pills per day*
a.	_____	_____	_____
b.	_____	_____	_____
c.	_____	_____	_____
d.	_____	_____	_____

   2   Please list all pain medications you have tried *in the past:*

	Drug	*Maximum Dose Used*	*Effect on Pain*
a.	_____	_____	_____
b.	_____	_____	_____
c.	_____	_____	_____
d.	_____	_____	_____

e. _____ _____ _____

f. _____ _____ _____

3 Please indicate which of the following treatments you have tried for your pain problem and the results of each. (Leave blank if not tried.)

Write: A . . . if tried and major relief.
B . . . if tried and some relief.
C . . . if tried and no effect.
D . . . if tried and the pain got worse.

_____ Tranquilizers   _____ Pain relievers

_____ Surgery   _____ Traction

_____ Nerve blocks   _____ Trigger point injections

_____ Braces or cast(s)   _____ Acupuncture

_____ Chiropractic   _____ Massage

_____ Physical therapy   _____ Psychotherapy

_____ Other counselling   _____ Biofeedback

_____ Relaxation training   _____ Hypnosis

_____ Exercise program   _____ Homeopathy

_____ Transcutaneous electrical nerve stimulator (TENS)

4 Are there other measures you have personally tried to decrease your

pain: _____

_____

_____

_____

_____

L *Past Pain History*

1 How many painful disorders have you been treated for in the past

other than your present problem? _____

2 How many times in the past have you been to a hospital emergency

room because of a pain problem? _____

3 How many times have you been admitted to a hospital for any

problems associated with pain? _____

4 List the *most recent* operations you have had for pain:

Use the numbered items here to describe the results of your surgery:

1. operation was a complete success
2. original pain was less after the operation (% relief)
3. original pain was same after the operation
4. original pain was relieved after surgery but came back
5. operation produced different pain problem (explain)
6. original pain was worse after the operation

Procedure	Hospital	Date	Result
1. _____	_____	____	_____
2. _____	_____	____	_____
3. _____	_____	____	_____
4. _____	_____	____	_____
5. _____	_____	____	_____
6. _____	_____	____	_____
7. _____	_____	____	_____

5 Has a close friend or relative ever had a significant pain

problem? YES / NO

M *General Medical History*

1 What other medical problems do you now have?

a. _____

b. _____

c. _____

d. _____

2 In what way do any of these have an effect on your pain?

_____

_____

3 Please list *all* the drugs (pills, creams, etc. whether prescription or not) *except pain medications* that you are taking now:

   Drug   *Dose*   *Reason*

a. _____

b. _____

c. _____

d. _____

e. _____

f. _____

4 Please list all operations and hospitalizations you have had (not including those for pain) and the dates (include tonsillectomy, appendectomy and hysterectomy).

_____

_____

_____

_____

5 Have you ever had or do you currently have any of the following?

_____ diabetes   _____ epilepsy   _____ heart disease

_____ liver disease   _____ kidney disease   _____ ulcers

_____ stroke   _____ cancer   _____ joint problems

_____ significant emotional problems

6 Are you sensitive or allergic (develop a rash or problem breathing or any significant problem) to any of the following?

_____ penicillin   _____ aspirin   _____ codeine

_____ novocaine   _____ sleeping pills   _____ iodine

_____ other (please list) _____

7 *Checklist of Problems*

Please check the items you feel are applicable to you:

_____ Has your health been poor much of your life?

_____ Do you have difficulty swallowing?

_____ Loss or change of voice?

_____ Deafness?

_____ Double vision?

_____ Blurred vision?

_____ Blindness?

_____ Fainting spells or loss of consciousness or blackouts?

_____ Memory loss?

_____ Seizures or convulsions?

_____ Trouble walking?

_____ Paralysis or muscle weakness?

_____ Urinary retention or difficulty urinating?

_____ Abdominal pain?

_____ Nausea?

_____ Vomiting spells (other than during pregnancy)?

_____ Bloating (gassy feeling)?

_____ Intolerance (e.g., get sick) of a variety of foods?

_____ Diarrhea?

_____ Do you feel uninterested/indifferent in sex?

_____ Do you experience an absence of pleasure during sex?

_____ Do you experience pain during intercourse?

_____ Do you have back pain?

_____ Do you have joint pain (knee, elbow, etc.)?

_____ Do you have pain in the arms and legs?

_____ Do you have genital pain (other than during sex)?

_____ Do you have pain on urination?

_____ Do you have other pain (other than headache)?

_____ Do you have shortness of breath?

_____ Do you have palpitations (awareness of fast heart)?

_____ Do you have chest pain?

_____ Do you frequently have dizziness?

_____ Has someone close to you recently died or become ill?

        If yes, who: _____

Women, do you feel the following occur more frequently and/or severely in you than in other women?

_____ Painful menstruation?

_____ Menstrual irregularity?

_____ Excessive bleeding?

_____ Severe vomiting throughout pregnancy?

N   Questions about your mood and functioning:

For each item circle the number which best fits how you feel.

	1 strongly agree	2 agree somewhat	3 disagree somewhat	4 strongly disagree

1 I worry a lot.	1	2	3	4
2 I feel hopeful about the future.	1	2	3	4
3 I'm frequently irritable.	1	2	3	4
4 I enjoy doing things as much as ever.	1	2	3	4
5 I sleep as well as ever.	1	2	3	4
6 I often feel depressed.	1	2	3	4
7 I often feel nervous or fearful.	1	2	3	4
8 I have lots of energy.	1	2	3	4
9 My memory and concentration seem fine.	1	2	3	4
10 My appetite has changed.	1	2	3	4
11 My weight has not changed much over the past couple months.	1	2	3	4
12 I feel like I have little control over much of what happens to me.	1	2	3	4
13 I have much to be angry about.	1	2	3	4

14 I don't feel like doing many of the things I used to enjoy.   1 2 3 4

15 I often feel guilty.   1 2 3 4

16 I feel like there are people in my life I can truly count on for support.   1 2 3 4

17 I'm under a lot of stress at this time.   1 2 3 4

18 I feel I'm lucky in life.   1 2 3 4

O *Addenda*

Is there any information *not* requested on this questionnaire that you think might be important or relevant to your case? If so, please use this space to give us your thoughts.

_____

_____

_____

_____

_____

_____

_____

_____

_____

_____

_____

_____

_____

P *Release of Information:*

May we release the information on this questionnaire to the referring physician and other physicians participating in your care?   YES / NO

If yes, please sign and date: _____

_____

APPENDIX B: PHYSICIAN INTERVIEW GUIDE

I   Purposes of Questionnaire
  A   The patient questionnaire is designed:
    1   To get basic information directly from patient and to make more efficient use of the physician's time.
    2   To serve as a guide to history and systems review.
    3   To screen for:
      a   somatization
      b   drug problems
      c   family problems
      d   work/compensation/financial disincentives for recovery
      e   pattern of health care overuse.
    4   To get graphic information on the time course and location of the pain.
    5   As a guide to the physical examination.
    6   To give the patient a chance to document his or her ideas about their pain.
  B   This separate physician-administered part is designed to supplement the patient questionnaire in those areas that may be sensitive for the patient. Obviously, more information will be obtained if a certain degree of rapport is established prior to asking the questions. Questions are in several categories listed below.
    1   *Events in history:* If the pain began with an injury, get the details. How did it happen? Where? Who was involved? Does patient hold someone responsible? Is there a long history of illness? Is patient angry at a certain physician? Does patient believe problem is iatrogenic?
    2   *Social situation*
      a   *Current family situation:* Inquire about marital adjustment; sexual adjustment, and frequency and comfort of intercourse. What is the impact of pain on relationships with family and/or close friends? Sexual or physical abuse by spouse?
      b   Death or painful disease in close friend or relative? If so, when did it occur in relation to patient's disease? Where was that person's pain? Relationship of that person to patient? Any reason for patient to feel guilty about that person's death or disease?
      c   *Employment:* If working now, are there problems? If not, were there problems? Is the patient angry toward former employer? What was the nature of the work? Job satisfaction level. Ever been fired?
      d   *Other aspects of life:* Satisfied with educational level? Disappointed in accomplishments?

  e *Childhood:* Relationship with parents. History of sexual or physical abuse. Any mental illness, depression, alcoholism, or suicide in family?

 3 *Evidence of mental illness in patient:* Psychiatric hospitalizations. Psychiatric care. Suicidal ideation or attempts. Frequent crying, persistent depressed mood? Treatment with antipsychotic or antidepressant medication?

 4 *Substance dependence*
  a Opiates, tranquilizers, analgesics: Effect on pain vs. mood. Schedule of taking medications (regular vs. sporadic). Need medications for sleep?
  b Alcohol use: Maximum. Does the patient drink more when anxious or when pain is worse? On weekends? Use it for sleep?
  c Tobacco: Current use. Lifetime.
  d Use of nonprescription drugs or street drugs.
  e Coffee, tea, or other stimulants.

 5 *Spouse interview:* Most prominent changes that the spouse has observed in the patient. How does spouse know when patient is in pain? Has patient been getting worse? What are the signs? How does patient's pain affect spouse? Social life. Income. Spouse's health?

II Special Points in the Physical Examination
 A *General Observations:* gait, guarding, facial expression, tearfulness, voice.
 B *Motor Exam:* muscle atrophy, weakness, loss of deep tendon reflexes.
 C *Sensory Exam:* sensory loss (light touch, temperature, stereognosis), allodynia, hyperalgesia, summation, spread of sensation,
 D *Myofascial Exam:* trigger points, limitation of range of motion.
 E *Sympathetic Function:* skin temperature, color, moisture.

APPENDIX C: DAILY PAIN AND
MEDICATION RECORD

Day _____   Date _____

	ACTIVITY (what you were doing)	MEDICATIONS (Name & Dose)	PAIN LEVEL (0–10)
11 pm | 2 am			
2 am | 5 am			
5 am | 8 am			
8 am | 11 am			
11 am | 2 pm			
2 pm | 5 pm			
5 pm | 8 pm			
8 pm | 11 pm			

Chapter 9

Analgesic Drugs

A primary goal of medical practice is to ease suffering. Ideally this is accomplished by accurate diagnosis and appropriate therapy leading to elimination of the cause of the patient's discomfort. However, many patients have significant pain despite the best available medical care. This occurs when the natural history of the disease includes a painful phase (e.g., passing a ureteral stone) or when there is a lag between the initiation of appropriate treatment and complete cure (e.g., bacterial pneumonia or meningitis). Sometimes the treatment itself is associated with severe pain (e.g., postoperative). In other circumstances there is a known somatic disease but the treatments available are inadequate (certain types of cancer or refractory arthritis). Finally, as discussed at length in Chapters 7 and 8, many patients have pain that is either of obscure origin or due primarily to psychosocial factors.

In these and other similar situations the physician is obligated to provide symptomatic relief. It should never be assumed that a patient's level of pain is tolerable. On the contrary, because most people do not seek medical attention for mild pains, all patients complaining of pain should be taken seriously unless there is good evidence that they are elaborating the complaint. No patient should be allowed to suffer any longer than is necessary for the physician to carry out an evaluation and decide on the best treatment. The strategy employed to provide the relief will depend on many factors, including the cause of the pain, its anticipated duration (and the patient's life expectancy), the general health of the patient, and his or her ability to comply with a given treatment.

At the present time most pain problems are managed with analgesic medications. It is thus important for everyone involved in direct patient care to have a good working knowledge of the properties of analgesic drugs. To this end, the present chapter will provide essential information on the most commonly used analgesics, the opiates, the nonsteroidal anti-inflammatory drugs, and acetaminophen. Chapter 10 will cover drugs that are not traditional analgesic agents but are commonly used to treat pain. I will briefly review in Chapter 11 the more specialized and controversial subject of the nonpharmacologic treatment of pain and, in Chapter 12, outline a general approach to the management of pain patients.

Opioid Analgesics

For at least 2500 years, preparations of the juice from the seed capsule of the opium poppy (*Papaver somniferum*) have been used to ease pain (8). In 1806, Serturner purified one of the constituent alkaloids and named it morphine, after Morpheus, the Greek god of dreams (18). Morphine subsequently became one of the most widely used drugs for the treatment of severe pain, and it remains the standard against which all other analgesic drugs are compared.

MORPHINE

Distribution, Absorption, and Metabolism (7, 18, 40)

Morphine is available clinically as the sulfate salt. In the bloodstream about one-third of it is bound to plasma proteins. Unbound morphine is predominantly ionized at physiological pH and it is very hydrophilic. It distributes rapidly to most of the body tissues. Although morphine crosses the blood-brain barrier relatively poorly, clinically effective levels in the brain can be achieved within a few minutes of an IV bolus (40).

Morphine is inactivated in the liver by glucuronidation and then eliminated by the kidney. The plasma half-life after an IV bolus injection is 2–3 hours. A significant fraction of the morphine absorbed from the gut after oral administration is inactivated on its first pass via the portal circulation to the liver. Thus, although morphine is well absorbed from the gut, it is significantly less potent when given orally. Compared to parenteral administration, a sixfold greater PO dose is required to produce the same level of analgesia (16). Furthermore, when morphine is given PO, the onset of analgesia is slower. The peak analgesic effect after PO administration is at about 90 minutes, compared to approximately 30 minutes for IV and 45 minutes for IM injection.

Mechanism of Morphine Analgesia

As discussed in Chapter 5, morphine acts in the central nervous system (CNS) to block the transmission of the nociceptive message. It activates pain-modulating neurons that project to the spinal cord and inhibit transmission from primary afferent nociceptors to dorsal horn sensory projection cells. Morphine also has a direct action on pain transmission at the spinal cord. Morphine analgesia depends upon a specific class of receptor (the mu opiate receptor), which is present in brainstem pain-modulating nuclei and in the spinal cord dorsal horn. The presence at these sites of opiate receptors and endogenous opioid peptides, plus the fact that local application of morphine produces analgesia, indicates that systemically administered morphine produces analgesia by mimicking the action of endogenous opioid peptides. The presence of a CNS pain-modulating circuit that can be selectively activated by opiates provides a compelling explanation for morphine's most striking and clinically important property: its ability to reduce pain with little impairment of other CNS functions (18). There are no other analgesic agents as selective as the opioids.

Because it acts in the CNS to block pain transmission, morphine produces effective analgesia for a broad range of painful conditions, provided a sufficient dose is given. In fact, short of regional or general anesthesia, morphine and its congeners are the most effective analgesics available. In theory, morphine should reduce the perceived intensity of all sensations that are generated by nociceptor activation of normal pain transmission pathways. Morphine might be less effective for pains associated with CNS lesions because such pains are not necessarily produced by normal activity in pain transmission pathways. For similar reasons, one might expect certain types of psychogenic pain to be resistant to morphine.

OTHER MORPHINE-LIKE DRUGS

There are numerous drugs in the morphine class (Table 9.1). They all produce analgesia by the same CNS mechanism (see Chapter 5), and all are effective for the treatment of a broad range of acute pain problems. Although they differ in potency—for example, 75 mg of meperidine (Demerol) produces about the same

Table 9.1   Opioids Commonly Used for Acute-Severe Pain (16, 18)

	Equianalgesic initial IM dose (mg)	Average duration of effect	Approx. oral/ parenteral ratio	Approx. plasma $t_{1/2}$ (hours)
Morphine	10	4.5	1/6	3
Meperidine (Demerol)	75	3	1/4	3.5
Hydromorphone (Dilaudid)	1.5	4.5	1/5	2.5
Methadone (Dolophine)	10	4.5[a]	1/2	24
Codeine	130	4.5	1/2	3
Levorphanol (Levodromoran)	2	4.5	1/2	14

[a]This may depend on the type of pain problem. A recent study indicates that a single dose of methadone can provide analgesia lasting 12–24 h (14).

average analgesic effect as 10 mg of morphine—all the drugs of this type have similar efficacy. In other words, at the highest doses tolerated, all of the drugs produce the same degree of pain relief. By the same token, if an adequate dose of one of these drugs does not work, it is unlikely that an equivalent dose of any of the others will provide relief.

In addition to having about the same analgesic efficacy, the morphine-like drugs all have a very similar pattern of side effects. Unfortunately, all produce nausea and vomiting, respiratory depression, sedation, constipation, and other side effects. Furthermore, they all have the potential to induce tolerance and dependence, and there is significant (although incomplete) cross-tolerance between them.

Meperidine (Demerol)

Meperidine is one of the most commonly prescribed opiate analgesic agents for hospitalized patients with moderate to severe pain. Although it is just as effective and has a somewhat faster onset of action than morphine, it is not clear why meperidine is such a popular drug. Its most distinctive feature is its relatively short duration of action. This can be a useful property if the anticipated duration of the pain is less than 2 hours. However, it can create serious problems for patients whose pain lasts longer because physicians commonly order it on a q3h or q4h schedule.

The principal metabolite of meperidine is normeperidine, which has a plasma half-life of over 14 hours. Normeperidine is a CNS excitant and can cause seizures. It is especially likely to accumulate in patients with renal failure (see Table 9.4, below).

Heroin

Despite the fact that heroin is not presently available for clinical use in the United States, it is worth discussing because its value in pain patients has been the subject of controversy. There has been some desire expressed to make it available, mainly because of its high solubility and potency and the rapid onset of its analgesic effect (30). In fact, on a milligram-per-milligram basis, heroin is a more potent analgesic agent than morphine. However, as discussed above, one can simply use a higher dose of morphine to achieve the same level of analgesia. Heroin does pass the blood-brain barrier more readily than morphine and this is probably a major reason for its more rapid onset of action.

Heroin appears to produce its analgesic effect indirectly. Current evidence indicates that it has no direct action at the opiate receptor. Following absorption, heroin is rapidly metabolized to 6-acetylmorphine and morphine, both of which have analgesic efficacy. Thus heroin is probably a pro-drug, whose analgesic effect is produced by its metabolites (11). Heroin is a potentially useful analgesic drug, and the arguments against its reintroduction are flimsy. However, since its properties are not that different from drugs that are already available, it is unlikely that more than a few patients would benefit if it were more widely available.

Methadone

When used parenterally in hospitalized patients, methadone is remarkably similar to morphine in terms of dose- and time-effect curve. It is curious that, despite methadone's very long plasma half-life, some studies have indicated that its analgesic effect is not significantly longer than that of morphine (but see ref. 14). Sedation and respiratory depression, however, may outlast the analgesia. Thus, if given acutely at the usual 4-hour interval, methadone can accumulate and place the patient at risk for sedation and respiratory depression.

Because of its high oral-to-parenteral ratio, methadone has been used extensively in situations where oral administration is desirable (e.g., cancer patients who may have severe pain but do not otherwise need to be hospitalized) (11). With careful adjustment of dose, methadone can be a useful alternative for ambulatory patients who have problems with other opiates (11, 14).

Table 9.2   CNS Actions of Morphine and Morphine-like Drugs

Analgesia

Mood changes

Nausea and vomiting

Sedation, mental clouding

Respiratory depression

Cough suppression

Pupillary constriction

SIDE EFFECTS OF MORPHINE
AND MORPHINE-LIKE DRUGS (18)

Central Nervous System Actions

Table 9.2 lists the major CNS effects of morphine and morphine-like drugs. Some of these actions limit their clinical usefulness as analgesic agents. For example, although many patients initially enjoy the euphoria and relaxation that accompany the pain relief, there are those who complain that they "aren't themselves" or "cannot think straight" and prefer the pain to the mental clouding.

Although the mental impairment produced by morphine is usually minimal, in some patients, especially those with severe pain who require higher doses for adequate relief, there may a significant degree of sedation. At higher doses, opiates produce profound obtundation. In fact, very high doses of morphine (e.g., above 1 mg/kg IV) are sometimes used for general anesthesia. Rapidly acting synthetic opioids such as fentanyl are particularly useful for this purpose (22).

Respiratory depression is a very prominent and consistent effect of morphine-like drugs. Even at typical analgesic doses (8–15 mg/70 kg) there may be some slowing of the respiratory rate. Morphine depresses respiration by reducing the brainstem respiratory center's sensitivity to CO_2. Because the respiratory centers retain their sensitivity to O_2, administration of O_2 without respiratory support may induce apnea. Although not usually a problem in healthy patients at typical analgesic doses, morphine-like drugs should be used with caution in patients with any form of respiratory compromise that has the potential to cause CO_2 retention.

Morphine acts directly on the medullary chemosensitive trigger zone to produce nausea and vomiting, the most common acute side effects of opioids. Input from the vestibular system exacerbates this problem, so that nausea and vomiting are more frequent among patients who are ambulatory. They are less common if the patients are recumbent and can be treated with a phenothiazine antiemetic

Table 9.3   Peripheral Actions of Morphine and Morphine-like Drugs

Decreased gastrointestinal tract motility

Increased biliary duct pressure

Pruritis

Histamine release

Urinary retention

(e.g., prochlorperazine (Compazine) or promethazine). Pretreatment with pro-chlorperazine 30 minutes before parenteral morphine is a reasonable approach to preventing this problem. Nausea and vomiting decrease with repeated adminis-tration of morphine, and patients usually do not need to be treated for them after the first day or two. There is no evidence that other opiates at equianalgesic doses are less likely to produce nausea than morphine.

Peripheral Actions

Table 9.3 lists some of the peripheral actions of morphine and morphine-like drugs. Prominent among these are effects on the gastrointestinal (GI) tract. Gut motility is slowed and sphincter tone is increased. These actions are primarily due to a direct effect on the intrinsic neurons of the GI tract; however, there is some evidence that decreased peristalsis can be produced by a direct action of morphine on the CNS (32). Because of these actions, opioids produce consti-pation in almost all patients with normal bowel function. Although not life threatening, this is a significant problem in patients who need them on a long-term basis. It should be anticipated in all patients and managed prophylactically with stool softeners and cathartics. On the other hand, one of the major thera-peutic indications for opioids is for patients with diarrhea. The synthetic com-pound diphenoxylate (Lomotil) is an example of an opioid used specifically for this purpose.

Morphine-like drugs should be used with caution in patients with acute abdominal pain. In addition to the slowing of gut motility, the increase in biliary tract pressure produced by opiates may lead to epigastric distress and biliary colic. This can create increased distress and diagnostic confusion in patients with abdominal pain.

THE THERAPEUTIC USE
OF MORPHINE-LIKE DRUGS

The guiding principle in the management of pain is that the physician should make the patient as comfortable as possible consistent with good medical judgment. If a sufficient dose is given, morphine-like drugs should relieve moderate to severe pain. When given parenterally, analgesia is rapid and reliable. Almost all patients will obtain significant relief. Although the relief obtained is often incomplete, most patients report that their pain has been reduced to a tolerable level. From a clinical standpoint, this may be preferred to complete analgesia because the patient is much more comfortable but can still report on the location of the pain and tenderness. Thus the diagnostic and prognostic value of the pain (i.e., its sensory aspects) seem to be at least partially preserved. This clinical impression is supported by experimental studies indicating that morphine produces a relatively greater reduction in the affective or unpleasantness aspect of pain than on its purely sensory component (36).

Once the decision has been made to use opioid analgesics it is critical that the patient be given an adequate dose. Because patients vary greatly in the amount of morphine they require for adequate analgesia, each individual should be carefully titrated to a level of drug that provides pain relief with minimal sedation. **The most common mistake that is made in treating acute pain with opioid analgesics is to order too small a dose.** The undertreatment of hospitalized patients with moderate to severe pain is an extremely common problem (27). A recent survey found that at least one-third of acute postoperative patients received inadequate doses of analgesic medications despite experiencing marked pain (5). Physicians tend to order too small a dose or to order it at intervals that are too long. When administration is made discretionary, nurses tend to give patients less than the maximum dose ordered. The problem stems from a lack of knowledge of the usual range of doses and an exaggerated fear that the patient will become addicted (5). In fact, addiction is *extremely* unusual in people who have been treated with opioids in a medical setting (35). Clearly, the administration of inadequate doses of opioids is an unnecessary cause of suffering that could easily be corrected.

To obtain rapid pain relief, start with a parenteral dose of 8–10 mg of morphine (or its equivalent). Then return to the patient at the time of the drug's expected peak effect (about 45 minutes after an IM injection). Ask specifically whether the medication has helped the pain and try to have the patient estimate the percent relief. By 45 minutes the patient should have significant (approximately 50 percent) relief. If the patient has not obtained significant relief and is alert, an additional 8-mg dose should be given.

This procedure should be repeated until a dose is achieved that either gives relief or produces excessive sedation. Because the analgesic effect of morphine increases as the log of dose, it is occasionally necessary to double the dose more than once to achieve relief. **The key to successful treatment is to ask the patient how much relief he or she obtained from the drug.** The only way to determine whether a sufficient dose of morphine has been given is by assessing the patient's response. If the physician cannot return to assess the drug effect, the orders should be written so that the nurse will return to the bedside at the time of the expected peak drug effect, ask the patient if he or she has had significant relief from the drug, and if not, give the patient additional morphine.

The other important step for optimal treatment of hospitalized patients with pain is to determine the duration of action of the drug being used. Because the duration of morphine analgesia is variable in different people and for different pain problems, the interval between doses must be adjusted for each individual. To do this, instruct the patient to call for the nurse as soon as he or she feels that the pain is returning. The interval between doses can then be adjusted so that future doses are given *before* the pain begins to increase. This procedure will minimize patient suffering and anxiety.

Tolerance and Route of Administration

There are a variety of morphine-like drugs used in the treatment of acute pain (16, 18, 39). Although the principles for optimal use are the same for all drugs in this class, certain patients may not tolerate one of the drugs (Table 9.4) or a particular route of administration. This becomes a major problem in patients with cancer, who are potentially ambulatory but who require high levels of opiates. In situations where repeated injections are not feasible, the physician should consider alternative routes of administration. Rectal suppository preparations may be of particular value in patients with nausea and vomiting. Furthermore, first pass elimination in the liver can be partially avoided by rectal administration. Morphine, hydromorphone, and oxymorphone are presently available in rectal suppository form. Morphine appears to be about equieffective when given PO and per rectum (9). Theoretically, hydromorphone (Dilaudid) should be more potent than morphine when given by the rectal route since it is more lipophilic.

The logical problems of morphine analgesia posed by the need for carefully timed nurse or doctor visits can be overcome by using one of several newly developed methods for analgesic drug delivery. The first of these is **patient-controlled analgesia** (PCA) (21). As the name indicates, the PCA apparatus delivers a preset dose of morphine through an indwelling IV line when the patient pushes a button. The apparatus is loaded with sufficient drug to cover the patient's needs for 12–24 hours. The device is usually programmed so that there is a minimum interval of 15–30 minutes between doses. Newer devices permit the physician to specify a maximum total dose per 4-hour period to prevent overmedication. Preliminary reports indicate that PCA devices are safe and reliable for patients with postoperative pain (11) and cancer pain (4). It is of interest that patients differ as much as four-fold in their self-maintained opioid plasma levels. PCA seems to be a remarkably efficient way to adjust the opioid dose precisely to the patient's needs. One hopes that these devices find widespread acceptance in the near future.

Table 9.4 Undesirable Drug or Disease Interactions of Narcotic-type Analgesics*

Drug	Interaction	Result
Meperidine	Cirrhosis	↑ Bioavailability and ↓ clearance = accumulation
Pentazocine	Cirrhosis	↑ Bioavailability and ↓ clearance = accumulation
Propoxyphene	Cirrhosis	↑ Bioavailability and ↓ clearance = accumulation
Meperidine	Renal failure	↑ Normeperidine, a toxic metabolite = accumulation
Propoxyphene	Renal failure	↑ Norpropoxyphene, a toxic metabolite = accumulation
Morphine	Older than 50 years	↓ Clearance = accumulation
Meperidine	Phenytoin	↑ Biotransformation = faster elimination
Methadone	Rifampin	↑ Biotransformation = faster elimination
Meperidine	Monoamine oxidase inhibitors	Excitation, hyperpyrexia, and convulsions
Any narcotic	Alcohol or other central nervous system depressants	Enhanced depressant effects

*Reprinted by permission from Inturrisi, C. E.: Role of opioid analgesics. *Am. J. Med.* **77(Suppl. 3A)**:33, 1984.

Another way to administer opioids is by **continuous infusion.** This can be done by the intravenous (33) or subcutaneous (43) route. Neither of these methods of administration should be used unless the more traditional approaches are not working. Continuous IV infusion is used in patients who require large doses of opioids and need to receive them at frequent intervals. This is a situation that applies primarily to cancer patients who are partially tolerant to opioids. The main advantage of the continuous IV infusion is that it allows one to avoid the very high peak plasma levels associated with bolus administration. Such high peak levels usually produce unwanted sedation. Continuous subcutaneous infusion has also been used in situations where parenteral drug is required but multiple injections are not feasible.

Opioids can be injected directly at the level of the spinal cord, either intrathecally or epidurally (3, 6). The advantage of direct **spinal administration** is that the analgesic effect is restricted to the region that is the source of the noxious input and that a lower total dose is required to produce the same degree of analgesia. Morphine is a particularly useful drug for intrathecal use because it is hydrophilic and thus very slowly absorbed from the cerebrospinal fluid (CSF). It is not unusual to observe up to 24 hours of analgesia following a single lumbar intrathecal dose (0.5–4 mg) of morphine. The bad news is that morphine slowly ascends to the brainstem in the CSF, placing patients at risk for delayed (7–12 hours) respiratory depression. This is a particular menace to patients with pulmonary disease. More lipophilic agents such as methadone, hydromorphone, and fentanyl produce a much briefer and more localized analgesic effect (3, 6).

Spinal administration of opioids is now an accepted procedure for the treatment of acute postoperative pain (3, 38). However, the technique should be used only by experienced personnel and only if the patient can be continuously monitored. Only preservative-free preparations should be injected intrathecally.

In addition to its usefulness in patients with acute pain, spinal infusion of opioids has been used for prolonged periods in patients with lower body cancer pain (31). Respiratory depression seems to be less of a problem with chronic use, but close observation is mandatory when initiating treatment or when changing drug or dose.

PROLONGED USE OF MORPHINE-LIKE DRUGS

One of the thorniest issues in the treatment of patients with pain is the advisability of prolonged use of opioid analgesics. The problem is a confused tangle of political, moral, psychological, and medical issues. Although there are many patients who are functional only because they are taking morphine-like drugs on a regular basis, others endure daily pain because either they or their doctor have serious reservations about the long-term use of potentially addicting drugs.

Morphine-like drugs are the most effective painkillers available and, with prolonged use, their major side effects (i.e., constipation and sedation) are mild. The use of these drugs in ambulatory patients with pain due to cancer is now well accepted; there is simply no justification for withholding adequate doses of opiates from cancer patients who need and can tolerate them. The controversy is mainly over whether to use morphine-like drugs in patients with persistent pain that is not associated with malignancy. Some view opioids as harmful for patients with chronic pain and advocate that patients be withdrawn from them as a prerequisite for successful treatment (15, 28). Others take a sharply opposing view, citing numerous patients with significant pain problems who are able to lead productive lives for years while being treated with stable doses of morphine-like drugs (34, 41).

There is some merit to both of these points of view. Although there is no doubt that some pain patients do well on long-term opioid treatment, in others the drugs are more of a problem than a help. Because patients with chronic benign (noncancer) pain are such a varied group, it is clearly inappropriate to generalize about the value of morphine-like drugs in their treatment. It is just as bad a mistake to deny morphine to a patient who has no better alternative as it is to ignore the fact that drug abuse is a major problem for some patients.

Tolerance, Dependence, Abuse, and Addiction

Tolerance When the magnitude of the biological action of a drug is reduced following repeated administration of a fixed dose, tolerance is said to have occurred. Another way to look at it is that larger and larger doses of the drug are required to produce the same magnitude of effect. Tolerance may develop at a different rate for each of a drug's biological actions. For morphine-like drugs, tolerance develops relatively rapidly for the respiratory depressant action and very slowly for pupillary constriction and inhibition of gut motility. For clinical analgesia, the time course of tolerance development is unpredictable. Frequently, the first manifestation of tolerance is that the duration of analgesia produced by a fixed dose of opioid shortens. Patients complain that their pain is beginning to return before their next scheduled dose.

The mechanism of tolerance is unknown. It could represent reduced absorption, increased metabolic degradation, a change in the opiate receptor, or a change in the neural networks that modulate pain transmission. Whatever the mechanism, there is cross-tolerance between all of the morphine-like analgesics. A patient tolerant to one will be at least partially tolerant to all.

Dependence Physical dependence refers to the situation in which removal of the drug creates discomfort for the patient beyond what can be accounted for by the return of pain. People who are physically dependent on morphine-like

Table 9.5   Opioid Abstinence Syndrome

Early-mild	Late-severe
Anxiety	Nausea and vomiting
Drug requests	Diarrhea
Lacrimation	Fever
Yawning	Abdominal pain
Piloerection	Hypertension
Rhinorrhea	Tachycardia
Dilated pupils	Leukocytosis
Anorexia	Insomnia
Tremor	

drugs experience a characteristic abstinence syndrome when the drugs are stopped or when an antagonist is given (Table 9.5). The abstinence syndrome varies from mild to severe depending on the pharmacokinetics of the drug, the amount the patient has been taking, and how abruptly the drug is stopped. Slowly tapering the dose (by 20 percent every 3 or 4 days) will prevent the full-blown abstinence syndrome. Clonidine can also be used to ameliorate the symptoms of opioid withdrawal (39).

Abuse and Addiction   We live in a society in which the use of certain drugs for enjoyment is acceptable. Caffeine and ethanol are accepted by the majority as fairly harmless when used in moderation. Occasional use of amphetamines and minor tranquilizers, although somewhat less widely accepted, rarely meets with strong disapproval. Habitual use of certain other drugs (e.g., marijuana, cocaine), although acceptable to some people, is avoided by others who think they are dangerous. Clearly, there is a gray area of drug use that some consider valid recreational use and that others consider drug abuse. Beyond this gray area, there is general agreement on the signs that indicate that the "recreational" use of drugs has become incompatible with normal life: when the use of drugs impairs a person's ability to carry out his or her daily activities, when the acquisition of drugs becomes the major focus of a person's life, when loss of access to the drug causes significant disruption to the person's life, and when the need for money to buy drugs leads to illegal activity. The majority of people strongly disapprove of this level of drug use and most would consider that a person who is affected to this degree is a drug addict. Jaffe (17) defined addiction as "a behavioral pattern of drug use, characterized by overwhelming involvement with the use of a drug (compulsive use), the securing of its supply, and high tendency to relapse after withdrawal." How much of a problem is drug abuse in patients with chronic pain complaints?

The very definition of drug abuse is at issue when one attempts to apply it to chronic pain patients. There are some patients who have a history of frequent "recreational" drug or alcohol use that antedates their contact with the medical profession. These patients have learned that the complaint of pain is a way to assure themselves a relatively cheap, legal, and reliable supply of opioids, anxiolytics, and/or barbiturates. Some of these "patients" may even sell their legally obtained drugs on the street. Such patients have a drug abuse problem that requires a specialized treatment program. In other cases, the problem may have begun with a pain of somatic origin but at some point the pleasant effect of the drug rather than its pain-relieving action became the major reason for the patient's pain complaint (see Chapter 7). Technically, these people are not drug abusers. However, the drug-taking behavior complicates the evaluation of their pain complaint. In these cases, opioid withdrawal may be very useful if carried out in the setting of a behaviorally oriented treatment program.

Although there is no question that drug abuse is a potential risk factor for the use of opioid analgesics in patients with chronic non-malignant pain, it is not clear how big a risk it is for them. There are actually very few data on the incidence of drug abuse following opioid exposure in chronic pain patients.

Perhaps the most relevant data on the risk of abuse in "normal people" exposed to opioids come from surveys of Vietnam veterans (37). Twenty percent of all Vietnam veterans were psychologically dependent on opioid drugs while in Vietnam. However, of this group, less than 4 percent continued regular drug use after returning home. These data show that even people who use opioids regularly for pleasure can quit when the drugs are no longer freely available. In contrast to this relatively low risk of addiction in normal people following prolonged exposure to high-dose opioids, interviews with addicts suggest that 5–10 percent had their first exposure to opioids in a medical setting (17). Thus, although only a small percentage of people are at serious risk for opioid abuse, in those who are at risk, exposure in the medical setting can initiate a long-term problem.

Whether patients with chronic pain are like the normal population and thus at low risk for drug abuse or are a special high-risk subpopulation is still an open question. Part of the difficulty in resolving this question is that the judgment about whether a patient is abusing a drug depends on the point of view of the physician as well as the patient's behavior. For example, some treatment programs include termination of analgesic intake in their definition of success. Since they intentionally de-emphasize the patient's subjective judgments of pain they are less likely to see the value of using opioids. Consequently, they would tend to view any use of opioids as abuse. On the other hand, those who take the patient's pain complaint at face value might come to a different conclusion. If the patient says the medicine relieves his or her pain, it is an appropriate medical use of the drug and therefore, by definition, it is not drug abuse.

As mentioned above, there are several clinical reports of the use of opioids in patients with chronic non-malignant pain. The reports are anecdotal but they do show that some patients can be maintained for years on a stable low dose of opioids (equivalent to 20 mg or less of morphine, daily) (34). A significant number of the patients were able to lead apparently normal lives. Drug abuse did occur in a few patients, but there was some evidence that they had a pre-existing drug abuse problem. In conclusion, the weight of current evidence indicates that opioids can be helpful for selected patients with chronic non-malignant pain.

Guidelines for the Long-Term Use of Morphine-Like Drugs

At the present time, long-term treatment with opioid analgesics cannot be undertaken lightly. Although the drugs are safe at the usual doses needed for pain relief, there are three major problems. The first is the development of tolerance and subsequent escalation of dose. The second is the small but real risk of drug abuse by the patient. The third is the possibility of legal action by state agencies against a physician who prescribes controlled drugs inappropriately. These problems are unlikely to occur when good medical judgment is used. The guidelines recently published jointly by the California Medical Association and the California Board of Medical Quality Assurance (Appendix A) are very useful if a physician is in doubt about how to proceed with a given patient. Briefly discussed below is my approach to patients in this situation.

Evaluation   The first thing to do is a thorough evaluation of the patient, both medically and psychologically. If the patient has a clear-cut medical problem such as cancer or intractable arthritis, further diagnostic workup is not necessary. In other patients, I have found that the approach outlined in Chapter 8 is a useful screening procedure. Multidisciplinary evaluation of chronic pain patients should be carried out to determine whether the pain problem fits into a well-described syndrome, to decide if further diagnostic studies are indicated, and to suggest treatment strategies that have a higher benefit/risk ratio than chronic opioid use. Common sense dictates that patients should not be treated with opioids if they have a major psychiatric disturbance or a history of drug or alcohol abuse. Proper evaluation will obviate the need for long-term opioid treatment in many patients.

Treatments   An accurate record of the treatments tried in any given patient is an important part of the documentation needed to support the use of morphine-like drugs. Other types of potent drugs, behavioral methods, physical therapy, nerve blocks, transcutaneous electrical nerve stimulation, and biofeedback are among the approaches that can be used before instituting long-term opioid treatment (see Chapter 11). Documenting these treatments and their effect (or lack of effect) should be part of the evaluation of all pain patients.

Before instituting long-term opioid therapy, the patient should be informed that there is a small risk of psychological dependence. The signs of tolerance should be stated and it should be emphasized that the end point is adequate analgesia, not sedation or euphoria. Patients also should be informed about the drug's side effects and possible reactions, but the risks should not be overstated. Many patients already have an exaggerated fear of the consequences of taking morphine-like drugs. They are afraid that taking the drug will inevitably turn them into addicts with consequent loss of control over their own behavior. The physician can use this opportunity to reassure the patient that the use of opioids will not make him or her violent or prone to criminal action, and that their use is not incompatible with normal mental function. The point is for the patient to know what the risks and benefits are so that they can make an informed decision and not endure unnecessary pain.

It is very helpful to discuss with the patient what the goals of therapy are. Try to define some activities (household, work, recreation) that the patient can attempt with improved pain control. Inform the patient that complete relief from pain may not be possible but that it is often possible to bring the pain down to a level the patient can live with. Once this is understood, the drug should be titrated to a dose and interval that keeps the patient reasonably comfortable. After the optimal dosage schedule is established it should be recorded and the patient given a month's supply.

The physician should be prepared for an extended relationship with the patient because the problem may last for years. Having a single responsible physician is critical for successful long-term treatment (34). The patient should agree that there will only be one physician writing the prescription for the pain medication and that he or she will try to use no more than the amount prescribed each month. The physician should assure the patient that he or she will continue to write the prescription but only if the patient abides by the above conditions. Most patients will comply with this arrangement.

Patients should be re-evaluated periodically and an attempt made to lower their dose of opioid analgesic. If the pain returns when the dose is lowered, an alternate strategy is to add a nonopioid analgesic to the patient's drug regimen (see below). Adding a nonsteroidal anti-inflammatory agent, acetaminophen (see below), or tricyclic antidepressant (see Chapter 10) may permit the same level of analgesia to be maintained with a lower dose of the opioid.

In conclusion, morphine-like drugs are the most potent drugs available for the management of patients with severe pain resulting from ongoing tissue-damaging processes. They are most useful for patients with acute pain but, if necessary, they can also be used on a long-term basis in carefully selected patients.

Provided the patients have a clear-cut focal pain syndrome, no major psychiatric disturbance, and no previous history of drug abuse, I have rarely found drug abuse to be a problem.

Aspirin and Other Nonsteroidal Anti-inflammatory Drugs

Along with acetaminophen, aspirin and the other nonsteroidal anti-inflammatory drugs (NSAIDs) are by far the most commonly used analgesic drugs. Aspirin was introduced at the turn of the century and its use is currently very widespread. A recent survey found that over 60 percent of the adult population in the United States has used aspirin (42). The popularity of aspirin is well deserved because it is very effective for the mild to moderate headaches or musculoskeletal pains that are so common in everyday life. Furthermore, with occasional use at the doses required for pain relief (600–1200 mg), serious side effects are unusual. The NSAIDs are considered as a group with aspirin because they produce analgesia across a similar range of conditions, possibly by a similar mechanism.

MECHANISM OF ANALGESIA

In contrast to morphine-like drugs, which act at specific receptor sites in the CNS to block pain transmission, the aspirin-like compounds are thought to act primarily in the periphery (20, 26). As reviewed in Chapter 2, tissue damage initiates a complex set of events leading to activation of primary afferent nociceptors. In addition to direct activation of the nociceptor, tissue-damaging stimuli cause the release or synthesis of chemical mediators that can also activate or sensitize nociceptors. Many of the same compounds also play an important role in triggering other phenomena associated with inflammation (vasodilatation, edema, attraction of leucocytes, etc.). With the evolution of the inflammatory response there is further accumulation of substances that activate or sensitize nociceptors. Consequently, any treatment that reduces inflammation will *pari passu* reduce the accompanying pain.

One important process underlying inflammation is the breakdown of arachidonic acid to prostaglandins by the enzyme cyclooxygenase. Injection of prostaglandins can induce inflammation and directly sensitizes the terminals of primary afferent nociceptors. NSAIDS inhibit cyclooxygenase, which explains their anti-inflammatory effect and at least partially accounts for their analgesic action (10, 20). Accordingly, NSAIDS should be more effective for pains associated with peripheral tissue-damaging processes, particularly those that have a relatively greater inflammatory component.

Table 9.6   Pharmacologic Actions of Aspirin*

Low dose	High dose
Analgesia	Anti-inflammatory effect
Antipyresis	Erosion of gastric mucosa
Prolonged bleeding time	Tinnitus (ototoxicity)
Gastric irritation	Metabolic acidosis (children)
Nausea and vomiting	Stimulation of respiration

*Data from ref. 10.

THE PHARMACOLOGY OF ASPIRIN

Table 9.6 lists the common pharmacologic actions of aspirin. The analgesic and antipyretic effects and the prolongation of bleeding time are actions of therapeutic significance and can be produced by a single dose of aspirin. The other actions listed are generally unwanted side effects that are seen with high doses or with prolonged use.

Effect on Platelets   Even a low dose of aspirin (less than 100 mg) causes the irreversible acetylation of platelet cyclooxygenase. This blocks platelet aggregation and elevates bleeding time. It takes about 1 week for the platelets to regenerate, so aspirin should be stopped a week prior to any surgical procedure or blood donation. Aspirin is contraindicated in any patient with a bleeding or clotting abnormality.

Gastrointestinal Effects   From a practical standpoint, GI toxicity is the major limitation to the use of aspirin. Nausea and epigastric burning are very common, even with low doses. Aspirin has a direct destructive action on the gastric mucosa. In addition, by inhibiting prostaglandin synthesis, aspirin indirectly causes a decrease in mucus production and an increase in acid production, leading to further gastric irritation. The combination of gastric erosion and defective blood clotting makes GI hemorrhage the most dangerous risk to the long-term use of aspirin. Massive GI bleeding occurs in about 15 of 100,000 patients each year (19). The risk is greater in elderly patients.

The problem of gastric erosion can be largely obviated by the use of an enteric-coated form of aspirin (23). Therefore, an enteric-coated form should be considered in all patients when aspirin treatment of more than a few days is anticipated.

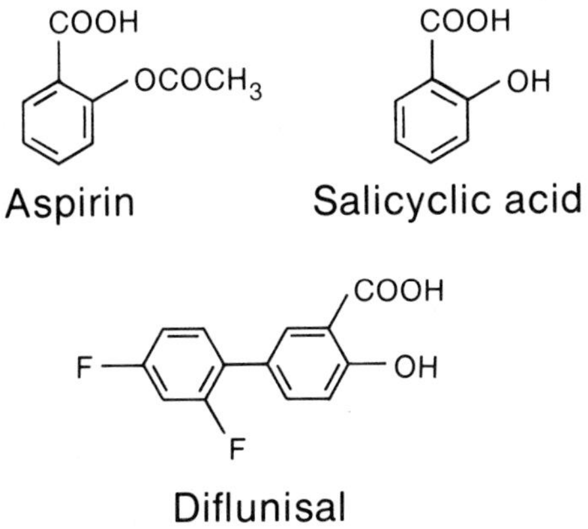

Aspirin   Salicyclic acid

Diflunisal

Figure 9.1 The salicylates.

Absorption, Distribution, and Metabolism

Aspirin is completely absorbed from the GI tract, reaching a peak plasma concentration in about 2 hours. The actual plasma concentration of aspirin is low because it is rapidly hydrolyzed to salicylic acid, 90 percent of which is bound to plasma protein (Figure 9.1). Salicylic acid is metabolized primarily in the liver to salicyluric acid, which is excreted by the kidneys (see ref. 10). When patients are given repeated high doses of aspirin, the metabolic pathways become saturated and the plasma salicylate half-life is greatly prolonged. Whereas the plasma half-life of salicylate following a single dose of aspirin is 2–3 hours, it is about 12 hours after a day or two at anti-inflammatory doses (4–6 g total daily dose).

Therapeutic Use of Aspirin for Analgesia

Because of its long record of safety and efficacy for common pains and its widespread use, aspirin has developed a reputation as a relatively weak analgesic agent that should be used primarily for mild to moderate pains. In fact, the aspirin-like drugs can relieve pains that are considered to be severe. Clinical studies indicate that, in addition to its accepted efficacy for such common problems as headache, osteoarthritis, and dysmenorrhea, aspirin can provide significant relief for postoperative, postpartum, and cancer pain (1, 20).

In adults, 650 mg every 4 hours is the usual starting dose. If this is not effective, the dose can be raised in 325 mg steps to 1300 mg every 4 hours. There is no good evidence that doses above this level confer an additional analgesic effect, although higher doses are often helpful in the treatment of rheumatic diseases (20). As the dose is raised, the incidence of side effects rises and

Table 9.7   Common Nonopioid Analgesic Agents*

Drug	Peak effect (hours)	Plasma $t_{1/2}$ (hours)	Average analgesic dose (mg)	Dose interval (hours)
Aspirin	2.0	4–6[a]	625	4–6
Diflunisal	2.5	10	500	10
Ibuprofen	1.5	3	400	4–6
Naproxen	3.0	12	250	12
Fenoprofen	2.0	2.5	200	4–6
Acetaminophen	1.0	2.0	500	3–5

*Data from refs. 1, 10, and 20.
[a]For active metabolite, salicylic acid.

the margin of safety diminishes. The major benefit of aspirin in long-term use is that it is significantly less expensive than any other drug in its class.

For those patients who do not tolerate long-term high-dose aspirin, or in whom there are contraindications, other peripherally acting drugs should be considered. In this situation, enteric-coated aspirin, diflunisal, acetaminophen, or one of the other NSAIDs should be considered.

DIFLUNISAL

In patients who have a good response to aspirin but cannot tolerate high doses, diflunisal (Dolobid) is a possible alternative. It is a salicylate (Figure 9.1) and has a range of actions and side effects similar to that of aspirin. As a result of strong protein binding, diflunisal has a significantly longer plasma half-life than salicylic acid (Table 9.7). Since it can be given q12h, patient compliance is likely to be better than with aspirin. In contrast to aspirin, diflunisal's action on cyclooxygenase is reversible so it does not irreversibly impair platelet aggregation. Thus the impairment of coagulation it produces is of shorter duration (48 hours) than that due to aspirin (about 1 week). Diflunisal also seems to have less of an erosive effect on the upper GI mucosa.

PROPIONIC ACID DERIVATIVES (1, 10, 20)

The propionic acid derivatives so far approved for analgesic use include ibuprofen (Motrin, Nuprin, Advil), naproxen (Naprosyn), and fenoprofen (Nalfon) (Figure 9.2). Except for aspirin, they are the most commonly used NSAIDs.

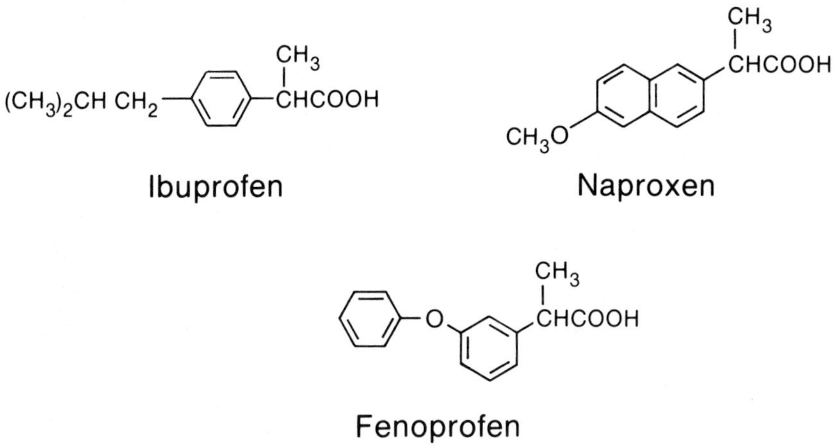

Figure 9.2 The proprionic acid derivatives.

Although they differ from each other in potency, absorption, and duration of action (Table 9.7), they have the same range of efficacy and side effects. All have been shown to provide relief for a wide variety of pains, especially those of musculoskeletal origin. They seem to be particularly effective for dysmenorrhea.

Like diflunisal, the inhibition of cyclooxygenase produced by the proprionic acid derivatives is reversible. Thus their inhibition of platelet function is short-lived compared to aspirin. Although GI irritation is the most common side effect (about 15 percent incidence), this does not occur as frequently as with aspirin. Gastric erosion is also less common and GI bleeding is rare. Although these drugs act by the same mechanism as aspirin and have the same range of therapeutic and toxic effects, they are safer than aspirin and are tolerated better by most patients. Their relative safety is indicated by the fact that ibuprofen was approved for over-the-counter sale.

The common analgesic doses for the proprionic acid derivatives are shown in Table 9.7. The doses required for optimal analgesia have not been established. As with all analgesics, the goal is to determine the minimum dose required for adequate patient comfort. This occasionally requires building up the dose to near toxicity.

OTHER NSAIDS

In the past two decades there has been an explosive growth of new NSAIDs introduced by the pharmaceutical industry. Almost all have the same basic mechanism of action (cyclooxyenase inhibition), and all seem to have the same range of pharmacologic actions. They differ primarily in their time-effect curves and their cost. As of this writing, none are available for parenteral administration in the United States. Although only the drugs discussed above and mefenamic acid (Ponstel) have FDA approval for use as analgesic agents, it is very likely that most, if not all NSAIDs have analgesic efficacy at doses lower than required for their anti-inflammatory action.

SUMMARY AND GENERAL CONSIDERATIONS

Aspirin and the other NSAIDs have a broad range of efficacy for the symptomatic treatment of pain. They all inhibit cyclooxygenase in peripheral tissues, thus interfering with the mechanism of transduction in primary afferent nociceptors. Although the NSAIDs are considered by many to be useful as analgesics only in patients with mild to moderate pain, they are often very effective for severe pain. How effective they are depends more on the mechanism of the pain than its severity. If there is a significant inflammatory component, NSAIDs can provide potent relief. The NSAIDs all have a similar range of actions and side effects, although aspirin by virtue of its direct erosive action on the gastric mucosa and its irreversible effect on platelets places patients at increased risk of GI symptoms and hemorrhage. All NSAIDs, including aspirin, can elicit an acute hypersensitivity reaction, with hives and respiratory distress. Individuals with a history of asthma and nasal polyps are at high risk (20).

   In contrast to opioid analgesics, which relieve pain to some extent in almost all patients, the NSAIDs often provide no relief, even when pushed to toxicity. It is not easy to predict which patients will respond to NSAIDs. Even in a group of patients with what appears to be the same painful condition, some will get good relief and others will not be helped at all (20). The reasons for this are not clear. The practical implication is that NSAIDs should be tried in any patient with identifiable tissue damage whose pain is expected to last for more than a day or two.

Acetaminophen

Next to aspirin, acetaminophen is the most commonly used analgesic agent (42). It is useful for the same types of pain as aspirin. It is widely used by the general public for self-treatment of headache and common musculoskeletal pains. It has a reputation for being a safe drug and many people prefer it because it produces less gastric irritation than aspirin.

   Although it shares antipyretic and analgesic efficacy with aspirin, it differs from aspirin and the other NSAIDs. It has only minimal anti-inflammatory action. Furthermore, its anti-inflammatory action is not due to inhibition of cyclooxygenase (13, 44). On the other hand, acetaminophen does inhibit brain cyclooxygenase. This has been proposed to account for its antipyretic action and possibly for its analgesic effect as well (10).

Acetaminophen is rapidly absorbed from the GI tract and reaches its peak plasma concentration in 30–60 minutes. Its plasma half-life is about 2 hours (Table 9.7). The major serious side effect is hepatic necrosis, which is dose dependent and is potentially fatal in an individual who ingests a single dose of 25 g or more.

At the usual analgesic doses, acetaminophen is well tolerated. In contrast to aspirin and the other NSAIDs, side effects are uncommon. If an anti-inflammatory effect is not important, acetaminophen should be tried before the NSAIDs. A typical analgesic dose is 500 mg q4h. The total daily dose should be kept under 4 g.

Combining Analgesic Drugs

The availability of several classes of drugs that produce analgesia by different mechanisms raises the possibility that combining them might produce a clinically beneficial effect. Using a single drug at its usual analgesic dose often provides unsatisfactory relief. The physician is then faced with the alternatives of raising the dose of that drug, changing to another drug, or adding a second drug. Although there is appropriate concern among many physicians about the routine use of drug combinations, there is good evidence that giving relatively low doses of two drugs can provide an adequate level of analgesia with fewer side effects than using one drug at a relatively high dose (2).

This potential benefit is less when the two drugs used have a similar mechanism of analgesia. For example, typical analgesic doses of two different NSAIDs would not be expected to bestow any greater benefit than increasing the dose of a single NSAID. There may be some additive effect when a lower dose of acetaminophen is combined with an NSAID, but this is not always seen (2). In contrast, combinations that include an effective dose of an opioid and either acetaminophen or an NSAID are significantly more effective than the same dose of either drug alone. Numerous clinical studies of patients with acute postoperative pain or cancer pain have consistently demonstrated an additive effect when the two different types of drugs are given together (2) (Figure 9.3).

When such combinations are used it is important to give the patient a dose of acetaminophen or NSAID that is in the effective range for analgesia (e.g., 625 mg aspirin or 500 mg acetaminophen). The opioid is then titrated to obtain the optimal balance between analgesia and side effects. Obviously, the common use of fixed-dose combination tablets (e.g., aspirin plus oxycodone (Percodan) or acetaminophen plus codeine) makes such individual adjustments of dose awk-

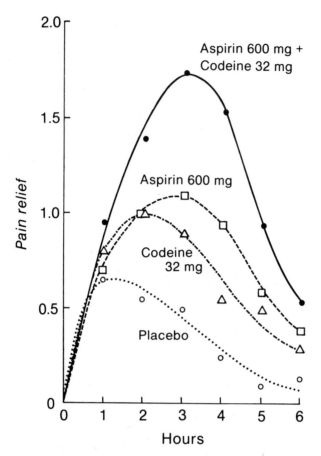

Figure 9.3 Additive analgesic effect of aspirin and codeine. Comparative time-effect curves for 600 mg aspirin, 32 mg codeine, and the two combined. (Adapted from ref. 2).

ward. On the other hand, once the appropriate dose of both drugs is determined, the combination tablets may make the patient's life simpler and improve compliance.

SEDATING DRUGS

There is a long history of combining standard analgesics with sedatives, anxiolytics, and major tranquilizers. The efficacy of such combinations is doubtful (2, 29). There is no question that patients with pain are anxious and have difficulty sleeping. They may feel more relaxed and sleep better with sedating drugs of any category, including barbiturates, benzodiazepines, and phenothiazines. Furthermore, sedating drugs produce a degree of muscle relaxation and may consequently relieve some patients who have a significant component of acute muscle spasm. However, despite the fact that these sedative-analgesic combinations provide relief for some patients, the rationale for their use is questionable. Muscle spasm, anxiety, and insomnia, although clearly related to pain, should be viewed as distinct problems. Treatment of several problems that may or may not exist by fixed-dose combination drugs is a shotgun approach. It is a poor substitute for the appropriate evaluation and treatment of each of the various problems of the pain patient.

MISCELLANEOUS ADJUVANT DRUGS

There are other drugs that have been shown to have analgesic efficacy in certain situations and to potentiate the analgesic action of opioids, NSAIDs, or acetaminophen. The antihistamines and tricyclic antidepressants are among them and will be discussed in the next chapter. The final group to be discussed in this chapter are the CNS stimulants.

Caffeine

Numerous clinical studies have indicated that caffeine significantly enhances the analgesic effect of both aspirin and acetaminophen. This enhancement occurs for a variety of patients including those with cancer, headache, and postoperative pain. A pooled analysis of published studies indicates that patients who receive at least 65 mg of caffeine require 40 percent less aspirin or acetaminophen for the same level of relief as patients not receiving caffeine (24). Most of the studies have only documented a short-term effect. However, since 65 mg of caffeine is relatively harmless, it may be useful to add it to the regimen of patients who are not obtaining adequate relief with acetaminophen or NSAIDs alone.

Amphetamines

The use of opioids for severe pain is often attended by significant sedation. The use of CNS stimulants is a logical way to overcome this problem. Forrest and his colleagues (12) examined this possibility in a multicenter study of 450 patients with postoperative pain. The results were quite dramatic: dextroamphetamine (10 mg) not only reversed the sedating effect of morphine, it markedly potentiated the analgesia. Ten milligrams of dextroamphetamine cut the median effective dose for morphine approximately in half. Thus at the same dose of morphine patients receiving dextroamphetamine were not only more alert, they were more comfortable. Although the benefit of this combination seems clear-cut, it should be stressed that the pain problem being treated was short-lived.

There is no evidence that amphetamine-opioid combinations are of value for long-term use.

The mechanism of amphetamine potentiation of opioid analgesia is unknown. Amphetamines stimulate the release of catecholamines in the CNS, and it is possible that they enhance analgesia by potentiating the action of the noradrenergic limb of the pain-modulating network (Chapter 5). Tricyclic antidepressants (Chapter 10), which enhance the action of CNS biogenic amines by blocking their reuptake, also potentiate morphine analgesia (25).

Summary

Despite the bewildering array of compounds and combinations of compounds used to treat pain patients, the principles of their use are straightforward. They involve careful observation and clinical judgment. Pain should not be treated before at least a tentative diagnosis and clear-cut goals of therapy are established. Whenever possible, a single drug should be used, at the lowest effective dose. The effective dose can only be determined by asking the patient how much relief was obtained and how long it lasted. For acute pain requiring parenteral therapy, opioids are the drugs of choice because of their rapid onset of action and their reliability. If side effects appear it should be possible to lower the dose by adding acetaminophen, an NSAID, or amphetamine.

Because of the potential problems of tolerance and abuse, opioids should be considered for long-term use only after therapeutic trials of single nonopioid drugs have shown them to be inadequate or poorly tolerated. If the decision is made to use opioids chronically, they should be initially tried in combination with either acetaminophen or an NSAID so that a lower dose of the opioid can be used. The nonopioid can be withdrawn if it does not add to the analgesic effect of the opioid. The majority of patients who need analgesic medication can be managed reasonably well using this approach.

References

1   Amadio, P., Jr.: Peripherally acting analgesics. *Am. J. Med.* **77(3A):**17–25, 1984.

2   Beaver, W. T.: Combination analgesics. *Am. J. Med.* **77(3A):**38–53, 1984.

3   Bromage, P. R.: Clinical aspects of intrathecal and epidural opiates. In H. L. Fields et al. (eds.), *Advances in Pain Research and Therapy, Vol. 9*. Raven Press, New York, 1985, pp. 733–748.

4   Citron, M. L., Johnston-Early, A., and Boyer, M.: Patient-controlled analgesia for severe cancer pain. *Arch. Intern. Med.* **146:**734–736, 1986.

5   Cohen, F. L.: Postsurgical pain relief: Patients' status and nurses' medication choices. *Pain* **9**:265–274, 1980.

6   Cousins, M. J., and Mather, L. E.: Intrathecal and epidural administration of opioids. *Anesthesiology* **61**:276–310, 1984.

7   Dahlstrom, B., Hedner, T., Mellstrand, T., Nordberg, G., Rawal, N., and Sjostrand, U.: Plasma and cerebrospinal fluid kinetics of morphine. In K. M. Foley and C. E. Inturrisi (eds.), *Advances in Pain Research and Therapy, Vol. 8.* Raven Press, New York, 1983, pp. 37–44.

8   Ellis, E. S.: *Ancient Anodynes.* William Heinemann, London, 1946.

9   Ellison, N. M., and Lewis, G. O.: Plasma concentrations following single doses of morphine sulfate in oral solution and rectal suppository. *Clin. Pharm.* **3**:614–617, 1984.

10 Flower, R. J., Moncada, S., and Vane, J. R.: Analgesic-antipyretics and the anti-inflammatory agents; drugs employed in the treatment of gout. In A. G. Gilman et al. (eds.), *The Pharmacological Basis of Therapeutics,* (7th ed.). MacMillan, New York, 1985.

11 Foley, K. M., and Inturrisi, C. E.: *Opioid Analgesics in the Management of Clinical Pain.* Raven Press, New York, 1986.

12 Forrest, W. H., Brown, B. W., Brown, C. R., Defalque, R., Gold, M., Gordon, H. E., James, K. E., Katz, J., Mahler, D. L., Schroff, P., and Teutsch, G.: Dextroamphetamine with morphine for the treatment of postoperative pain. *N. Engl. J. Med.* **296**:712–715, 1977.

13 Glenn, E. M., Bowman, B. J., and Rohloff, N. A.: Anti-inflammatory and PG inhibitory effects of phenacetin and acetaminophen. *Agents Actions* **6**:513–516, 1977.

14 Gourlay, G. K., Cherry, D. A., and Cousins, M. J.: A comparative study of the efficacy and pharmacokinetics of oral methadone and morphine in the treatment of severe pain in patients with cancer. *Pain* **25**:297–312, 1986.

15 Gildenberg, P. L., and DeVaul, R. A.: *The Chronic Pain Patient.* Karger, Basel, 1985.

16 Inturrisi, C. E.: Role of opioid analgesics. *Am. J. Med.* **77(Suppl. 3A)**:27–36, 1984.

17 Jaffe, J. H.: Drug addiction and drug abuse. In A. G. Gilman et al. (eds.), *The Pharmacological Basis of Therapeutics* (7th ed.). Macmillan, New York, 1985, pp. 532–581.

18   Jaffe, J. H., and Martin, W. R.: Opioid analgesics and antagonists. In A. G. Gilman et al. (eds.), *The Pharmacological Basis of Therapeutics* (7th ed.). Macmillan, New York, 1985, pp. 491–531.

19   Jick, H.: Effects of aspirin and acetaminophen in gastrointestinal hemorrhage. *Arch. Intern. Med.* **141:**316–321, 1981.

20   Kantor, T. G.: Peripherally-acting analgesics. In M. Kuhar and G. Pasternak (eds.), *Analgesics: Neurochemical, Behavioral and Clinical Perspectives.* Raven Press, New York, 1984.

21   Keeri-Szanto, M.: Drugs or drums: What relieves postoperative pain? *Pain* **6:**217–230, 1979.

22   Kitihata, L. M., and Collins, J. G.: *Narcotic Analgesics in Anesthesiology.* Williams & Wilkins, Baltimore, 1982.

23   Lanza, F. L., Royer, G. L., and Nelson, R. S.: Endoscopic evaluation of the effects of aspirin, buffered aspirin, and enteric-coated aspirin on gastric and duodenal mucosa. *N. Engl. J. Med.* **303:**136–138, 1980.

24   Laska, E. M., Sunshine, A., Mueller, F., Elvers, W. B., Siegel, C., and Rubin, A.: Caffeine as an analgesic adjuvant. *JAMA* **251:**1711–1718, 1984.

25   Levine, J. D., Gordon, N. C., Smith, R., and McBryde, R.: Desipramine enhances opiate postoperative analgesia. *Pain* **27:**45–50, 1986.

26   Lim, R. K. S., Guzman, F., Rodgers, D. W., Goto, K., Braun, C., Dickerson, G. D., and Engle, R. J.: Site of action of narcotic and non-narcotic analgesics determined by blocking bradykinin-evoked visceral pain. *Arch. Int. Pharmacodyn.* **152:**25–58, 1964.

27   Marks, R. M., and Sachar, E. J.: Undertreatment of medical inpatients with narcotic analgesics. *Ann. Intern. Med.* **78:**173–181, 1973.

28   Maruta, T., Swanson, D. W., and Finlayson, R. E.: Drug abuse and dependency in patients with chronic pain. *Mayo Clin. Proc.* **54:**241–244, 1979.

29   Moertel, C. G., Ahmann, D. L., Taylor, W. F., and Schwartau, N.: Relief of pain by oral medications. *JAMA* **229:**55–59, 1974.

30   Mondzac, A. M.: In defense of the reintroduction of heroin into American medical practice and H.R. 5290—The Compassionate Pain Relief Act. *N. Engl. J. Med.* **311:**532–535, 1984.

31   Moulin, D. E., and Coyle, N.: Spinal opioid analgesics and local anesthetics in the management of chronic cancer pain. *J. Pain Sympt. Manag.* **1:**79–86, 1986.

32 Porreca, F., and Burks, T. F.: The spinal cord as a site of opioid effects on gastrointestinal transit in the mouse. *J. Pharmacol. Exp. Ther.* **227:**22–27, 1983.

33 Portenoy, R. K., Moulin, D. E., Rogers, A. G., Inturrisi, C. E., and Foley, K. M.: Intravenous infusion of opioids in cancer-related pain: Review of cases and guidelines for use. In K. M. Foley and C. E. Inturrisi (eds.), *Opioid Analgesics in the Management of Clinical Pain.* Raven Press, New York, 1986, pp. 413–424.

34 Portenoy, R. K., and Foley, K. M.: Chronic use of opioid analgesics in non-malignant pain: Report of 38 cases. *Pain* **25:**171–186, 1986.

35 Porter, J., and Jick, H.: Addiction rare in patients treated with narcotics. *N. Engl. J. Med.* **302:**123, 1980.

36 Price, D. D., Von der Gruen, A., Miller, J., Rafii, A., and Price, C.: A psychophysical analysis of morphine analgesia. *Pain* **22:**261–269, 1985.

37 Robins, L. N., Davis, D. H., and Goodwin, D. W.: Drug use by U.S. Army enlisted men in Vietnam: A follow-up on their return home. *Am. J. Epidemiol.* **99:**235–249, 1974.

38 Stenseth, R., Sellevoid, O., and Breivik, H.: Epidural morphine for postoperative pain: Experience with 1085 patients. *Acta Anaesthesiol. Scand.* **29:**148–156, 1985.

39 Stimmel, B.: *Pain, Analgesia and Addiction. The Pharmacologic Treatment of Pain.* Raven Press, New York, 1983.

40 Swerdlow, M.: General analgesics used in pain relief: Pharmacology. *Br. J. Anaesth.* **39:**699–712, 1967.

41 Taub, A.: Opioid analgesics in the treatment of chronic intractable pain of non-neoplastic origin. In L. M. Kitihata and J. D. Collins (eds.), *Narcotic Analgesics in Anesthesiology.* Williams & Wilkins, Baltimore, 1982, pp. 199–208.

42 Taylor, H., and Curran, N. M.: *The Nuprin Pain Report.* Louis Harris & Assoc., New York, 1985.

43 Ventafridda, V., Spoldi, E., Caraceni, A., Tamburini, M., and De Conno, F.: The importance of continuous subcutaneous morphine administration for cancer pain control. *The Pain Clinic* **1:**47–55, 1986.

44 Vinegar, R., Truax, J. F., and Selph, J. L.: Quantitative comparison of the analgesic and anti-inflammatory activities of aspirin, phenacetin and acetaminophen in rodents. *Eur. J. Pharm.* **37:**23–30, 1976.

Appendix A: Guidelines for Prescribing Controlled Substances for Chronic Conditions—A Joint Statement by the BMQA and the CMA*

The California Medical Association [CMA] and the Board of Medical Quality Assurance [BMQA] believe that the best medical care occurs within the context of the physician-patient relationship, where the treating physician is familiar with the details of the patient's condition, medical history and life circumstances. That knowledge of the patient's individual circumstances makes the physician the most appropriate person to make clinical interpretations and treatment decisions, including the decision of whether to prescribe medications. Prescribing drugs, particularly controlled substances, requires the thoughtful application of clinical judgment. In the practice of medicine, physicians are often confronted with difficult situations—particularly in the treatment of chronic conditions involving pain, insomnia, anxiety or depression—that require carefully balanced judgment as to whether, when and where prescription of controlled substances is appropriate.

In our view, the best protection for the physician against allegations of inappropriate prescribing lies in the physician's knowledge of and close adherence to the existing standards of appropriate prescribing. Similarly, the best protection for the patient against the development of avoidable drug dependence is adherence to these same standards.

It is important to recognize that the standard for treatment of an **acute** clinical condition is quite different from the standard for treatment of a **chronic** condition. These guidelines discuss treatment and on-going care of chronic conditions.

Guidelines

When used within the context of a comprehensive treatment plan, the pharmaceuticals now available for pain, insomnia, anxiety and depression are safe and effective therapeutic agents and can safely be used for treatment of a chronic condition when these guidelines are followed.

1 History and Medical Examination A diagnostic examination must be performed and a medical history taken—appropriate for the clinical circumstances—sufficient to establish diagnosis, allow the formulation of a treatment

*Reprinted by permission from Department of Consumer Affairs Action Report Board of Medical Quality Assurance **29:** 5–6, 1985.

plan and rule out presence of any contraindications to the use of any medication contemplated.

2   Diagnosis/Medical Indication   A working diagnosis should be delineated including the presence of a recognized and accepted medical indication for the continued prescription of controlled substances. The quantity and strength of a controlled substance prescribed must be reasonably necessary and must meet the patient's needs. When the decision is being made whether to use medication, consideration should be given to avoiding, wherever possible, overutilization of controlled substances and minimizing iatrogenic dependence problems.

3   Written Treatment Plan with Recorded Measurable Objectives   A written treatment plan should be prepared to include clearly stated measurable objectives, further planned diagnostic evaluation and alternative treatments contemplated. When the decision has been made to use medication, the physician should record the expected dosing schedules and the expected duration of treatment with medications.

4   Informed Consent   There should be a discussion with the patient of the risks and benefits of the treatments contemplated. When the treatment includes a controlled substance, there should be discussion of the addiction potential, possible adverse reactions to the drug, likely therapeutic end points, and the risks and benefits of this drug as compared with other drugs and other treatment methods. The discussions should be recorded in the patient record.

5   Periodic Reviews and Modification as Indicated   Periodically, the physician should review all aspects of the patient's treatment plan in light of response to treatment and progress toward treatment goals. The physician should consider the effect of any new information which has developed during the course of treatment.

For patients who have not improved despite continuation of controlled substances, the physician should consider (and document) the appropriateness of a new trial of less dangerous treatment.

During these periodic reviews, the physician should

- assess and record the patient's response to treatment, both specific target signs and symptoms;
- assess and record compliance with the medication schedule;
- evaluate the patient for clinical or laboratory evidence of toxicity or adverse reactions to treatment, including the development of tolerance or psychological or physical dependence.

Adequate monitoring includes communication with pharmacists, nurses and other health professionals in an effort to assure that the patient is adhering to the intended treatment plan and that prescribed controlled substances are not being diverted or abused. After such a review, the physician should make any modifications indicated.

6   Consultation   In situations where treatment is not producing the desired improvement or where medication is required on an on-going basis, and other modalities are inappropriate or have failed, the physician should obtain appropriate consultation and/or refer the patient to specialists in the clinical problem area.

In geographic areas where specialists are not available, the independent opinion of any other physician with experience with this clinical condition would be helpful in ensuring (and documenting) appropriate care.

Consultation reports should be made a part of the patient's medical record.

7   Records   The physician should keep accurate and complete records documenting dates and clinical findings for all evaluations, consultations, treatments, medications, and patient instructions. The failure to maintain entries which fully disclose the type, extent and basis for therapy is one of the major factors in physician liability. In a situation where a physician decides on an approach which departs from customary practice, documentation justifying such a course of treatment is a critical prerequisite to continuing treatment.

In addition to following a comprehensive treatment plan based on these guidelines, the physician should incorporate two elements into his/her professional practices: 1) being watchful for any indications of manipulation or illegal conduct by the patient, and 2) staying abreast of current medical information pertinent to the treatment of chronic conditions.

1   Patient Manipulation   The physician should be alert to the possibility of manipulation (which can be either consciously or unconsciously motivated) by the drug-seeking patient and ready to withhold potentially harmful treatments from a patient who fails to cooperate with prudent treatment recommendations. Physicians should never accept as a rationale for prescribing controlled substances the argument that, if the physician refuses to prescribe, the patient will buy drugs from the street or obtain them from another physician.

In cases where a manipulative patient refuses to cooperate with the physician's treatment plan, the physician should take the appropriate steps to refuse to continue treatment. (See "Basic Legal Principles: Discontinuing Treatment with the Problem Patient.") At that point referral to a specialty program is generally the most appropriate course of action.

2   Current Information   The physician should keep current on new developments, approaches, and recommendations in prescribing. The physician should select continuing medical education activities which address his/her clinical practice. The physician should use the opportunities for informal consultation which are provided by contact with colleagues at hospital medical staff meetings and county medical society and specialty society meetings.

Conclusion

This document reiterates the principles of good medical practice which guide physicians in the treatment of all patients. When the treatment is for a chronic condition, these principles take on additional significance for the protection of both the patient and the physician.

Basic Legal Principles: Discontinuing Treatment with the Problem Patient

Physicians are not required to continue treatment of a patient who is uncooperative, refuses to follow treatment advice and/or presents difficulties in the doctor-patient relationship. A patient has no legal right to force a physician to continue a particular course of treatment.

Three overriding legal obligations, however, must be meticulously honored when discharging the potential problem patient. These are the obligations to provide for continuity of patient care; to inform and make the patient aware of the consequences of following or *not* following the recommended treatment; and to give reasonable notice of intent to discontinue treatment.

Six areas of physician conduct should be emphasized:

1 Medical Review The physician should review with the patient his medical history and treatment progress leading to his current medical condition. Where a problem patient is involved, emphasis should be placed upon compliance problems and the adverse medical implications of the patient's past lack of cooperation.

2 Recommend A proposed course of treatment should be proposed to the patient explaining how the particular treatment plan presents the most acceptable approach to dealing with the patient's current medical condition.

3 Warn/Inform The patient must be informed and warned about not only the risk of proposed treatment and available alternatives, if any, but the risks of *not* following the treatment plan and/or discontinuing treatment. The physician must make the patient aware of all material risks which may result if a patient refuses or discontinues treatment.

4 Continuity The physician should offer to implement the chosen treatment plan. If the patient refuses, he should be provided with a list of names and addresses of area physicians qualified to deal with the patient's unique needs. An offer to assist the patient by consulting with any new physician should be made. Where the patient has become chemically dependent, needed medications should be prescribed only for a time period reasonably necessary to allow for the establishment of a new doctor-patient relationship.

5 Confirm with Patient Where the medical risks associated with discontinuance of treatment are significant, the physician should confirm all of the above procedural steps by registered mail to the patient. This is an excellent way of documenting the "reasonable notice" requirements imposed by California law.

6 Documentation Thorough documentation of the performance of all relevant procedural steps must appear in the physician's records. This is particularly true where the chemically dependent or high risk patient is involved.

Chapter 10

Anticonvulsants, Psychotropics, and Antihistaminergic Drugs in Pain Management

Analgesic drugs are thought to act by one of three mechanisms: by interfering with nociceptive transduction in the peripheral tissues, by directly inhibiting pain transmission at central synapses, or by enhancing the action of pain modulating systems. The drugs to be discussed in this chapter, although useful in the treatment of certain painful conditions, have not traditionally been classified as analgesic drugs. To be classified as an analgesic, a drug should have demonstrated antinociceptive action in animal models of pain. In addition, clinically, it ought to relieve pain caused by a variety of different diseases. Opiates and nonsteroidal anti-inflammatory drugs clearly fulfill these criteria, but the evidence is less clear for the anticonvulsants and the psychotropic drugs discussed below.

The usefulness of anticonvulsants, for example, has only been established for the treatment of neuropathic pains such as trigeminal neuralgia that have a paroxysmal component. It may be that, in such cases rather than acting as analgesics, the drugs are actually ameliorating the pathophysiological abnormality

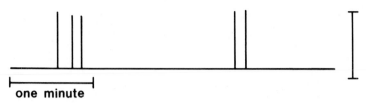

one minute

Flashing, Shooting, Stabbing, Paroxysmal

Figure 10.1 Time course and descriptive terms for lancinating pains. The pains are very brief, about 1 second or less, and often occur in clusters.

that produces the pain. Thus the drugs would not be expected to be useful in managing other types of pain. In contrast, the antidepressant drugs are effective for subacute or chronic pain caused by a variety of diseases such as arthritis and headache as well as certain neuropathic conditions like postherpetic neuralgia. These drugs may actually have a general analgesic action that is distinct from that of the opiates or nonsteroidal anti-inflammatory drugs.

Anticonvulsants

Trigeminal neuralgia is the most common painful condition for which anticonvulsants are effective. For epilepsy, the most commonly used anticonvulsant drug is phenytoin. Shortly after phenytoin was established as an effective and relatively nonsedating antisesizure medication, it was found to be useful in the treatment of trigeminal neuralgia (5). Following the report of Iannone et al. (25) confirming phenytoin's efficacy, it came into widespread use for this condition. In 1962, carbamazepine was reported to be useful for patients with trigeminal neuralgia, and it was subsequently found to be more effective than phenytoin for this condition (6). Trigeminal neuralgia has also been reported to respond to other anticonvulsant drugs such as clonazepam (36).

The syndrome of trigeminal neuralgia is very distinct. It occurs in an older population (mean age about 50) and consists of intermittent clusters of momentary electric shock–like stabs of pain (Figure 10.1). The pain is restricted to one side of the face, usually in the maxillary or mandibular division of the trigeminal nerve. The patients characteristically have trigger points where light touch will cause pain. Eating and talking may be extremely painful. The sensory examination is otherwise unremarkable. The pain may remit spontaneously for months or even years, during which time there is no obvious sensory disturbance. A similar condition occurs in the sensory distribution of the glossopharyngeal nerve. Other syndromes and locations for lancinating neuropathic pain are uncommon; however, they do occur and they respond to anticonvulsants.

The efficacy of anticonvulsants for lancinating neuropathic pain syndromes

Table 10.1   Conditions Responsive to Anticonvulsants

Trigeminal neuralgia

Glossopharyngeal neuralgia

Tabetic lightning pains

Paroxysmal pains of multiple sclerosis

Miscellaneous lancinating pains
  Postlaminectomy
  Postamputation
  Postherpetic neuralgia

Diabetic neuropathy

is indicated by Table 10.1, which lists conditions that consistently respond to anticonvulsants (11, 12, 14, 50). All of the listed conditions involve nerve damage as a prominent feature and, in all, a lancinating or shooting component is present. Even diabetic neuropathy, which is characteristically steady and burning, has been reported to have a "shooting" component in a large percentage of cases (46). A very provocative report along these lines is that from Swerdlow and Cundill (54), who reported their clinical experience treating 170 patients with "lancinating" pain. Although the study was uncontrolled, the observations are relevant to this discussion. The pains were due to a wide variety of causes. Only three patients had trigeminal neuralgia. The one common feature, other than nerve damage, was the lancinating nature of the pain. These authors used four anticonvulsants: phenytoin, carbamazepine, clonazepam, and valproic acid. Although clonazepam seemed to be the most consistently effective drug, each of the drugs seemed to be helpful in a significant number of patients.

It is unlikely that we will understand how anticonvulsants relieve pain until we know the mechanism of the lancinating neuropathic pains that respond to them. Trigeminal neuralgia is the most common of these syndromes, and because of its characteristic temporal pattern and location it presents no diagnostic problem. The momentary duration of the pain, its occurrence in clusters, and the fact that it can be elicited by peripheral stimulation of a trigger point make it different from most other neuropathic pain.

There is no agreement about the pathology of trigeminal neuralgia, but in a small number of cases it is caused by tumors of the cerebellopontine angle, and it has also been seen in patients with multiple sclerosis. It has been observed that the majority of trigeminal neuralgia patients have tortuous blood vessels that abut part of the trigeminal nerve or ganglion (26). Placing a small pledget between the artery and the nerve usually provides immediate and long-lasting relief (27). Relief may also be obtained by lesions of the sensory root of the trigeminal nerve. These clinical observations indicate that the neural activity giving rise to the pain of trigeminal neuralgia arises in the periphery and that compression and/ or demyelination of the nerve are predisposing factors. As discussed in Chapter 6, demyelinated patches of primary afferent axons become loci of ectopic impulse generation (58). Furthermore, damaged primary afferents develop ectopic sites of increased mechanical sensitivity and impulse generation both at the site of damage and near the dorsal root ganglion. Kerr (29) has proposed that demyelinated regions of the trigeminal nerve are sites of ephaptic spread and that pain triggered from the periphery is due to the short circuiting of impulses from non-nociceptive to nociceptive afferents at the site of damage (see Figure 6.5). According to this theory, spontaneous pains would be due to mechanical stimulation of the nerve or ganglion, possibly by the pulsating vessel (29).

Whether or not ephaptic spread is involved, it seems likely that trigeminal neuralgia involves ectopic impulse generation. In animal studies, anticonvulsant drugs have been shown to reduce discharge from sites of ectopic impulse generation in damaged nerve (63). This would be an attractive explanation for anticonvulsant pain relief because it would explain the clinical observation that these drugs are only effective for lancinating pain associated with nerve damage.

In summary, clinical observations have established that anticonvulsants are effective for the treatment of lancinating pains associated with nerve damage. Furthermore, it appears that any drug with anticonvulsant action is likely to be helpful for such conditions. Their efficacy for other types of pains is questionable, although there is some evidence that nonlancinating neuropathic pains may respond (36). Animal studies suggest that the anticonvulsants are specifically valuable for neuropathic pains because they suppress ectopic sites of impulse generation that develop in damaged peripheral nerve.

TREATMENT OF LANCINATING NEUROPATHIC PAINS

At the present time, carbamazepine is the first-line drug for the treatment of lancinating neuropathic pain. Because of individual variations in absorption and metabolism of carbamazepine and the fact that signs of toxicity appear near the upper range of plasma concentrations required for control of pain, it is very important to carefully adjust the dose when initiating long-term therapy. Therapy is begun with a dose of 100 mg twice daily. The dose should be increased by 100 mg per day until relief is obtained or signs of toxicity appear. For most patients relief is obtained at plasma concentrations between 5 and 10 μg/ml and side effects usually appear at levels above 8 μg/ml (56). In a given patient there is a very sharp threshold for the plasma level required to obtain relief. For example, in one patient a plasma level of 5.6 μg/ml gave no relief, whereas a level of 6.4 μ/ml gave complete relief.

The most common dose-related side effects are sedation, ataxia, vertigo,

Table 10.2   Anticonvulsants Used in Pain Management

	Plasma half-life (hours)	Therapeutic plasma concentration	Dose range
Carbamazepine	10–20	4–10 µg/ml	100–600 mg bid
Phenytoin*	6–24	10–15 µg/ml	200–400 qhs
Clonazepam*	18–30	5–70 ng/ml	0.5–6 mg tid

*Available as injectable drug.

and blurred vision. These subside somewhat with continued use and are another reason to build the dose gradually. Nausea and vomiting are also common. A mild leukopenia occurs in about 10 percent of patients and persists in 24 percent. In rare cases there is irreversible aplastic anemia. Regular monitoring of hematologic function is recommended. Because of these side effects and the fact that trigeminal neuralgia undergoes spontaneous remissions, it is probably worthwhile tapering the drug after 3 to 6 months and then reinstituting therapy if the pain returns.

The anticonvulsants most commonly used for pain are listed in Table 10.2 with their therapeutic plasma levels. Except for carbamazepine, these levels have been established for epilepsy control. In the case of carbamazepine, the range of plasma levels required for therapy of trigeminal neuralgia and epilepsy are the same. There is no reason to think that this is not the case for the other anticonvulsants. Readers are referred to Rall and Schleifer (43) for a detailed account of the pharmacology of anticonvulsants.

Although for long-term treatment of trigeminal neuralgia phenytoin is not as effective as carbamazepine, phenytoin is available for parenteral administration. This can be useful in patients who are having severe and frequent attacks. In such patients, intravenous administration of phenytoin often provides immediate relief. For intravenous administration, phenytoin should be diluted by half in normal saline immediately before use and injected in boluses of 50 mg or less each minute, to a total dose of 600–1000 mg.

Because the benzodiazepines have few side effects other than sedation, clonazepam should be considered as an alternative drug for lancinating neuropathic pain, especially in patients who require plasma levels of phenytoin or carbamazepam in the toxic range to obtain pain relief.

Baclofen is another drug that has been shown to be effective for the treatment of trigeminal neuralgia (15). Baclofen is a γ-aminobutyric acid analog that has been used in the treatment of spasticity, and shares some therapeutic actions with the benzodiazepines. Baclofen is of some interest since it is the only drug shown to be effective for trigeminal neuralgia that is not known to be an anticonvulsant drug.

Tertiary Amines

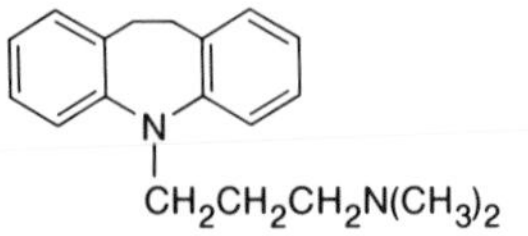

CH$_2$CH$_2$CH$_2$N(CH$_3$)$_2$ CHCH$_2$CH$_2$N(CH$_3$)$_2$ CHCH$_2$CH$_2$N(CH$_3$)$_2$

Imipramine 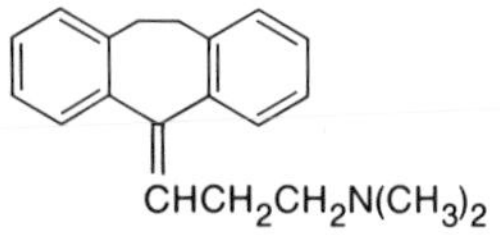   Amitriptyline 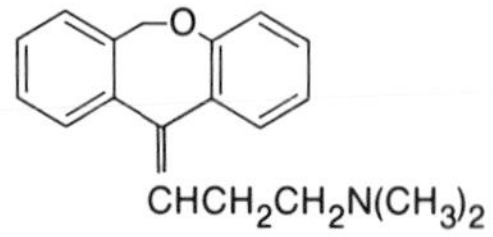   Doxepin

Secondary Amines

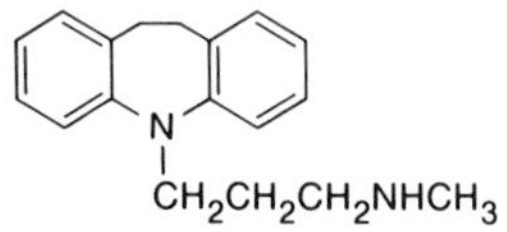

CH$_2$CH$_2$CH$_2$NHCH$_3$ CHCH$_2$CH$_2$NHCH$_3$

Desipramine 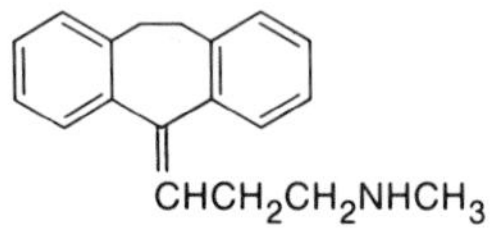   Nortriptyline

Atypical Antidepressant

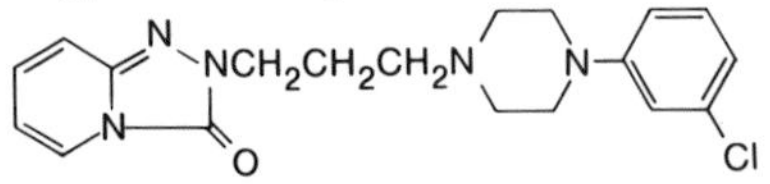

Trazodone

Figure 10.2   Structures of common antidepressants. The tertiary amines, imipramine and amitriptyline are demethylated in the body to desipramine and nortriptyline, respectively.

In summary, anticonvulsant drugs are dramatically effective for neuropathic pains that have a lancinating component. Trigeminal neuralgia is the most common pain of this type and carbamazepine is the drug of choice. Other anticonvulsants, including phenytoin and clonazepam, are also effective in this condition. A variety of other conditions associated with nerve damage and lancinating pain also respond to anticonvulsants. It is unclear whether any nonlancinating pains respond to anticonvulsants. The mechanism of anticonvulsant pain relief is unknown, but it seems likely to involve limitation of the generation of impulses at ectopic sites on primary afferents.

Antidepressants

In the past two decades tricyclic antidepressants have assumed an important role in the treatment of patients with pain (Figure 10.2). In contrast to the anticonvulsants, which are effective primarily for neuropathic pain with a lancinating component, clinical studies indicate that tricyclics are useful for patients having

Table 10.3 Painful Conditions that Respond to Tricyclic Antidepressants

Postherpetic neuralgia**

Diabetic neuropathy**

Tension headache**

Migraine headache**

Rheumatoid arthritis*

Chronic low back pain*

Cancer

*Controlled studies indicate benefit but not analgesia.
**Controlled trials demonstrate analgesia.

a variety of painful diseases. Tricyclics have come into widespread use for several reasons. In the doses necessary for pain control, toxicity is rarely a problem. Furthermore, although there are usually unpleasant side effects such as dry mouth, constipation, and dizziness, most patients tolerate them quite well. Imipramine and amitriptyline (Figure 10.2) are quite sedating; however, because chronic pain patients often have insomnia, the sedation may be helpful. In fact, the drugs are usually given at bedtime, both to induce sleep and to minimize daytime drowsiness. Finally and perhaps most important, since the drugs do not produce euphoria and tolerance does not develop with long term use, abuse is not a problem.

Table 10.3 lists the conditions for which there is reasonably good clinical evidence that tricyclic antidepressants (imipramine or amitriptyline) are beneficial. Controlled therapeutic trials have indicated a beneficial effect of tricyclics for postherpetic neuralgia (60), diabetic neuropathy (20, 32, 57), arthritis (23, 49) and both migraine (8, 19) and tension (9, 33) headache. There are a number of reports of success using tricyclic antidepressants to treat cancer pain; however, they were uncontrolled studies (30, 59). Tricyclics have also been used in the treatment of low back pain. Although a significant effect on the severity of low back pain has not been demonstrated, there are two controlled studies that indicate that there is some benefit from antidepressants in this condition. One found a reduced analgesic intake among patients while taking amitriptyline (42), and the other demonstrated an increase in activity and ability to work while taking imipramine (1).

The following case report is an example of a patient's response to the pain-relieving action of antidepressants:

Mrs. S., a 46-year-old shorthand typist, had generalized osteoarthrosis for thirteen years with pain mostly in hips and hands. She had become easily tired; otherwise no other comments on her home or her work. There was increasing pain in her hands in spite of phenylbutazone, 100 mg. four times a day, and paracetamol, 3 g. or more daily. Clinically there was little systematic upset. Radiological signs of osteoarthrosis were present in the hips and in the hands: proximal interphalangeal and distal interphalangeal joints. On trial during the first three weeks there was a dramatic and marked improvement in pain which began about four days after starting the new pills. Subsequently, during the second three weeks, there was a slow deterioration with return of pain. On final interview, this lady, always cheerful previously, suddenly burst into tears, stating that she had not realized how worried she had been and how upsetting it was to feel better for the first time in three years, and then to feel worse again.

On checking the code, it was noted that imipramine had been the drug in the first three weeks and the placebo in the second three weeks. During the following two months she has been maintained with imipramine hydrochloride, 25 mg. thrice daily, with a return of virtual freedom from pain and improvement in morale. (49)

This case is typical of many patients who obtain significant pain relief from tricyclic antidepressants. The rapid response and relatively low dose of imipramine required for dramatic relief makes it unlikely that the pain relief was secondary to resolution of the patient's depression. However, this cannot be ruled out with certainty.

Although the clinical response to tricyclics is often dramatic, most patients obtain only partial relief and some patients do not respond at all, even at relatively high doses. In fact, there are controlled clinical studies that have failed to demonstrate a significant benefit of tricyclics in rheumatoid arthritis (21) and diabetic neuropathy (38). Nonetheless, the weight of current clinical evidence and my own experience indicates that amitriptyline and imipramine are useful for patients with a broad range of chronic painful conditions (2, 24, 30, 36, 59).

This broad range of analgesic efficacy in well-defined diseases suggests that tricyclic antidepressants have a general analgesic action. This possibility is supported by animal studies (reviewed below) demonstrating an antinociceptive effect of tricyclics, either alone or in combination with opiates. However, the clinical studies that demonstrate tricyclic efficacy are largely limited to chronic conditions that are characteristically associated with depression (see Chapter 7). In such cases, it is not always clear whether the depression is reactive or primary. Furthermore, if the depression and pain are both relieved it is difficult to know whether the relief of depression is secondary to an analgesic effect or, as some have suggested, the pain is a "depressive equivalent" and disappears because the tricyclics relieve depression (57).

This question has been addressed clinically using quantitative scales for rating depression in patients with postherpetic neuralgia. In this condition, Watson and his colleagues (60) were able to show that amitriptyline produces significant pain relief without a significant antidepressant effect. Of the 23 patients in their study, 14 were not measurably depressed, and, of these 14, 11 obtained good pain relief. This suggests that the pain relief was not secondary to a clini-

Table 10.4   Tricyclics Used in Pain and Depression Management

	Maintenance dose (mg)	Plasma level (μg/L)		Time to Respond
		Imipramine	Amitriptyline	
Pain	75	150	70	4–5 days
Depression	150	100–300	60–220	2–3 weeks

cally measurable improvement in depression. In a subsequent uncontrolled study of patients with postherpetic neuralgia (61) amitriptyline was compared to zimelidine, a newer antidepressant with a somewhat different range of pharmacologic properties. Only patients receiving amitriptyline obtained pain relief. Furthermore, in three patients who were rated as significantly depressed, the depression improved while on zimelidine but there was no effect on their pain. This study supports the idea that the analgesic effect of amitriptyline is independent of its antidepressant action.

Further support for this concept comes from studies of the dose, plasma concentration, and time course of the analgesic effect of imipramine and amitriptyline (Table 10.4) (3, 17). It seems quite clear that the usual effective dose for tricyclics in pain management is at the lower end of the range required for effective treatment of depression. For painful conditions, daily doses of 75 mg or less of amitriptyline or imipramine are sufficient. Interestingly, there is some evidence for a ceiling effect of amitriptyline in the treatment of postherpetic neuralgia. For some patients the pain was *exacerbated* by amitriptyline at doses above 100 mg per day (60). In contrast, a clinical response in depression usually requires a dose above 125 mg for either amitriptyline or imipramine (3). The effective plasma levels reflect this, those required for pain relief being at the lower end of the range for management of depression. Finally, the response time for relief in painful conditions seems to be more rapid than for depression. Patients usually have significant relief within 4–5 days of reaching an effective dose.

Table 10.5 lists the commonly used antidepressant drugs. Of these, only imipramine and amitriptyline have been shown to be effective analgesics in controlled clinical trials. However, there is no reason to believe that the other listed drugs would not be effective.

A POSSIBLE MECHANISM FOR THE ANALGESIA PRODUCED BY TRICYCLIC ANTIDEPRESSANTS

In addition to the clinical evidence that they produce analgesia, experiments using animal models of acute pain have consistently demonstrated an antinociceptive effect of tricyclic antidepressants (35, 44, 48). This antinociceptive ef-

Table 10.5   Commonly Used Antidepressant Drugs

	Injection form available	Usual daily dose (mg)	Extreme range (mg)
✗ Amitriptyline HCl (Elavil)	*	75–150	40–300
✗ ✚ Desipramine HCl (Norpramin, Pertofrane)		75–200	25–300
Doxepin HCl (Adapin, Sinequan)		75–150	25–300
✗ Imipramine HCl (Janimine, Tofranil)	*	50–200	30–300
✗ Nortriptyline HCl (Aventyl, Pamelor)		75–100	20–150
Trazodone HCl (Desyrel)		150–200	50–600

fect is apparently due to an action on the central nervous system because injection of very low doses of tricyclics directly into the brain inhibits nociceptive responses (51).

One of the most prominent pharmacologic actions of the tricyclics is inhibition of the uptake of biogenic amine neurotransmitters into nerve terminals. Since reuptake into the terminal from which they are released is the major mechanism for terminat'ng the action of biogenic amine transmitters, inhibiting uptake increases their concentration and their duration of action at the synapse (Figure 10.3). As outlined in Chapter 5, both serotonergic and noradrenergic neurons in the brainstem project to and inhibit nociceptive transmission cells in the spinal cord. The presence of these biogenic amine links in the pain-modulating circuit raises the possibility that the tricyclic antidepressants produce analgesia by enhancing the inhibitory action of serotonin and noradrenalin upon spinal pain transmission neurons.

Experimental studies are consistent with this hypothesis. Tricyclics administered systemically (35, 44) or intrathecally at the spinal level enhance the antinociceptive action of morphine given systemically (7, 55). This effect is blocked either by depletion of biogenic amines or by spinally administered biogenic amine antagonists (7, 55). Presumably, the morphine activates brainstem biogenic amine neurons projecting to the spinal cord and the tricyclics potentiate the action of the released biogenic amine transmitters (Figure 10.3). Both serotonin and noradrenaline are apparently involved, because antagonists of either transmitter partially block the antinociceptive action of the tricyclics (55).

Studies with other drugs are also consistent with the idea that enhancing the synaptic action of biogenic amines leads to analgesia. Cocaine, which blocks biogenic amine reuptake but is not known to be an effective antidepressant (3), has analgesic efficacy. Phenelzine, a monoamine oxidase inhibitor, enhances the

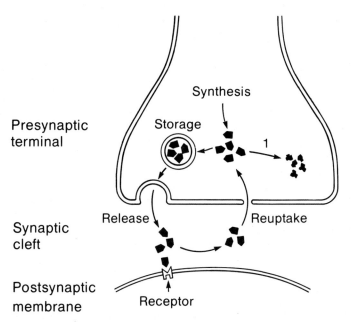

Figure 10.3 Typical biogenic amine synaptic terminal. Transmitters, including serotonin and norepinephrine, are synthesized in the presynaptic terminal and stored in vesicles. When the terminal is depolarized, the vesicle fuses with the terminal membrane and releases transmitter into the synaptic cleft, where it combines with receptor on the postsynaptic membrane to produce the biological action. The action of the transmitter is terminated mainly by its being removed from the synaptic cleft by reuptake into the presynaptic terminal. Tricyclic antidepressants block this step.

After reuptake, the transmitter is either taken back into vesicles for storage and rerelease, or is metabolically degraded (*1*), by monamine oxidase (MAO) inhibitors. MAO inhibitors may also have some analgesic action.

synaptic action of the biogenic amines, not by blocking reuptake but by slowing their catabolism. Phenelzine has analgesic potency in animal models of acute pain (35). Iprindole, an "atypical" tricyclic that is an effective antidepressant but produces very little reuptake blockage (45), does not potentiate morphine analgesia (7). This latter observation suggests that the antidepressant and analgesic actions of the tricyclic drugs have different mechanisms and that the analgesia is due to reuptake blockade.

In summary, both clinical and experimental evidence indicates that tricyclic antidepressants have an analgesic action that is distinct from their effect on depression. They are effective for a broad range of painful conditions and appear to ameliorate pain whether or not the patients are clinically depressed. The tricyclics relieve pain at lower doses, at lower plasma levels, and in a shorter period of time than required to produce a remission of endogenous depression. Current evidence is consistent with the hypothesis that antidepressants relieve pain by blocking biogenic amine reuptake and thus enhancing the action of serotonin and noradrenalin released by pain-modulating neurons.

CLINICAL USE OF ANTIDEPRESSANTS IN PAIN MANAGEMENT

Imipramine and amitriptyline have very similar dose ranges, plasma half-lives, side effects, and toxicity (Table 10.4). There are no data to indicate a preference for one or the other. It is best to start with a very low dose, especially in patients over the age of 60. With amitriptyline, an initial dose of 10 mg is reasonable. The dose should be increased by 10 mg every other day. The gradual build up of the dose minimizes side effects and avoids the possibility of giving a dose that is above what is needed (and possibly too high, if there is a window effect). Since they have a long plasma half-life, imipramine and amitriptyline can be given in a single daily dose. Because the drugs are sedating they are best given at bedtime. This sedating effect is actually a desirable feature for many patients whose pain is frequently most severe at night and causes insomnia. The dose should be increased until the patient reports maximum pain relief or the side effects are intolerable. In some cases doses in the analgesic range are ineffective. In such cases, the dose should be built up into the antidepressant range (150 mg/day or greater). It is probably also worthwhile to continue the drug for at least a month at high doses (i.e., to use the drug as an antidepressant), in case depression is a major factor. Sometimes patients will improve in their mood and say that they feel much better even though their pain is no less severe. In such cases, one can retrospectively assume that it was the depression that responded.

Side effects are extremely common, even at the low doses required for pain relief. In fact, the lack of side effects should raise the possibility of noncompliance and would be an indication to obtain plasma levels of the drug. The most common side effects are apparently due to the anticholinergic actions of the drugs. These are dry mouth, orthostatic hypotension, constipation, and urinary retention. More serious are the cardiac side effects, which are due to depression of excitability, an especially threatening problem for patients with preexisting conduction defects. One of the newer antidepressant drugs, trazodone (Desyrel), (Figure 9.2) produces significantly fewer anticholinergic and cardiac side effects; however, its efficacy as an analgesic is unknown.

The most important concern with regard to the tricyclics is that an overdose can be fatal (3). It is important that the patient's emotional status be assessed thoroughly before instituting tricyclic medication. If there is any indication that the patient is suffering from Major Depression, no more than 1000 mg of imipramine or amitriptyline should be dispensed. [See Baldessarini (3) for a discussion of the treatment of tricyclic overdose.]

Despite these problems, the tricyclics are extremely useful for a variety of chronic pain patients. Because they are nonaddicting and do not lose their effectiveness over time, they are preferable to opiates for long-term use. Furthermore, they are helpful for conditions such as painful neuropathies that do not respond to nonsteroidal anti-inflammatory agents, the other major class of drugs commonly used for the management of chronic pain. It is possible that combinations of tricyclics with other analgesics will be useful (see Chapter 9). Experimental studies show a facilitating interaction with opiates

Major and Minor Tranquilizers

The phenothiazines do not have a well-established place in the management of pain. The clinical evidence for the analgesic efficacy of this class of drugs is controversial at best. Despite this, their use, especially in combination with opiates or tricyclics, is not uncommon.

The most extensive study of this problem examined patients with perioperative pain (10, 40). Of nine different phenothiazines administered by intramuscular injection five were consistently beneficial: promazine, trimeprazine, methotrimeprazine, triflupromazine, and propiomazine. However, in subsequent studies only methotrimeprazine has been confirmed as an effective analgesic, either by itself or in combination with other drugs (37). Methotrimeprazine (Levoprome) has a broad range of efficacy, including postoperative pain, cancer pain, and chronic pain of various causes. To my knowledge it has only been shown to be effective when given by parenteral injection. The most extensive experience with methotrimeprazine is in the treatment of postoperative pain, for which 10 mg of methotrimeprazine was found to be equianalgesic to 10 mg of morphine sulfate by subcutaneous injection (34).

Methotrimeprazine has the usual phenothiazine side effects, including sedation, hypotension, and extrapyramidal syndromes. At the present time it can only be recommended for hospitalized patients with acute pain if there are compelling reasons to avoid opiates.

In addition to the studies reviewed above there are isolated reports of phenothiazine efficacy for certain chronic painful conditions. Chlorprothixene has been reported to be effective for the treatment of pain in postherpetic neuralgia (13, 41), and other phenothiazines have been used, mostly in combination with tricyclics, for a variety of chronic pains including diabetic neuropathy and postherpetic neuralgia (see refs. 24 and 36 for reviews). At the present time, however, the use of phenothiazines for the treatment of pain remains controversial and, because of prominent side effects, they should be reserved for selected individuals when more established therapies have not been helpful. Even the common practice of using phenothiazines such as promethazine (Phenergan) as routine adjunctive therapy with narcotics either to promote sedation or prevent vomiting is not of proven value and may even be harmful (37).

BENZODIAZEPINES

Although frequently used in situations that are acutely painful, there is no convincing evidence to support an analgesic effect for the benzodiazepines. Benzodiazepines have little or no effect on perceived pain intensity, but do alter the unpleasantness of the painful situation (22). They are used routinely as preoperative medication and there is no question that many painful procedures that do not require general anesthesia are made less stressful and consequently easier by the use of benzodiazepines at doses causing moderate sedation. Because of the relatively high safety margin between effective and toxic doses, their use as an adjunct to opiates in the acute pain situation is reasonable. However, their use for chronic pain is questionable. Many patients become dependent on benzodiazepines and undergo withdrawal when therapy is terminated.

As mentioned at the beginning of this chapter, the benzodiazepine clonazepam has demonstrated anticonvulsant action and is useful for lancinating neuropathic pains. It may be that the other benzodiazepines would also be useful in such conditions. Diazepam, for example, does have anticonvulsant efficacy and would be a reasonable drug to try. In addition, benzodiazepines are useful in the treatment of spasticity and may have some muscle relaxant action. In cases where pain is associated with either spasticity (e.g., spinal cord injury) or muscle spasm secondary to acute injury these drugs may be of help.

Antihistamines

Another class of drugs that has some analgesic potency is the antihistamines. Although the therapeutic indications for the use of this class of drugs are not well defined, clinical trials have shown that they are effective, either alone or in combination with standard analgesics, across a broad range of painful conditions.

Table 10.6 lists the conditions that have been shown to respond to antihistamines. The two antihistamines that have been most thoroughly evaluated with respect to their analgesic action are orphenadrine and hydroxyzine. Orphenadrine has been used primarily for the treatment of mild to moderate musculoskeletal pain (18, 47) and there is evidence that it is effective for postoperative pain (39, 62). The usual dose of orphenadrine is 50 mg by mouth up to four times daily.

Table 10.6   Painful Conditions Responding to Antihistamines

Condition	Drug (reference)	Dose and route
Headache	Phenyltoloxamine (16)*	60 mg PO
Low back pain	Orphenadrine (18)**	50 mg PO
Postoperative pain	Orphenadrine (39, 62)	50 mg PO
	Hydroxyzine (4)†	50–150 mg IM
Cancer pain	Hydroxyzine (52)	100 mg IM

Adapted from Rumore, M. M., and Schlichting, D. A.: Clinical efficacy of antihistamines as analgesics. *Pain* **25**:7–22, 1986.
In these products: *Percogesic, sinubid, poly-histine-D. **Norflex, norgesic, disipal, myotrol. †In these products: Vistaril, atarax.

It seems to be more consistently effective when given in combination with standard analgesic medications (47).

Hydroxyzine is in widespread use as an adjuvant for operative anesthesia. When administered by intramuscular injection (50–100 mg), it is quite effective for cancer pain (52) and for postoperative pain (4). It has an additive effect when given with 8 mg of morphine (Figure 10.4). It is of interest that hydroxyzine has little effect on this type of pain when given by mouth (28).

Despite the fairly extensive clinical literature documenting that several different antihistamines have analgesic effects over a range of painful conditions, there is very little understanding of how they work. Not all antihistamines have been shown to have analgesic potency. Furthermore, the critical studies relating analgesic potency to affinity of histamine receptor binding for a series of these compounds has not yet been carried out. Thus it must be kept in mind that these drugs may produce analgesia by an action unrelated to histamine antagonism.

Antihistamines were originally introduced for pain treatment because of their sedative and muscle-relaxing actions. These actions are fairly nonspecific and there is no direct evidence linking the sedation and muscle relaxation to the analgesia. It is not even clear whether antihistamine analgesia is due to an action on the CNS or an action in the peripheral tissues. Although there are histamine-containing neurons in the CNS, it is not known whether they are involved in pain transmission. As outlined in Chapter 2, histamine has an important role in peripheral nociceptive mechanisms. Animal studies, although supporting the analgesic efficacy of antihistamines (53), have not resolved the issue of whether they act in the periphery, the CNS, or both sites.

One very important study of experimental headache has related histamine antagonism to pain relief in human subjects. Krabbe and Olesen (31) confirmed that histamine could provoke and maintain throbbing headaches in patients who had a history of migraine. In a group of such patients, the headache was main-

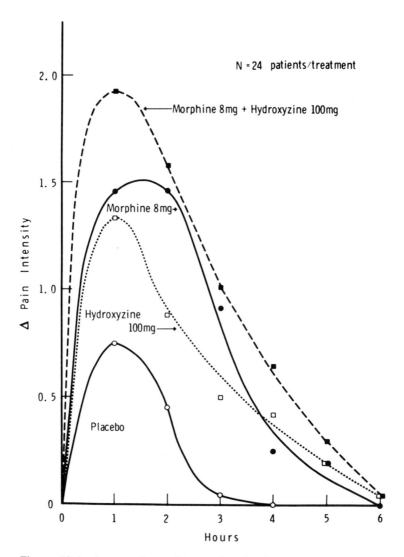

Figure 10.4 A comparison of the analgesic efficacy of hydroxyzine, morphine, and the combination. These are time-effect curves using a pain intensity difference scale to assess relief in patients with acute postoperative pain. (From Beaver, W. J., and Feise, G.: Comparison of the analgesic effect of morphine, hydroxyzine and their combination in patients with postoperative pain. *Adv. Pain Res. Ther.* **1:**553–557, 1976.)

tained by continuous infusion of histamine. During the histamine infusion, injection of the antihistamine mepyramine relieved the pain. Another antihistamine, cimetidine, was also effective. This study indicates that histamine can reproduce a clinically significant pain syndrome and that antihistamines can relieve the pain, presumably by blocking histamine's action.

In summary, the available evidence supports the notion that antihistamines have an analgesic action over a broad range of clinical conditions. At the present time, hydroxyzine appears to be a second-line parenteral drug in patients for whom narcotics would be appropriate but undesirable or contraindicated. Orphenadrine and other antihistamines may have some effectiveness in this situation and may also be of use on a subacute or chronic basis for mild to moderate pain of musculoskeletal origin.

References

1   Alcoff, J., Jones, E., Rust, P., and Newman, R.: Controlled trial of imipramine for chronic low back pain. *J. Family Pract.* **14:**841–846, 1982.

2   Atkinson, J. H., Jr., Kremer, E. F., and Garfin, S. R.: Psychopharmacological agents in the treatment of pain. *J. Bone Joint Surg.* **67:**337–342, 1985.

3   Baldessarini, R. J.: Drugs and the treatment of psychiatric disorders. In A. G. Gilman et al. (Eds.): *The Pharmacological Basis of Therapeutics* (7th ed.), Chapt. 19. Macmillan, New York, 1985.

4   Beaver, W. J., and Feise, G.: Comparison of the analgesic effect of morphine, hydroxyzine and their combination in patients with postoperative pain. *Adv. Pain Res. Ther.* **1:**553–557, 1976.

5   Bergouignan, M.: Successful cure of essential facial neuralgias by sodium diphenylhydantoinate. *Rev. Laryngol. Otol. Rhinol. (Bord.)* **63:**34–41, 1942.

6   Blom, S.: Tic douloureux treatment with new anticonvulsant. *Arch. Neurol.* **9:**285–290, 1963.

7   Botney, M., and Fields, H. L.: Amitriptyline potentiates morphine analgesia by a direct action on the central nervous system. *Ann. Neurol.* **13:**160–164, 1983.

8   Couch, J. R., and Hassanein, R. S.: Amitriptyline in migraine prophylaxis. *Arch. Neurol.* **21:**263–268, 1979.

9   Diamond, S., and Baltes, B. J. Chronic tension headache treated with amitriptyline—a double blind study. *Headache* **11:**110–116, 1971.

10 Dundee, J. W., Love, W. J., and Moore, J.: Alterations in response to somatic pain associated with anesthesia, Part XV: Further studies with phenothiazine derivatives and similar drugs. *Br. J. Anaesth.* **35**:597–609, 1963.

11 Dunsker, S. B., and Mayfield, F. H. Carbamazepine in the treatment of the flashing pain syndrome. *J. Neurosurg.* **45**:49–51, 1976.

12 Espir, M. L. E., and Millac, P.: Treatment of paroxysmal disorders in multiple sclerosis with carbamazepine (Tegretol). *J. Neurol. Neurosurg. Psychiatry* **33**:528–531, 1970.

13 Farber, G. A., and Burks, J. W.: Chlorprothixene therapy for herpes zoster neuralgia. *South. Med. J.* **67**:808–812, 1974.

14 Fields, H. L., and Raskin, N. H.: Anticonvulsants and pain. In H. L. Klawans (Ed.): *Clinical Neuropharmacology.* Raven Press, New York, 1976, pp. 173–184.

15 Fromm, G. H., Terrence, C. F., and Chatta, A. S.: Baclofen in the treatment of trigeminal neuralgia: Double-blind study and long-term follow-up. *Ann. Neurol.* **15**:240–244, 1984.

16 Gilbert, M. M.: Analgesic/calmative effects of acetaminophen and phenyltoloxamine in treatment of simple nervous tension accompanied by headache. *Curr. Ther. Res.* **20**:53–58, 1976.

17 Glassman, A. H., Perel, J. M., Shostak, M., Kantor, S. J., and Fleiss, J. L.: Clinical implications of imipramine plasma levels for depressive illness. *Arch. Gen. Psychiatry* **34**:197–204, 1977.

18 Gold, R. H.: Treatment of low back syndrome with oral orphenadrine citrate. *Curr. Ther. Res.* **23**:271–276, 1978.

19 Gomersall, J. D., and Stuart, A.: Amitriptyline in migraine prophylaxis. *J. Neurol. Neurosurg. Psychiatry* **36**:684–690, 1973.

20 Gomez-Perez, F. J., Rull, J. A., Dies, H., and Guillermo, J.: Nortriptyline and fluphenazine in the symptomatic treatment of diabetic neuropathy. A double-blind cross-over study. *Pain* **23**:395–400, 1985.

21 Grace, E. M., Kassam, Y., and Buchanan, W. W.: Controlled, double-blind, randomized trial of amitriptyline in relieving articular pain and tenderness in patients with rheumatoid arthritis. *Curr. Med. R. Opinion* **9**:426–429, 1985.

22 Graceley, R. H., McGrath, P., and Dubner, R.: Validity and sensitivity of ratio scales of sensory and affective verbal pain descriptors: Manipulation of affect by diazepam. *Pain* **5**:19–29, 1978.

23 Gringras, M.: A clinical trial of Tofranil in rheumatic pain in general practice. *J. Int. Med. Res.* **4:**41–49, 1976.

24 Hallett, M., Tandon, D., and Berardelli, A.: Treatment of peripheral neuropathies. *J. Neurol. Neurosurg. Psychiatry* **48:**1193–1207, 1985.

25 Iannone, A., Baker, A. B., and Morrell, F.: Dilantin in the treatment of trigeminal neuralgia. *Neurology* **8:**126–128, 1958.

26 Jannetta, P. J.: Arterial compression of the trigeminal nerve at the pons in patients with trigeminal neuralgia. *J. Neurosurg.* **26:**159–162, 1967.

27 Jannetta, P. J.: Microsurgical approach to the trigeminal nerve for tic douloureux. *Prog. Neurol. Surg.* **7:**180–200, 1976.

28 Kantor, T. G., and Steinberg, F. P.: Studies of tranquilizing agents and neperidine in clinical pain. In J. J. Bonica (Ed.): *Advances in Pain Research and Therapy* (Vol. 1), Raven Press, New York, 1976, pp. 567–572.

29 Kerr, F. W. L.: Craniofacial neuralgias. *Adv. Pain Res. Ther.* **4:**283–295, 1979.

30 Kocher, R.: The use of psychotropic drugs in the treatment of cancer pain. *Recent Results Cancer Res.* **89:**118–126, 1984.

31 Krabbe, A. A., and Olesen, J.: Headache provocation by continuous intravenous infusion of histamine. Clinical results and receptor mechanism. *Pain* **8:**253–259, 1980.

32 Kvinesdal, B., Molin, J., Froland, A., and Gram, L. F.: Imipramine treatment of painful diabetic neuropathy. *JAMA* **251:**1727–1730, 1984.

33 Lance, J. W., and Curran, D. A.: Treatment of chronic tension headache. *Lancet* **1:**1236–1239, 1964.

34 Lasagna, L., and DeKornfeld, T. J.: Methotrimeprazine—a new phenothiazine derivative with analgesic properties. *JAMA* **178:**119–122, 1961.

35 Lee, I., Chalon, J., Ramanathan, S., Gross, S., and Turndorff, H.: Analgesic properties of meperidine, amitriptyline and phenelzine in mice. *Can. Anaesth. Soc. J.* **30:**501–505, 1983.

36 Maciewicz, R., Bouckoms, A., and Martin, J. B.: Drug therapy of neuropathic pain. *Clin. J. Pain* **1:**39–49, 1985.

37 McGee, J. L., and Alexander, M. R.: Phenothiazine analgesia—fact or fantasy? *Am. J. Hosp. Pharm.* **36:**633–640, 1979.

38 Mendel, C. M., Klein, R. F., Chappell, D. A., Dere, W. H., Gertz, B. J., Karam, J. H., Lavin, T. N., and Grunfeld, C.: A trial of amitriptyline and fluphenazine in the treatment of painful diabetic neuropathy. *JAMA* **255:**637–639, 1986.

39 Mok, M. S., Lippman, M., and Steen, S. N.: Drug combinations with orphenadrine. *Clin. Ther.* **2:**188–193, 1979.

40 Moore, J., and Dundee, J. W.: Alterations in response to somatic pain associated with anesthesia, Part VII: The effects of nine phenothiazine derivatives. *Br. J. Anaesth.* **33:**422–431, 1961.

41 Nathan, P. W.: Chlorprothixene (Taractan) in post-herpetic neuralgia and other severe chronic pain. *Pain* **5:**367–371, 1978.

42 Pheasant, H., Bursk, A., Goldfarb, J., Azen, S. P., Weiss, J. N., and Borelli, L.: Amitriptyline and chronic low-back pain—a randomized double-blind crossover study. *Spine* **8:**552–557, 1983.

43 Rall, T. W., and Schleifer, L. S.: Drugs effective in the treatment of the epilepsies. In A. G. Gilman et al. (Eds.): *The Pharmacological Basis of Therapeutics.* Macmillan, New York, 1985, pp. 446–472.

44 Rigal, F., Eschalier, A., Devoize, J.-L., and Pechadre, J.-C.: Activities of five antidepressants in a behavioral pain test in rats. *Life Sci.* **32:**2965–2971, 1983.

45 Ross, S. B., and Renyi, A. L.: A comparison of the inhibitory activities of iprindole and imipramine on the uptake of 5-hydroxytryptamine and noradrenaline in brain slices. *Life Sci.* **10:**1267–1277, 1971.

46 Rull, J. A., Quibrera, R., Gonzalez-Millan, H., and Castaneda, O. L.: Symptomatic treatment of peripheral diabetic neuropathy with carbamazepine (Tegretol): Double blind crossover trial. *Diabetologia* **5:**215–218, 1969.

47 Rumore, M. M., and Schlichting, D. A.: Clinical efficacy of antihistaminics as analgesics. *Pain* **25:**7–22, 1986.

48 Saarnivaara, L., and Mattila, J. M.: Comparison of tricyclic antidepressants in rabbits: Antinociception and potentiation of the noradrenalin pressor response. *Psychopharmacologia* **35:**221–236, 1974.

49 Scott, W. A. M.: The relief of pain with an antidepressant in arthritis. *Practitioner* **202:**802–807, 1969.

50 Shibasaki, H., and Kuroiwa, Y.: Painful tonic seizure in multiple sclerosis. *Arch. Neurol.* **30:**47–51, 1975.

51 Spiegel, K., Kalb, R., and Pasternak, G. W.: Analgesic activity of tricyclic antidepressants. *Ann. Neurol.* **13**:462–465, 1983.

52 Stambaugh, J. E., and Lane, C.: Analgesic efficicay and pharmacokinetic evaluation of meperidine and hydroxyzine, alone and in combination. *Cancer Invest.* **1**:111–117, 1983.

53 Sun, C.-L., J., Hui, F. W., and Hanig, P. P.: Effect of H_1 blockers alone and in combination with morphine to produce antinociception in mice. *Neuropharmacology* **24**:1–4, 1985.

54 Swerdlow, M., and Cundill, J. G.: Anticonvulsant drugs used in the treatment of lancinating pain. A comparison. *Anaesthesia* **36**:1129–1132, 1981.

55 Taiwo, Y. O., Fabian, A., Pazoles, C. J., and Fields, H. L.: Potentiation of morphine antinociception by monoamine reuptake inhibitors in the rat spinal cord. *Pain* **21**:329–337, 1985.

56 Tomson, T., Tybring, G., Bertilsson, L., Ekbom, K., and Rane, A.: Carbamazepine therapy in trigeminal neuralgia, clinical effects in relation to plasma concentration. *Arch. Neurol.* **37**:699–703, 1980.

57 Turkington, R. W.: Depression masquerading as diabetic neuropathy. *JAMA* **243**:1147–1150, 1980.

58 Wall, P. D.: Changes in damaged nerve and their sensory consequences. In J. J. Bonica et al. (Ed.): *Advances in Pain Research and Therapy,* Volume 3. Raven Press, New York, 1979, pp. 39–52.

59 Walsh, T. D.: Antidepressants in chronic pain. *Clin. Neuropharmacol.* **6**:271–295, 1983.

60 Watson, C. P., Evans, R. J., Reed, K., Merskey, H., Goldsmith, L., and Warsh, J.: Amitriptyline versus placebo in postherpetic neuralgia. *Neurology* **32**:671–673, 1982.

61 Watson, C. P. N., and Evans, R. J.: A comparative trial of amitriptyline and zimelidine in post-herpetic neuralgia. *Pain* **23**:387–394, 1985.

62 Winter, L.: Analgesic combinations with orphenadrine in oral post-surgical pain. *J. Int. Med. Res.* **7**:240–246, 1979.

63 Yaari, Y., and Devor, M.: Phenytoin suppresses spontaneous ectopic discharge in rat sciatic nerve neuromas. *Neurosci. Lett.* **58**:117–122, 1985.

Chapter 11

Nondrug Methods for
Pain Control

For most physicians, analgesic medications are the mainstay of pain control. The reasons are obvious: they are of proven efficacy, widely available, and convenient for patients to use. Furthermore, not only is it quick and easy for the physician to write a prescription but, if there is a question about the dose or the side effects, one need only look in the *Physician's Desk Reference* (56).

Despite the convenience of analgesic drugs, many patients and most physicians are dissatisfied with their long-term use for non-malignant pain. One problem is the patient's feeling that the pain is still present, that the drugs merely cover it up or take the edge off. A more widespread problem is that many patients obtain little relief or experience intolerable side effects with nonsteroidal anti-inflammatory drugs, acetaminophen, or tricyclic antidepressants, and they are intimidated by the problems associated with long-term use of opioid analgesics.

This situation has led to the development of a variety of nondrug treatment techniques for pain control. Some of the most frequently used methods are listed in Table 11.1. At the present time, none of these methods has been established as effective for chronic, non-malignant pain. Because there are no generally agreed upon specific indications for their use, nondrug methods tend to be employed on a trial-and-error basis for a variety of pain problems. Each of the listed treatments has both adherents and critics. Although superficially quite different, they have much in common with each other. Each requires special training to

Table 11.1 Nondrug Treatments for Pain Control

Transcutaneous electrical nerve stimulation (TENS)

Neuroaugmentative surgery

Acupuncture

Cognitive-behavioral methods
  Hypnosis
  Relaxation
  Guided imagery, distraction
  Biofeedback

Ablative procedures
  Neurolytic blocks
  Ablative surgery

use, and, except for transcutaneous electrical nerve stimulation, they are all labor intensive and therefore expensive. Furthermore, they usually must be individually tailored to the patients needs and are therefore not standardized procedures. Because of this, their efficacy is highly dependent on the skill, experience, and personality of the person who employs them.

Another intriguing feature shared by most of these techniques is that the first reports of their use indicated remarkable success. However, as the initial wave of enthusiasm passed, they were subjected to more critical evaluation that often failed to confirm the dramatic success of the early reports (e.g., see ref. 7).

Despite mixed reviews, many of these treatments have gained widespread popularity, and it is not unusual for a chronic pain patient to have tried many or all of them. No matter which one you pick, some physicians swear by it and relate tales of occasional miraculous "cures," and others claim that their patients have tried one or more of the methods and obtained no lasting effect. Although these conflicting personal observations do not negate the possibility that these methods are useful, it is not yet possible to predict which chronic pain patient will respond to a given treatment. Furthermore, the clinical evidence for the efficacy of these treatments is derived from either uncontrolled or poorly controlled studies. This unsatisfactory state of affairs is likely to continue for the near future because of the difficulty in designing good clinical studies for these types of treatments. At the present time it is probably best to think of these approaches as being in a promising transitional phase. The efficacy and mechanism of action of each of these techniques are being studied and the specific indications for the use of each are evolving as experience accumulates.

Part of the difficulty in evaluating these approaches to pain control rests with the patient population. The patients who receive these treatments are usually those with chronic problems who have not responded to other, more traditional methods of pain management. As we have repeatedly pointed out, chronic pain patients are not a homogeneous group and they often have more than one factor contributing to their pain. Even patients with superficially similar complaints may have different underlying explanations for them. Thus, depending on its mechanism of action, a treatment that works for one patient's back pain may not help another patient.

Each of the methods under consideration has its proponents, including physicians and patients who have had success with it. The treatment apparently "worked" for them. But what does it mean to say that a treatment has worked? At first glance, it seems obvious. If the patient gets better, it means the treatment has worked. In clinical practice this is the bottom line. The patient does not really care how a treatment works as long as the pain is better, and if a physician has seen some patients improve with a given treatment he or she will be inclined to use it again. Although much of clinical practice is guided by such personal anecdotes, they do not provide a firm basis for conclusions about the efficacy of a treatment. Any of the treatments may have a specific analgesic action; however, it is also possible that the pain relief observed is not a specific effect of the treatment per se. To understand this, it is necessary to know how the natural history of a disease and the placebo effect can contribute to pain relief. Knowledge of the placebo effect provides insight into the tremendously important role of expectation and the physician-patient relationship in determining therapeutic outcomes, and it helps to explain why physicians differ in the success they have with different treatments.

Placebo Analgesia

There are several reasons why a patient may improve following a treatment. The treatment may be specifically helpful for the disease or injury that is producing the pain (e.g., an antibiotic for a bacterial infection) or it may be an effective treatment for pain (e.g., morphine). Another important possibility, illustrated by Figure 11.1, is that the natural course of the illness producing the pain is to improve and that, by coincidence, the treatment was given just before the improvement phase. The remaining possibility is that the pain relief is due to a placebo effect. Placebo analgesia occurs when some aspect of the treatment situation causes the patient to expect pain relief and the patient's expectation of relief, rather than any specific action of the treatment, triggers a neurally mediated reduction in pain.

There is a great deal of confusion about placebos and placebo responses. This is unfortunate because placebo responses have the potential to enhance or diminish analgesia, even in patients receiving treatments of proven efficacy. As a first step, it is important to define placebo. The derivation of the term is from the latin verb *placere,* to please. Placebo is the future indicative, meaning "I

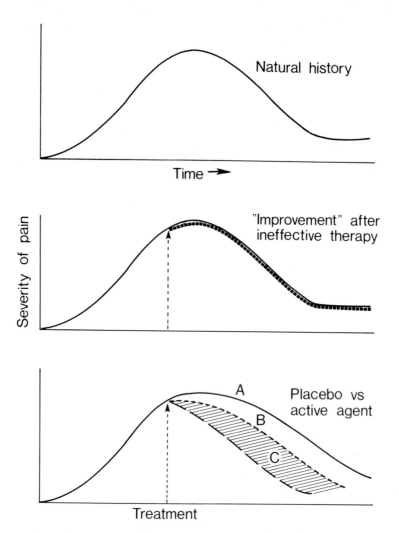

Figure 11.1 Natural history and the placebo effect. The pain associated with many diseases fluctuates in the absence of treatment (natural history; e.g., **top panel**). In such conditions, the effect of any intervention on pain must be evaluated relative to the expected natural history.

The **middle panel** illustrates a common situation that often leads to confusion. In this case a treatment was given that had no effect; however, since the patient improved following treatment both patient and physician might mistakenly attribute the improvement to the treatment. If the patient were given a placebo, the physician might mistakenly conclude that the patient was a placebo responder.

The **bottom panel** illustrates what happens if there is a placebo effect. Patients receiving placebo (*interrupted line, B*) do better than the untreated control group (*A*). In order to prove that a treatment is effective for pain or for the disease causing the pain, it is necessary to show that there is an effect (*C*) that cannot be attributed to the natural history and that is greater than the placebo effect.

Reproduced with permission from Fields, H.L., and Levine, J.D.: Placebo analgesia—a role for endorphins? *Trends in Neuroscience* **7**:271–273, 1984.

shall please." In the past, placebo was a nonpejorative term for palliative treatments. In modern medicine, the term placebo has taken on a different meaning; it is a "dummy" treatment meant to resemble a real treatment but known to be ineffective for the patient's condition. Placebo is used as the control in clinical trials designed to determine the efficacy of another treatment. Placebos are also employed in clinical practice to make the patient feel better by tricking him or her into believing something helpful has been done. Placebos are commonly used by physicians and nurses who are suspicious about the authenticity of a patient's complaints, the thinking being that if the patient responds to an imaginary treatment their pain must be imaginary (18).

NATURAL HISTORY VERSUS THE PLACEBO EFFECT

Although it may be obvious to the person who gives it that a treatment is a placebo, whether the patient responds to it is usually not obvious. This is illustrated by Figure 11.1. Most patients with chronic problems experience "spontaneous" fluctuations in the intensity of their pain. Migraine headache is a good example of this. Patients with migraine are free of pain most of the time. Their headaches are intermittent. When they do occur, the headaches build in severity over a period of from 30 minutes to several hours and then slowly decline. If the patient were to receive a treatment near the time of the peak severity of the headache (*arrow, middle trace,* Figure 11.1), the treatment would be followed by improvement. In the case illustrated, it would be erroneous to conclude that the relief was due to the treatment because the pain level would have declined without the treatment (because of the natural history of the disease). Similarly, if a placebo is given near the time of the peak severity, improvement will also be observed (*middle trace,* Figure 11.1). However, in this case, there is no placebo effect because the patient would have improved anyway. This example illustrates the difficulty of determining the occurrence of a treatment effect for a painful condition that fluctuates in severity without treatment. In order to demonstrate a placebo effect it is necessary to show that a *group* of patients who receive placebo differ from a group that has received no treatment (Figure 11.1, *bottom*). A very important corollary of this is that the occurrence of a placebo response in an individual is an inference because it is not known what would have happened if the placebo had not been given. To demonstrate that a treatment has a specific analgesic effect it is necessary to show that a group of patients receiving that treatment has less pain than a group that has received placebo (Figure 11.1, *bottom*). The placebo group controls both for placebo effects and for fluctuations in pain severity that are spontaneous.

If progress is to be made in the care of patients with chronic pain, it is necessary to establish the efficacy of the different treatments currently in use. Unfortunately, it is extremely difficult to prove the efficacy of complex, multistep treatments that are individually adjusted for different patients. The problem

Table 11.2   Features of Placebo Analgesia

Broad range of painful conditions respond

Any person can respond under the right circumstances

More severe pain predicts positive response

Greater anxiety predicts positive response

Physician attitude and communication influences patient expectation

is to exclude the possibility that the pain relief such treatments produce is largely a placebo effect. To see why this is a serious possibility a discussion of the features of placebo analgesia (Table 11.2) is required.

Potency of Placebo Analgesia

One common misconception about placebo analgesia is that placebos act only upon mild pains. In fact, placebo treatment can produce significant relief in conditions characterized by severe pain. This has been demonstrated directly for patients with postoperative pain (19, 34) and labor and postpartum pain (38). There is also anecdotal evidence for placebo efficacy across a wide range of painful conditions (6). Furthermore, we have shown that patients who report more intense pain are more likely to respond to a placebo (35).

Factors That Affect Placebo Analgesia

Are There Placebo Responders?   In trying to determine the mechanism of placebo analgesia it is important to identify those factors that predict the likelihood that a patient will respond. Because suggestion seems to be an integral part of the process, attempts have been made to correlate placebo analgesia with suggestibility and hypnotizability (16, 61). So far, however, it has not been possible to correlate the probability of responding to a placebo with any personality trait. Furthermore, there is some evidence to suggest that, under the right circumstances, anyone may respond. If placebos are repeatedly given to a group of patients, different individuals appear to respond at different times (26). Liberman's study (38) is particularly interesting in this regard. He recorded the effect of placebo administration on labor pain, postpartum pain, and experimental pain in 50 women on an obstetric service. Placebo analgesia was observed in each of the three situations. However, an analgesic response by an individual in one of the situations was not predictive for a response in the other two. The clinical situation is thus an important determinant of patient responsiveness to placebo.

Anxiety and Pain Intensity   As mentioned above, pain intensity is one predictor of placebo analgesia. Another reliable predictor is anxiety (16, 61). Although it is likely that pain will produce anxiety, the anxiety level prior to experimentally induced pain is predictive of a positive response to placebo (16). Thus the presence of anxiety seems to be an independent factor contributing to the placebo response.

Expectation   Obviously, the patient's expectation is a major factor leading to a placebo response (80). Expectation is a complex amalgam of the patient's past experience and current situational factors, including what the treating physician communicates. A series of failed attempts to provide pain relief would be expected to make a patient skeptical about future success. On the other hand, initial success would raise his or her expectation of continued success. This commonsense view was convincingly confirmed by the demonstration that a placebo is more likely to relieve pain if the patient's previous treatment was an effective analgesic drug (30).

Patients' expectations, and consequently their subjective response to a placebo, can be dramatically affected by what is communicated to them. For example, subjects receiving a placebo or an energizing drug such as caffeine will experience a sedating effect if led to believe that they have been given a tranquilizer (15, 80). The possibility should also be kept in mind that suggestion can be negative. The effectiveness of an active analgesic drug might be diminished if doubt is communicated to the patient.

The communication need not be a direct verbal suggestion. The tone of voice, gestures, or facial expression of the physician can communicate either confidence or doubt to the patient (78).

Another potentially important factor is the presence of side effects produced by the treatment (e.g., sedation, nausea, and dizziness). These side effects might serve as a cue to reinforce the idea that a powerful treatment has been given. It may be that the noxious side effects of ancient treatments like bleeding, emetics, cathartics, and burning the skin served to reinforce a placebo response.

Because of the differences between individual patients, situational cues, physician beliefs, and what is communicated by the physician to the patient, patients will have different expectations for different types of treatments. Consequently, different treatments will vary in their ability to induce placebo analgesia. One treatment may "work" for a patient in whom another treatment fails even if neither treatment has any intrinsic therapeutic efficacy. A treatment may be effective in the hands of a physician who is enthusiastic and positive about it but fail when used by a skeptic (7). The tension and drama of employing state-of-the-art diagnostic technology, consulting several specialists, undergoing a 3-hour surgical procedure, and spending 3 weeks in the hospital might provide a more convincing level of suggestion than a 10-minute encounter in the office of a young primary care physician who recommends two aspirin.

MECHANISM OF PLACEBO ANALGESIA

The mechanism of placebo analgesia can be approached at several different levels of analysis. At one level is the investigation of the psychological factors that contribute to patient expectation. A discussion of these factors, although important, is beyond the scope of this book. At another level, one can envision that the expectation of relief reduces anxiety. The reduction in anxiety could lead to an increase in pain tolerance (16). Reduced anxiety could also reduce muscle tone and sympathetic outflow. If muscle contraction or sympathetic tone were contributing to the pain this relaxation effect could reduce nociceptor input.

Another possibility is that the expectation of relief somehow leads to activation of the pain modulation network discussed in Chapter 5. The observation that the narcotic antagonist naloxone can at least partially block placebo analgesia (20, 34, 36) supports the notion that endogenous opioid peptides are involved and is consistent with the idea that activation of the endogenous pain modulation system contributes to placebo analgesia.

USE OF PLACEBOS IN CLINICAL PRACTICE

It is clear from the evidence discussed above that the use of placebos as a punitive measure or diagnostic test for patients suspected of malingering or exaggerating their complaints is unethical and, furthermore, that the "information" derived is misleading. Patients with more severe pain are more likely to respond to a placebo. A complaining, uncooperative patient who feels his or her needs are not being met is less likely to respond. On the other hand, it is good medical practice to exploit the full potential of the placebo as long as it is clearly in the patient's best interest. There is probably a placebo component to most treatments, including those proven to be effective analgesics. A physician who communicates interest and concern about the patient has taken a major step toward building the type of therapeutic alliance that will both enhance compliance and maximize the placebo potential of any therapy.

To avoid communicating doubt to a patient, the physician should only use a treatment he or she believes has a specific beneficial effect. If the efficacy of the treatment has not been proven, a brief discussion of why the physician thinks it will work can be helpful. One approach is to tell the patient that other patients with a similar problem who received the treatment improved. The risks and benefits should be carefully weighed and discussed with the patient. However, unless the treatment has significant risk (e.g., a surgical procedure), after the decision is made to proceed with it, its potential benefit should be confidently, if not enthusiastically, stressed. Although reassurance is helpful, direct questions from the patient must be answered honestly, even if you do not think it is in the patient's best interest to tell him or her the full story.

SUMMARY

In summary, placebo administration can produce a powerful analgesic effect. The evidence indicates that, under the right circumstances, anyone can respond. Interrelated situational factors such as ongoing pain, anxiety, and expectation are far more reliable predictors of a positive response to placebo than are any known personality traits of the patient. The power of physician communication to influence patient expectations is a tool that can be used to exploit the therapeutic potential of the placebo response.

Assessment of Alternative Approaches to Pain Control

The treatments to be discussed below have all been used to treat large numbers of patients with chronic benign pain. However, at the present time, none has been clearly established as having a specific analgesic effect. The problem has been to design a way to control for nonspecific factors in the treatment situation. Differences between individuals, the complexity of the treatment procedure, and the powerful effect of physician communication make it very difficult to determine the contribution of the placebo response to the analgesic effect of any of these treatments. How does one do placebo hypnosis or sham acupuncture without the knowledge of either the therapist or the patient? Does application of an electrical stimulator without batteries have the same placebo effect as active stimulation in the "wrong" area? These questions cannot yet be answered. They are raised simply to put the clinical data to be discussed below in perspective.

Transcutaneous Electrical Nerve Stimulation

Transcutaneous electrical nerve stimulation (TENS) is a therapeutic modality that has come into widespread use since 1965, when interest in it was sparked by Melzack and Wall's gate control hypothesis (see Chapters 3 and 6). Melzack and Wall proposed, and it was later demonstrated, that large-diameter myelinated primary afferents exert a specific inhibitory effect on dorsal horn pain transmission neurons (22). They predicted that selective stimulation of large-diameter afferents in a peripheral nerve would alleviate pain.

Fortunately, it is possible to activate the large-diameter myelinated primary afferents selectively because they have the lowest threshold to externally applied electrical stimuli. Such stimulation is not painful because the smaller diameter myelinated and unmyelinated nociceptive primary afferents have a much higher electrical threshold and consequently are not activated. This fortuitous circumstance makes TENS an attractive clinical tool.

EFFICACY

The first clinical trials reported dramatically successful pain relief but they were small, uncontrolled studies (40, 48, 77). Because TENS is associated with (and may depend on) a specific sensation induced by stimulation of the large-diameter fibers, it is extremely difficult to design a placebo that would be subjectively similar to "appropriate" TENS. Some studies have used TENS contralateral to the pain as a control (81), but even this does not get around the problem of experimenter expectation and so would not provide a disguise adequate to make a trial of TENS truly double-blind. Thus, at the present time, it cannot be accepted as proven that TENS has a specific analgesic effect. Nevertheless, of the nondrug treatments discussed in this chapter, TENS has the firmest theoretical basis and the most convincing clinical studies to support its use for pain relief.

There is also experimental support for the analgesic efficacy of TENS (81). In addition to the animal studies showing that large-diameter primary afferents inhibit pain transmission (see above and Chapters 3 and 6), human psychophysical studies have shown that there are consistent elevations of both pain threshold and pain tolerance during TENS (12, 60). Furthermore, blockade of myelinated afferents increases the painfulness of cutaneous stimuli.

There are several clinical studies showing that TENS relieves postoperative pain (14, 81). Postoperative pain is a good model for the study of clinical analgesic efficacy because there is a straightforward somatic nociceptive input and the patients do not have a high incidence of psychological disturbance. Furthermore, postoperative pain has a consistent natural history and is known to respond well to standard analgesics. Several studies have shown TENS to be significantly better than "control stimulation" (dead battery) for postoperative pain (81). Some of these studies also reported that TENS-treated patients have a lower incidence of objective postoperative complications such as ileus, atelectasis, and decreased pulmonary function (2, 81).

Of particular interest with regard to the use of TENS for postoperative pain is that it seems to have a differential effectiveness for different types of pain. This was clearly shown in a single-blind study of postcesarean patients (63). Compared to a control group (dead-battery stimulator) the TENS group had significantly less movement-related cutaneous incisional pain. However, TENS did not significantly reduce the deeper visceral pain caused by uterine contraction. In a sense, this is a kind of control because there is no obvious reason why a placebo should affect superficial more than deep pain.

TENS has been reported to be effective for several other types of pain (68, 81), including that associated with arthritis, cancer, and acute trauma. One of the more interesting trials was a study of TENS in rheumatoid arthritis (42). This study showed that high-frequency TENS is significantly more effective than low-frequency TENS. This finding supports the idea that the analgesia produced by TENS depends on an effect that is specific to the stimulation (as opposed to distraction or a placebo effect). Unfortunately, the potential usefulness of low-frequency TENS as a control was mitigated in this study by the fact that the treating investigator knew which parameters were being used. Benefit from TENS has also been reported for pain associated with a variety of nervous system injuries (81), including peripheral neuropathies, traumatic nerve injuries, and spinal cord and spinal root lesions.

A recent study of patients with angina pectoris may have some relevance to the mechanism of TENS. TENS not only reduced the frequency of angina attacks and increased exercise tolerance, it significantly reduced the exercise-induced ST depression on the electrocardiogram (43). This latter finding raises the possibility of a direct effect of TENS on the sympathetic nervous system.

CLINICAL USE OF TENS

It is reasonable to try TENS in patients with chronic pain in whom drugs are either ineffective or undesirable. Other than the initial expense and the time required to train the patient, there are few problems with its use. One is the minor skin irritation from the electrodes and the other is that the device is awkward for some patients to use.

There are a variety of commercial stimulators currently available (44). The package includes several flexible electrodes, conducting gel to improve the electrical connection between the electrode and the skin, and instructions. The devices have adjustable stimulation frequency and intensity. Although most patients do best with frequencies between 50 and 100 Hz (81), patients should be instructed to find the best parameters through trial and error. Similarly, they must experiment with different placements. There is general agreement that the most effective placements are close to the area of pain. For example, when used for postoperative pain, the electrodes are most effective when placed on either side of the incision. If there is deafferentation of the skin near the painful area, stimulation may worsen the pain. In these cases the electrodes should be moved to adjacent normally innervated areas. For a complete review of electrode placements for different locations of pain I recommend the book by Mannheimer and Lampe (44).

It is important to emphasize that patients need verbal instruction and encouragement to use TENS devices optimally. To simply give them a device and tell them to read the instruction book rarely works. Although it is simple to learn, the use of the TENS device should be demonstrated by an experienced professional who will take the time required to instruct the patient. After they are

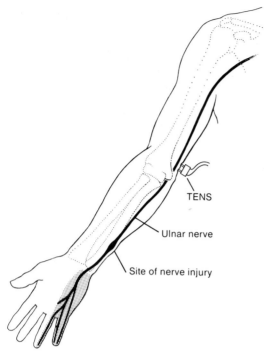

Figure 11.2 The use of TENS for treatment of painful nerve injury. In the example shown, the patient experienced pain in the hand secondary to a traumatic injury of the ulnar nerve in the forearm. In this case it was possible to stimulate the ulnar nerve above the medial epicondyle (TENS). Because the nerve is in a reliable position near the skin surface, it can be stimulated with minimal current. Paresthesias restricted to the ulnar-innervated surface of the hand (*stipple*) confirm that the ulnar nerve is being stimulated successfully.

shown how to use TENS, patients should be told to balance the comfort of the stimulator with the analgesic effect by changing stimulation parameters and electrode location.

Although as many as half of chronic pain patients report initial relief with TENS, the effect tends to wear off with time so that by 1 year only about 30% of patients continue to obtain significant benefit (81). On the other hand, for those patients who obtain continued relief it seems to be an ideal method of pain control. It is noninvasive, safe, and has only minor side effects. The onset of relief occurs within seconds to a few minutes. When used on a long-term basis it is inexpensive and, furthermore, places the patient in a position of control.

In my experience, the most dramatic successes with TENS have been in patients with pain due to traumatic injury of a peripheral nerve. This is not totally unexpected since, in these patients, part of the etiology of the pain is a predominant loss of large myelinated afferents. In these cases, TENS is most likely to succeed if an intact segment of nerve proximal to the site of injury can be stimulated (Figure 11.2). Presumably, this segment of nerve will have a full complement of normally functioning myelinated afferent axons. Successful stimulation is indicated by a tingling sensation that radiates into the cutaneous distribution of the nerve being stimulated. With this method, a few minutes of stimulation may provide hours of relief (48).

SUMMARY

In summary, TENS is a technique for pain control that has a convincing theoretical basis and is exceptionally safe. Although its efficacy for clinical pain is supported by both clinical and experimental observations, it has not been proven that the analgesia that is observed clinically is a specific effect of stimulation. Nevertheless, TENS is worth using in patients with postoperative pain, especially if opioids are a problem (e.g., in patients with pulmonary disease or post-thoracotomy). It also seems to be useful for painful nerve injuries, if a section of normal nerve proximal to the injury can be stimulated. Finally, because TENS is virtually free of side effects, it is appropriate to try it in any patient with chronic pain in whom long-term use of analgesic drugs is being considered.

Neurosurgical Procedures Involving Electrical Stimulation

PERIPHERAL NERVE IMPLANTS

There are two surgical procedures that grew out of the experimental and clinical evidence that activity in large-diameter myelinated afferents can have an analgesic effect. One of the procedures, the surgical implantation of stimulating electrodes on normal segments of a peripheral nerve, is a direct extension of transcutaneous stimulation (10, 31, 81). Because of the frequency of complications (57), this procedure has not gained general acceptance; consequently it is not possible to conclude whether it has any clinical value. There is no reason to believe that it would be any more effective than stimulating the nerve through the skin, but it is potentially useful as a way to stimulate nerves that are not accessible to transcutaneous stimulation.

DORSAL COLUMN STIMULATION

The other procedure that is a conceptual extension of TENS is dorsal column stimulation (DCS). This technique has been used extensively to treat non-malignant lower body pain. The procedure consists of a thoracic laminectomy with implantation of electrodes over the dorsal columns. The theoretical benefit of this electrode placement is that all primary afferents in the dorsal columns have large-diameter myelinated axons. Impulses elicited by DCS will propagate in both directions: rostrally to the dorsal column nuclei and antidromically back to the dorsal horn, where they should produce a predominantly inhibitory effect on pain transmission neurons (22). DCS produces a tingling, electric-like sensation (paresthesia) in most patients. This sensation is felt in the lower body, and pain relief depends on the patient's experiencing paresthesia in the same area as the pain (29).

The results of this procedure, although initially encouraging (51, 62), have been disappointing in long-term follow-up (29, 50, 54). There are many problems with the procedure and with its use. One of the major problems has been patient selection. As with most surgical procedures for pain, DCS is done as a treatment of last resort, in patients with long-standing pain who appear to have nothing to lose. Most of the patients who have had DCS have been patients with chronic low back pain (29, 50); however, selection and exclusion criteria for the procedures are vague. As with TENS, a high proportion of patients obtain good relief initially, only to have their pain return. Other patients are beset by complications including infection, cerebrospinal fluid leakage, or pain at the electrode implantation site. There is some evidence that, as with TENS, DCS is more effective in patients with chronic pain due to peripheral nerve injury than in other types of pain problems (53). However, in my opinion, because of the expense and risk of the procedure and the high incidence of return of the pain or development of a new pain problem, DCS should not be considered to be a routine procedure at the present time. Ideally, it should be carried out in the context of a protocol designed to determine its efficacy.

DEEP BRAIN STIMULATION

In addition to peripheral nerve and dorsal column stimulation, some patients with chronic pain have been treated by electrical stimulation through stereotaxically placed electrodes in the depth of the brain (23, 24, 72). Most of the patients who have undergone this type of procedure have had the electrodes placed either in the periventricular gray matter (PVG) of the caudal diencephalon or, more lateral and rostral, in the region of the sensory thalamus or internal capsule. These two placements appear to differ somewhat in their efficacy and will be discussed separately.

The PVG placement grew out of animal research demonstrating that midbrain stimulation suppresses responses to noxious stimulation. The PVG is the rostral extension of the periaqueductal gray, which has been shown by extensive animal experiments to be an important part of an intrinsic pain modulation system (see Chapter 5 for a complete discussion). Although not proven, the parsimonious view is that the pain relief produced by the PVG stimulation results from activation of this system. The best evidence supporting this view is that analgesia appears to be critically dependent on the electrode being placed correctly within the PVG (5, 9). This is particularly important as a control for a placebo effect, since neither the patient nor the surgeon would know the precise location of the electrode, and there is no sensory clue other than pain relief to reliably signal correct placement.

Despite its strong theoretical basis, and reasonable evidence that it can produce a clinically significant analgesic effect, PVG stimulation is still a procedure in search of an indication. There is presently no way to predict which patients will respond. Some neurosurgeons use a positive analgesic response to morphine infusion as a screening test for the procedure. If the patients get relief with morphine (10–30 mg IV), they are considered surgical candidates (23). One wonders whether such patients could have been managed equally well with analgesic drugs. Most patients undergo a period of trial stimulation before the electrodes are permanently implanted; however, even with this screening measure many patients cease to obtain relief within months of the implantation. As with DCS, PVG has been used as a treatment of last resort in chronic pain patients, mostly those with chronic low back pain (23), and its efficacy has never been compared to another type of treatment (e.g., a cognitive-behavioral approach). There has never been a controlled study of any sort.

The other major site that has been stimulated for pain control is the sensory thalamus. Thalamic stimulation has been used primarily for patients with deafferentation pains due to either central or peripheral nervous system damage (1, 25, 45, 72, 73). Thalamic stimulation is similar to TENS and DCS in that, in order for it to produce relief, the patients must obtain paresthesias in the area of pain. It is also similar to the other stimulation techniques in that it tends to lose its efficacy over time. In contrast to TENS and DCS, there is no clear explanation for the analgesic effect of thalamic stimulation. As with the other stimulation techniques, the efficacy of thalamic stimulation has not been proven and it is not yet possible to identify the patients who will respond.

At the present time I consider PVG and thalamic stimulation to be in an experimental phase. Their complications include infection and hemorrhage, and electrode movement is also a problem. Despite these potentially serious problems, thalamic and PVG stimulation offer promise of future therapeutic avenues for patients with intractable pain. If their efficacy and therapeutic indications can be established, they would represent a step that is intermediate between noninvasive modalities (e.g., drugs, TENS, hypnosis) and the more destructive ablative neurosurgical procedures.

Acupuncture

This method of treatment, which was known to the ancient Chinese, has enjoyed a surge of popularity in the West. Traditional acupuncture is a complete system of "medical" care that considers many diseases to be the result of disturbances in the balance of two basic universal forces, *yin* and *yang* (76). According to the classic teachings, such disturbances are detected primarily by an examination of the pulses (76). The yin and yang act in the body through 12 channels called meridians that connect the vital centers. To restore the balance to normal, acupuncture needles are placed along the meridians at sites (acupuncture points) appropriate for the particular abnormality. It is not clear how these sites were originally determined, but there is supposed to be a specific heavy aching sensation elicited when needles are twirled at the right acupuncture point (66).

Although the meridian system is quite elaborate and specific, it is quite clear that it is not necessary to use the traditional acupuncture points to obtain analgesia. Several careful studies have shown that needling provides equally good pain relief whether applied to specified acupuncture points or at sham sites (33, 41, 47). In fact, needling seems to be more likely to relieve pain when it is applied close to or in a segmental relationship to the pain (12, 46). Some of the acupuncture points are over sensitive sites in musculoskeletal tissues that may be myofascial trigger points (46), and it is interesting in this regard that "dry needling" is reported to be effective for some myofascial syndromes (69). Whether needling that is not done at traditionally specified points should be called acupuncture is debatable. What it is called depends more on who does it than on what it is they do.

The problems besetting the evaluation of the analgesic efficacy of needling are the same as for TENS. It really is very difficult to carry out a truly double-blind study. Thus one cannot rule out a major contribution to "acupuncture" analgesia by a placebo effect.

There has been some methodological convergence in the use of needling and TENS for pain management. Many acupuncturists now use electrical stimulation through their needles instead of twirling them. They have found empirically that brief trains of high-intensity stimulation are most effective (46). A similar effect of brief high-intensity stimulation is also seen when cutaneous electrodes instead of needles are used (46). Thus it does not seem to matter whether needles or skin stimulation is used. On the other hand there is evidence that the types of pain that respond to brief high-intensity TENS are different from those responding to the more commonly used low-intensity continuous TENS (42, 46, 64). If this is true, it would be important to conduct a clinical trial comparing the two types of TENS in a well-defined patient population (e.g., postoperative pain). In practice, both types of TENS should be tried in each patient to obtain an optimal effect.

Although it is premature to discuss the mechanism of "acupuncture" analgesia, it may be that, in addition to the TENS effect produced by low-intensity stimulation of large-diameter myelinated afferents, the high-intensity stimuli (and the needling) activate Aδ and C primary afferent nociceptors, which are known to have a widespread inhibitory effect on dorsal horn pain transmission cells. Such an inhibitory action could account for the apparent analgesic effectiveness of a variety of mildly painful manipulations generally referred to as counterirritation (32, 37, 46).

In summary, the term acupuncture applies to the use of needles or small skin electrodes that deliver intermittent mildly painful stimuli. There is evidence that such stimuli have a somewhat different analgesic effect than low-intensity continuous TENS; however, the specific indications for "acupuncture" have not been spelled out, nor has its analgesic efficacy been proven.

Cognitive and Behavioral Methods (20, 75)

Methods for distraction and relaxation have come into widespread use for pain control. Their appeal is obvious; they are noninvasive, harmless, and provide the patient with tools to deal not only with pain but with a variety of stressful life situations. The methods fall into three major categories: hypnosis, guided imagery, and direct relaxation techniques. Biofeedback, though originally developed as a way of manipulating autonomic and muscle function, may help pain patients primarily through relaxation or distraction (28).

With the possible exception of biofeedback, these methods are not standardized procedures. Therapists each have their own technique, which they will adjust depending on the patient's traits and the nature and location of the pain. Although it is certainly within the capacity of most clinicians to learn these methods, training and practice are required for optimal efficacy. I will briefly describe each type of approach in a very general way just to give the reader a flavor for what is done.

HYPNOSIS

Hypnosis was one of the first cognitive methods to be used for pain control. It consists of establishing rapport with patients, having them relax and attend to the therapist's voice, and then, through suggestion, manipulating their attention away from the sensation of pain (55). As usually practiced (4), hypnosis depends on the patient's ability to shift his or her attention to sensations, thoughts, and images that arise "spontaneously" or as a result of the therapist's suggestions. The patients' motivation for relief, their imagination, and their trust in the therapist are very important.

Hypnosis sessions are often initiated by direct suggestions of muscle relaxation (4). Relaxing a muscle is something a patient can do easily and it improves his or her ability to attend to the therapist's other suggestions. In modern hypnotic technique, suggestions are usually put forward indirectly as possibilities rather than commands. The suggestions are often determined by feelings or images that are relevant to the particular patient. For example, if the patient has a pain in his or her right hand, the therapist might enquire about how the left hand feels. If the patient indicates that the left hand feels comfortable, the therapist might ask if the patient is able to expand the region of comfort into part of the painful region. If the pain is burning, the therapist might ask whether the patient can remember or imagine the cool feeling of snow or an iced drink. If the pain has fluctuated during the day, the patient can be asked to remember those times when the pain was less severe or absent. During the session, suggestions can be made to the patient to notice future times at home when the pain is less severe without stating directly if or when those times will occur. Clearly, the hypnotherapist must be able to improvise based on the material raised in the session. In addition to these indirect suggestions, some patients may respond to "requests" to imagine sensations of comfort, numbness, or analgesia in the painful region. The point is that hypnotherapy involves relaxation and distraction (imagery), is very much guided by the patient's response, and is more like an educational process than a medical treatment. Successful treatment requires that the patient retain the ability to shift his or her attention away from the pain.

Hypnosis has been reported to relieve a broad variety of acute and chronic pain problems (21, 55, 75). Although not usually adequate for major surgical procedures, it has been used for minor, but distinctly painful ones such as burn debridement, bone marrow aspirations, and dental procedures (55). In addition, there are many anecdotal reports of rapid, dramatic, and complete relief in patients with chronic pain problems (4). This extensive clinical experience strongly supports the use of hypnosis for pain control. However, it is unclear whether hypnosis has a specific analgesic effect apart from distraction, relaxation, and the placebo effect (75). Patients differ widely in their ability to be hypnotized and, in practice, no two are treated in the same way. To try to standardize the treatment would rob it of much of its power. These problems make it difficult to design an adequate sham hypnosis treatment. Thus it has not yet been possible to show what it is about hypnosis that relieves pain.

In addition to its pain-relieving effect, hypnosis is a useful adjunct to psychotherapy (4). In some patients with chronic pain, the hypnotic session provides a shortcut to developing trust and changing the patient's expectations. Even though, as is often the case, the initial pain relief is transient, it demonstrates to the patient that the pain can be controlled by some inner mental mechanism. Restoring a sense of inner control is invaluable if the patient is to sustain any benefit. It is also frequently the case that during the hypnotic session, emotionally significant material is revealed by the patient, for example, grief or unresolved anger at a spouse that has died. Hypnosis is best done by a psychotherapist who is able to take advantage of this material to help the patient.

In summary, hypnosis is a cognitive method that depends on focusing the patient's attention away from his or her pain. It depends on the patient's imagination and the therapist's ability to guide the patient's attention to those images and feelings that are most constructive. In skilled hands, hypnosis can provide benefits beyond relaxation and distraction by identifying unresolved conflicts that are contributing to patients' preoccupation with their pain. I have found that a skilled hypnotherapist can be very helpful in the evaluation and treatment of patients with chronic non-malignant pain. If available, such a person should be involved in the initial evaluation process.

RELAXATION AND GUIDED IMAGERY

Although most methods emphasize either relaxation or imagery, in practice the two are almost inseparable. Methods that emphasize muscle relaxation instruct the patient to attend to the different muscle groups and to voluntarily contract and then relax them in sequence (see, e.g., ref. 8 or 27 for methodological details). The shift of attention to the particular muscles is in itself a kind of guided imagery. Other methods that are billed as relaxation techniques induce relaxation by having patients attend to respirations (71), meditate, count, repeat a word or phrase, or focus on specific sensations in different parts of the body. All of these tasks involve distraction. On the other hand, when the emphasis is on distraction via guided images, patients are often prepared by relaxation methods (70).

One of the benefits of relaxation and guided imagery methods is that they can be standardized to a certain extent. Their use does not require extensive training. Furthermore, instructions can be tape-recorded and the patients can use them at home (see ref. 17 for a sample script). This greatly decreases the cost and the logistical problems that pain patients have in getting to the clinician's office.

Outcome studies for relaxation and distraction methods are fraught with the same problems as for hypnosis. Although there is no question that chronic pain patients enrolled in treatment programs using these techniques do better than waiting list controls (74), it is not at all clear why. Furthermore, it is not yet possible to predict which patients will respond to these treatments. At the present time, these methods are mostly used as an alternative to drugs or surgical management. They are usually employed in the pain clinic setting as part of a comprehensive treatment program that includes drug withdrawal, psychotherapy, family counseling and behavior modification. Although such multimodality approaches increase the chance of helping the patient, they make outcome studies difficult to interpret in terms of the contribution of each of several concurrently employed approaches.

BIOFEEDBACK

Biofeedback is a technique that depends on providing measurements of certain physiological parameters to patients so that they can learn to control them. For pain patients, the parameters monitored have included skin temperature, electromyographically (EMG) recorded muscle activity, and electroencephalographic activity. For example, if EMG activity is to be controlled, electrodes are placed over the appropriate muscle and the amount of electrical activity is displayed to the patient. The patient is given some instructions or hints as to how to lower the reading (e.g., relaxation, imagery) and the displayed activity (feedback) gives the patient immediate and unequivocal information about the success of his or her efforts.

Although biofeedback has been used for a variety of chronic pain problems (28), its most common use is for the treatment of headache and most of the systematic studies of its efficacy have been carried out in headache patients. Originally, EMG biofeedback was used for muscle contraction headache, the reasoning being that if muscle contraction were causing the headache, patients that could learn to relax the appropriate muscles could abort their own headaches. In fact, patients treated with frontalis muscle EMG biofeedback do significantly better than those who receive either no treatment or placebo tablet controls (13, 74). However, the evidence indicates that this effect is not specific to the biofeedback procedure. First, the clinical improvement observed in headache patients receiving biofeedback is not superior to control groups who receive only relaxation training. Second, the observed improvement in headache with biofeedback is unrelated to whether the patient's EMG activity increases or decreases. This was elegantly demonstrated by Andrasik and Holroyd (3) using "pseudobiofeedback" controls. In their study, three groups of headache patients were given earphones and told that an increase in the audible tone meant that they had successfully reduced their frontalis EMG activity. This was true for only one group (EMG decrease). One of the other groups heard an increase in the tone when their frontalis EMG increased. The third group heard an increase in the tone if their frontalis EMG did not change. All three groups learned to increase the tone and, consequently either decrease, increase, or leave their frontalis EMG unchanged. A fourth group simply recorded their headaches but did not receive biofeedback. In this study all three groups had significant improvement in their headaches compared to the no-treatment controls. There were no differences between "real" biofeedback and pseudobiofeedback. Similar results have been obtained using skin temperature as the regulated parameter (28).

Thus, the available evidence indicates that the beneficial effect of biofeedback does not depend on a change in muscle contraction or sympathetic outflow. It is due to some change in the patient that accompanies but is not specific to the feedback signal. Possible factors that could contribute to the beneficial effect of biofeedback include distraction, muscle relaxation, reduced anxiety (58), and increased feelings of personal control over the symptoms (82). For some patients, the biofeedback approach may facilitate other relaxation and distraction methods (28), but it is not clear how to identify those individuals.

Ablative Procedures on
Nociceptive Pathways

Over the past two decades the use of ablative procedures has diminished markedly. There are many reasons for this, including a better appreciation of the large contribution of cognitive and behavioral factors to pain, the development of alternative noninvasive methods of pain management, the improved use of analgesic medications, and the recent development of neurostimulatory methods. The most important factor, however, is the growing awareness that ablative surgery often fails completely, or provides only transient relief. Furthermore, ablative procedures are frequently accompanied by unwanted and irreversible side effects. These include weakness and painful dysesthesias that can be as troublesome as the original pain (11).

At the present time, the indications for ablative procedures are few. They are used most often in cancer patients with a limited life expectancy who have pain despite optimal analgesic medications. The procedures that have been used include chemical or surgical neurolysis of peripheral nerves; lesions of the dorsal roots, dorsal root ganglia, and dorsal root entry zone; anterolateral cordotomy; spinothalamic tractotomy in the brainstem; thalamotomy; and cortical lesions (see reference 79 for details of these procedures). None of these ablative procedures are recommended for patients with a normal life expectancy. Although many of these procedures may be useful in patients with pain due to malignancy (67), few of them are currently done in sufficient numbers to draw firm conclusions about their efficacy.

An important exception is that lesions of the trigeminal root can give lasting relief for patients with trigeminal neuralgia (65). This effect on trigeminal neuralgia may have little applicability to other types of pains. Trigeminal neuralgia is a unique syndrome characterized by brief lancinating pains, and it responds to anticonvulsants, which are ineffective for other types of pains (Chapter 10).

Anterolateral cordotomy is the most common neurosurgical procedure for pain relief (see Chapters 3 and 6). It is suitable for terminally ill patients because it can be done percutaneously. Percutaneous cordotomy does not require a skin incision, can be done under local anesthesia, and gives excellent analgesia for up to 2 years (39, 49, 59). This procedure is only suitable for unilateral lower body pain (below the arm) in patients with a short life expectancy. In such patients, up to 80% may obtain significant benefit (59). Complications include weakness, respiratory depression, bowel and bladder dysfunction, and painful dysesthesias, the latter presumably due to deafferentation.

One other procedure worth noting is the dorsal root entry zone (DREZ) lesion, developed by Nashold and his colleagues (52). As discussed in Chapter 6, this is one of the few ablative procedures that seems to help chronic non-malignant pain. Although the numbers are small, DREZ lesions have been reported to be helpful for patients with deafferentiation-type pains due to brachial plexus avulsion, spinal cord injury, and postherpetic neuralgia (52). At the present time, however, the procedure is new and long-term results are not yet available.

In summary, neurolytic and ablative neurosurgical procedures should be used primarily in patients with limited life expectancy. If they are to be used for chronic non-malignant pain, the high rates of failure, of recurrence of pain, and of postoperative complications should be candidly discussed with the patient.

References

1   Adams, J. E., Hosobuchi, Y., and Fields, H. L.: Stimulation of internal capsule for relief of chronic pain. *J. Neurosurg.* **41**:740–744, 1974.

2   Ali, J., Yaffe, C. S., and Serrette, C.: The effect of transcutaneous electric nerve stimulation on postoperative pain and pulmonary function. *Surgery* **89**:507–512, 1981.

3   Andrasik, F., and Holroyd, K. A.: A test of specific and non-specific effects in the biofeedback treatment of tension headache. *J. Consulting Clin. Psychol.* **48**:575–586, 1980.

4   Barber, J., and Adrian, C.: *Psychological Approaches to the Management of Pain.* Brunner Mazel, New York, 1982.

5   Baskin, D. S., Mehler, W. R., Hosobuchi, Y., Richardson, D., Adams, J. E., and Flitter, M. A.: Autopsy analysis of the safety, efficacy and cartography of electrical stimulation of the central gray in humans. *Brain Res.* **37**:231–236, 1986.

6   Beecher, H. K.: *The Measurement of Subjective Responses: Quantitative Effects of Drugs.* Oxford University Press, New York, 1959.

7   Benson, H., and McCallie, D. P., Jr.: Angina pectoris and the placebo effect. *N. Engl. J. Med.* **300**:1424–1429, 1979.

8   Bernstein, D. A., and Borkovec, T. D.: *Progressive Relaxation Training: A Manual for the Helping Professions.* Research Press, Champaign, IL, 1973.

9   Boivie, J., and Meyerson, B. A.: A correlative anatomical and clinical study of pain suppression by deep brain stimulation. *Pain* **13**:113–126, 1982.

10 Campbell, J. N., and Long, D. M.: Peripheral nerve stimulation in the treatment of intractable pain. *J. Neurosurg.* **45**:692–699, 1976.

11   Cassinari, V., and Pagni, C. A.: *Central Pain*. Harvard University Press, Cambridge, MA, 1969.

12   Chapman, C. R., Chen, A. C., and Bonica, J. J.: Effects of intrasegmental electrical acupuncture on dental pain: Evaluation by threshold estimation and sensory decision theory. *Pain* **3**:213–227, 1977.

13   Chapman, S. L.: A review and clinical perspective on the use of EMG and thermal biofeedback for chronic headaches. *Pain* **27**:1–43, 1986.

14   Cooperman, A. M., Hall, B., Mikalacki, K., Hardy, R., and Sadar, E.: Use of transcutaneous electrical stimulation in the control of postoperative pain—Results of a prospective, randomized, controlled study. *Am. J. Surg.* **133**:185–187, 1977.

15   Dinnerstein, A. J., and Halm, J.: Modification of placebo effects by means of drugs: Effects of aspirin and placebos on self-rated moods. *J. Abnorm. Psychol.* **75**:308–314, 1970.

16   Evans, F. J.: Expectancy, therapeutic instructions, and the placebo response. In L. White et al. (eds.), *Placebo: Theory, Research and Mechanisms*. Guilford Press, New York, 1985.

17   Ferguson, J. E., Marquis, J. N., and Taylor, C. B.: A script for deep muscle relaxation. *Dis. Nerv. Syst.* **38**:703–708, 1977.

18   Goodwin, J. S., Goodwin, J. M., Vogel, A. V.: Knowledge and use of placebos by house officers and nurses. *Ann. Intern. Med.* **91**:106–110, 1979.

19   Gracely, R. H., Dubner, R., Wolskee, P. J., and Deeter, W. R.: Placebo and naloxone can alter postsurgical pain by separate mechanisms. *Nature* **306**:264–265, 1983.

20   Grevert, P., Leonard, H. A., and Goldstein, A.: Partial antagonism of placebo analgesia by naloxone. *Pain* **16**:129–143, 1983.

21   Hilgard, E. R., and Hilgard, J. R.: *Hypnosis in the Relief of Pain*. William Kaufman, Los Altos, CA, 1975.

22   Hillman, P., and Wall, P. D.: Inhibitory and excitatory factors influencing the receptive field of lamina 5 spinal cord cells. *Exp. Brain Res.* **9**:284–306, 1969.

23   Hosobuchi, Y.: Subcortical electrical stimulation for control of intractable pain in humans. *J. Neurosurg.* **64**: 543–553, 1986.

24   Hosobuchi, Y., Adams, J. E., and Linchitz, R.: Pain relief by electrical stimulation of the central gray matter in humans and its reversal by naloxone. *Science* **197**:183–186, 1977.

25   Hosobuchi, Y., Adams, J. E., and Rutkin, B.: Chronic thalamic stimulation for the
      control of facial anesthesia dolorosa. *Arch. Neurol.* **29:**158–161, 1973.

26   Houde, R. W., Wallenstein, M. S., and Rogers, A.: Clinical pharmacology of an-
      algesics. *Clin. Pharmacol. Ther.* **1:**163–174, 1960.

27   Jacobson, E.: *Modern Treatment of Tense Patients.* C. C. Thomas, Springfield, IL,
      1970.

28   Jessup, B. A.: Biofeedback. In P. D. Wall and R. Melzack (eds.), *Textbook of Pain.*
      Churchill Livingstone, Edinburgh, 1984, Chpt. 3.G.2.

29   Krainick, J. U., and Thoden, U.: Dorsal column stimulation. In P. D. Wall and R.
      Melzack, (eds.), *Textbook of Pain.* Churchill Livingstone, Edinburgh, 1984, Chpt.
      3.D.3.

30   Laska, E., and Sunshine, A.: Anticipation of analgesia, a placebo effect. *Headache*
      13:1–11, 1973.

31   Law, J. D., Swett, J., and Kirsch, W. M.: Retrospective analysis of 22 patients with
      chronic pain treated by peripheral nerve stimulation. *J. Neurosurg.* **52:**482–485,
      1980.

32   LeBars, D., Dickenson, A. H., and Besson, J. M.: Diffuse noxious inhibitory con-
      trols (DNIC) II. Lack of effect on non-convergent neurones, supraspinal involvement
      and theoretical implications. *Pain* **6:**305–327, 1979.

33   Lee, P. K., Andersen, T. W., Modell, J. H., and Saga, S. A.: Treatment of chronic
      pain with acupuncture. *JAMA* **232:**1133–1135, 1975.

34   Levine, J. D., and Gordon, N. C.: Influence of the method of drug administration
      on analgesic response. *Nature* **312:**755–756, 1984.

35   Levine, J. D., Gordon, N. C., Bornstein, J. C., and Fields, H. L.: Role of pain in
      placebo analgesia. *Proc. Natl. Acad. Sci. USA* **76:**3528–3531, 1979.

36   Levine, J. D., Gordon, N. C., and Fields, H. L.: The mechanism of placebo anal-
      gesia. *Lancet* **2:**654–657, 1978.

37   Levine, J. D., Gormley, J., and Fields, H. L.: Preliminary clinical observations on
      the analgesic effect of needle puncture (acupuncture). *Pain* **2:**149–159, 1976.

38   Liberman, R.: An experimental study of the placebo response under three different
      situations of pain. *J. Psychiatr. Res.* **2:**233–246, 1964.

39 Lipton, S.: Percutaneous cordotomy. In P. D. Wall and R. Melzack (eds.), *Textbook of Pain*, Churchill Livingston, Edinburgh, 1984, Chpt. 3.C.7.

40 Loeser, J. D., Black, R. D., and Christman, R. N.: Relief of pain by transcutaneous stimulation. *J. Neurosurg.* **42**:308–314, 1975.

41 Lynn, B., and Perl, E. R.: Failure of acupuncture to produce localized analgesia. *Pain* **3**:339–351, 1977.

42 Mannheimer, C., and Carlsson, C. A.: The analgesic effect of transcutaneous electrical nerve stimulation (TNS) in patients with rheumatoid arthritis. A comparative study of different pulse patterns. *Pain* **6**:329–334, 1979.

43 Mannheimer, C., Carlsson, C. A., Vedin, A., and Wilhelmsson, C.: Transcutaneous electrical nerve stimulation (TENS) in angina pectoris. *Pain* **26**:291–300, 1986.

44 Mannheimer, J. S., and Lampe, G. N.: *Clinical Transcutaneous Electrical Nerve Stimulation*. F. A. Davis, Philadelphia, 1984.

45 Mazar, G., Merienne, L., and Cioloca, C.: Comparative study of electrical stimulation of posterior thalamic nuclei, periaqueductal gray, and other midline mesencephalic structures in man. In J. J. Bonica et al. (eds.), *Advances in Pain Research and Therapy, Vol. 3*. Raven Press, New York, 1979.

46 Melzack, R.: Acupuncture and related forms of folk medicine. In P. D. Wall and R. Melzack, (eds.), *Textbook of Pain*. Churchill-Livingstone, Edinburgh, 1984, Chpt. 3.D.2.

47 Mendelson, G.: Acupunture analgesia. 1. Review of clinical studies. *Aust. N.Z. J. Med.* **7**:642–648, 1977.

48 Meyer, G. A., and Fields, H. L.: Causalgia treated by selective large fibre stimulation of peripheral nerve. *Brain* **95**:163–167, 1972.

49 Mullan, S.: Percutaneous cordotomy. *J. Neurosurg.* **35**:360–366, 1971.

50 Nashold, B. S., Jr.: Dorsal column stimulation for control of pain: A three-year follow-up. *Surg. Neurol.* **4**:146–147, 1975.

51 Nashold, B. S., and Friedman, H.: Dorsal column stimulation for control of pain: Preliminary report on 30 patients. *J. Neurosurg.* **36**:590–597, 1972.

52 Nashold, B. S., Jr., Ostdahl, R. H., Bullitt, E., Friedman, A., and Brophy, B.: Dorsal root entry zone lesions: A new neurosurgical therapy for deafferentiation pain. In J. J. Bonica et al. (eds.), *Advances in Pain Research and Therapy, Vol. 5*. Raven Press, New York, 1983.

53 Nielson, K. D., Adams, J. E., and Hosobuchi, Y.: Phantom limb pain. Treatment with dorsal column stimulation. *J. Neurosurg.* **42:**301–307, 1975.

54 Nielson, K. D., Adams, J. E., and Hosobuchi, Y.: Experience with dorsal column stimulation for relief of chronic intractable pain (1968–1973). *Surg. Neurol.* **4:**148–152, 1975.

55 Orne, M. T., and Dinges, D. F.: Hypnosis. In P. D. Wall and R. Melzack (eds.), *Textbook of Pain.* Churchill Livingstone, Edinburgh, 1984, Chpt. 3.G.6.

56 *Physicians Desk Reference* (41st ed.). Medical Economics Co., Inc., Oradell, NJ, 1987.

57 Picaza, J. A., Cannon, B. W., Hunter, S. E., Boyd, A. S., Guma, J., and Maurer, D.: Pain suppression by peripheral nerve stimulation. Part II. Observations with implanted devices. *Surg. Neurol.* **4:**115–126, 1975.

58 Plotkin, W. R., and Rice, K. M.: Biofeedback as a placebo: Anxiety reduction facilitated by training in either suppression or enhancement of alpha brainwaves. *J. Consult. Clin. Psychol.* **49:**590–596, 1981.

59 Rosomoff, H. L.: Percutaneous spinothalamic cordotomy. In R. H. Wilkins and S. S. Rengacharry (eds.), *Neurosurgery, Vol. 3.* McGraw-Hill, New York, 1985.

60 Satran, R., and Goldstein, M. N.: Pain perception: Modification of threshold of intolerance and cortical potentials by cutaneous stimulation. *Science* **180:**1201–1202, 1973.

61 Shapiro, A. K.: Factors contributing to the placebo effect. *Am. J. Psychother.* **18:**73–88, 1964.

62 Shealy, C. N., Mortimer, J. T., and Hagfors, N. R.: Dorsal column electroanalgesia. *J. Neurosurg.* **32:**560–564, 1970.

63 Smith, C. M., Guralnick, M. S., Gelfand, M. M., and Jeans, M. E.: The effects of transcutaneous electrical nerve stimulation on post-cesarean pain. *Pain* **27:**181–193, 1986.

64 Sjolund, B., and Eriksson, M.: The influence of naloxone on analgesia produced by peripheral conditioning stimulation. *Brain Res.* **173:**295–301, 1979.

65 Sweet, W. H., and Wepsic, S. G.: Controlled thermocoagulation of trigeminal ganglion and results for differential destruction of pain fibers. *J. Neurosurg.* **29:**143–156, 1974.

66 Tan, L. T., Tan, M., and Veith, I.: *Acupuncture Therapy, Current Chinese Practice.* Temple University Press, Philadelphia, 1973.

67 Tasker, R. R.: Surgical approaches to the primary afferent and the spinal cord. In H. L. Fields et al. (eds.), *Advances in Pain Research and Therapy, Vol. 9.* Raven Press, New York, 1985.

68 Thorsteinsson, G., Stonnington, H. H., Stillwell, G. K., and Elveback, L. R.: Transcutaneous electrical stimulation: A double-blind trial of its efficacy for pain. *Arch. Phys. Med. Rehab.* **58**:8–13, 1977.

69 Travell, J. G., and Simons, D. G.: *Myofascial Pain and Dysfunction, The Trigger Point Manual.* Williams & Wilkins, Baltimore, 1983.

70 Turk, D. C., and Meichenbaum, D.: A cognitive-behavioral approach to pain management. In P. D. Wall and R. Melzack (eds.), *Textbook of Pain.* Churchill Livingstone, Edinburgh, 1984.

71 Turk, D. C., Meichenbaum, D. H., and Genest, M.: *Pain and Behavioral Medicine: A Cognitive Behavioral Perspective.* Guilford Press, New York, 1983.

72 Turnbull, I. M.: Brain stimulation. In P. D. Wall and R. Melzack (eds.), *Textbook of Pain.* Churchill Livingstone, Edinburgh, 1984, Chpt. 3.D.4.

73 Turnbull, I. M., Shulman, R., and Woodhurst, B.: Thalamic stimulation for neuropathic pain. *J. Neurosurg.* **52**:486–493, 1980.

74 Turner, J. A., and Chapman, C. R.: Psychological interventions for chronic pain: A critical review. I. Relaxation training and biofeedback. *Pain* **12**:1–21, 1982.

75 Turner, J. A., and Chapman, C. R.: Psychological interventions for chronic pain: A critical review. II. Operant conditioning, hypnosis and cognitive-behavioral therapy. *Pain* **12**:23–46, 1982.

76 Veith, I.: *The Yellow Emperor's Classic of Internal Medicine* (new ed.). University of California Press, Berkeley, 1972.

77 Wall, P. D., and Sweet, W. H.: Temporary abolition of pain in man. *Science* **155**:108–109, 1967.

78 Watzlawick, P.: *How Real is Real?: Confusion, Disinformation, Communication.* Random House, New York, 1976.

79 White, J. C., and Sweet, W. H.: Pain and the Neurosurgeon, A Forty-year Experience. C. C. Thomas, Springfield, IL, 1969.

80 Wilson, C. W. M.: Suggestion and the placebo: An analysis of bias in clinical trials. In C. A. Keele and R. Smith (eds.), *The Assessment of Pain in Man and Animals*. Livingstone, London, 1962.

81 Woolf, C. J.: Transcutaneous and implanted nerve stimulation. In P. D. Wall and R. Melzack (eds.), *Textbook of Pain*. Churchill Livingstone, Edinburgh, 1984, Chpt. 3.D.1.

82 Zaichkowsky, L. D., and Kamen, R.: Biofeedback and meditation: Effects on muscle tension and locus of control. *Percept. Motor Skills* **46:** 955–958, 1978.

Chapter 12

Summary: A General Approach to Comprehensive Pain Management

The approach to patients with the complaint of pain has three conceptually distinct components. Because pain is a symptom rather than a disease, the first step consists of an effort to diagnose and, if possible, treat an underlying somatic cause. If this approach fails to provide adequate relief, the next step is to look for somatic or psychological factors that may be exacerbating or perpetuating the pain. However, even with adequate evaluation and management of any underlying disease or exacerbating factor, many patients continue to complain of pain. For these patients, it becomes necessary to direct one's efforts at direct symptom control. This third component of pain management consists of using therapeutic interventions that either reduce the pain intensity (e.g., with analgesic medications) or reduce its impact on the patient's life.

All three components of pain management are essential to optimal patient care. Even for apparently straightforward acute and subacute problems (e.g., musculoskeletal injuries, migraine headache, and postoperative pain), an approach that focuses on symptom control and bypasses the evaluation of potential exacerbating and perpetuating factors can result in needless patient suffering.

For purposes of treatment, pain patients should be divided into three groups: acute and subacute pain with an identified somatic cause, persistent pain with an identified somatic cause, and persistent pain with complicating factors. The approach to each of these types of patient is different.

Acute and Subacute Pain

The management of acute and subacute pain should not be a serious problem. The cause is usually obvious and the treatments available are effective and reliable. The major exacerbating factor in acute pain is anxiety. Often, simple reassurance or the use of anxiolytic medication can markedly reduce the patient's anxiety and consequently the suffering component of their pain. As discussed in Chapter 9, for those patients who require analgesic medication, it is essential that they receive an adequate dose and receive it at an interval short enough to keep them comfortable. If they expect that the pain will return before the painkiller arrives, their anxiety level will jump and their pain will be more difficult to control. The short-term use of opioid or nonsteroidal anti-inflammatory drugs (NSAIDs) carries little risk and is beneficial for the overwhelming majority of people. These drugs are effective, convenient, and relatively inexpensive. Furthermore, when used on an outpatient basis, they place a large degree of control in the patient's hands, which, in itself, helps to lower the patient's anxiety level.

Persistent Pain with an Identified Somatic Source

MEDICATIONS

Although many patients with persistent pain have complex psychological or behavioral disturbances, others are psychologically normal people with a clear-cut somatic source for their pain (e.g., arthritis, cancer, postherpetic neuralgia). For these patients the use of analgesics, even strong opiate analgesics, is justifiable. This is most obviously true for patients with cancer, where the risk of drug dependence is minor compared to the threat that the disease poses to the patient's life. The problem is more complicated in patients with chronic pain that is not due to malignancy. Most physicians are justifiably reluctant to use opioids in these patients, except as a last resort. Although the fear of addiction is overblown, these drugs do create problems in some patients (see Chapter 9) and should never be used as the first line of treatment for chronic non-malignant pain. On the other hand, it is my impression that there are many patients who could receive significant relief with judicious use of the opiate analgesics but who currently do not receive them.

Although there are no generally accepted rules for the use of opiates in patients with chronic non-malignant pain, I would suggest the following guidelines: First, a clear-cut somatic cause for their pain should be identified. Second, patients should have a comprehensive evaluation such as that outlined in Chapter 8 and opiates should not be used in patients who have significant psychiatric or behavioral problems until those problems are addressed. Finally, common sense dictates that opiates not be used in patients who have a history of compulsive drug or alcohol use, unless there is no other way to control their pain. Using these guidelines and the methods described in Chapter 9, opiates can provide an important treatment option for many patients, if other modalities fail.

Once the decision is made to use analgesic drugs, patients should be started on a low dose of acetaminophen or an NSAID. The dose should be built to maximal effect or until the side effects become intolerable. If that does not provide acceptable relief, the next stage should be to use a tricyclic antidepressant, again beginning with a low dose and building to maximal effect or tolerance.

Patients should be questioned closely about drug effects, including analgesia, sedation, and other side effects. If these drugs are not effective or not tolerated, opiates may be required. With opiates, the strategy is somewhat different. Because of the potential of patients to develop tolerance and dependence, it is critical to find the lowest effective dose and insist on not escalating it. Patients should be warned that opiates are to be used to reduce pain, not for relaxation or mood elevation. Combining an opiate with a tricyclic, an NSAID, or acetaminophen is often an effective way to keep the opioid dose down and thus delay the onset of tolerance.

ALTERNATIVE TREATMENT APPROACHES

Although most physicians prefer medications as the first line of treatment for pain control, alternative approaches (Chapter 11) may be preferable for some patients. Even a patient with a somatic nociceptive focus who is doing reasonably well with analgesic medication should be considered for one of the noninvasive methods discussed in Chapter 11. Transcutaneous electrical nerve stimulation (TENS), guided imagery, relaxation, or self-hypnosis training may provide the patient with coping skills that will permit a reduction in his or her medication intake. In the hands of a skilled therapist, hypnosis also holds the potential to uncover unsuspected emotional problems. Alternative methods should always be considered in patients prior to initiating opiate analgesic therapy, or, in patients that are already taking them, prior to increasing the dose. In this way, it may be possible to delay or prevent tolerance.

SURGERY

In some patients, none of these strategies provides adequate pain control and their pain demands an escalation of the opiate dose. In cancer patients this usually indicates extension of the tumor. In other patients, the cause is unclear and a reevaluation is indicated. If nothing treatable is turned up, more invasive approaches may be considered. In patients with cancer, or those who have a short life expectancy for other reasons, peripheral or central ablative procedures (e.g., dorsal root lesions or spinothalamic tractotomy) are a reasonable option. In patients with a normal life expectancy, ablative procedures should be avoided. Neurostimulation methods may be employed (e.g., periventricular gray matter stimulation or thalamic stimulation for chronic deafferentation); however, a candid discussion of their experimental nature is advisable.

Neurosurgical procedures for pain relief should only be considered if a thorough evaluation indicates that there is a somatic source for the patient's pain. The ideal surgical candidate is one for whom there is a reasonable expectation that relief of the pain will enable him or her to return to a normal life, in other words, that he or she has no major problems that cannot be directly attributed to the pain. Even when these requirements are met, some patients will not benefit.

Persistent Pain with Complicating Factors

Although some chronic pain patients have a straightforward somatic nociceptive source, a very large number have several interacting problems that complicate their care. For such patients, a thorough evaluation, although time consuming, is an absolute necessity, if only to prevent the physician from making the patient worse. Patients with chronic pain need an evaluation of both somatic and psychological factors. However, because many patients communicate desperation about their somatic pain and deny major psychological problems, their physicians tend to focus on the somatic symptom and delay psychological referral. Probably the most frequent clinical error in dealing with chronic pain patients is to assume that their pain is due to a persistent somatic source of nociceptive input.

Because of this assumption, the physician initially (and appropriately) prescribes mild analgesics (e.g., an NSAID or acetaminophen) and counsels patience, in the expectation that the natural healing processes will resolve the problem. More often than not, however, patients either do not improve or worsen. When this happens, the physician orders a variety of diagnostic studies looking for the somatic source of the pain. If this search is unsuccessful, the next step is to refer the patient to one or more specialists. Patients with back pain are usually sent to orthopedic or neurological surgeons, those with headaches or painful neuropathies to a neurologist, those with abdominal pains to gastroenterologists or general surgeons, and so forth. Although these referrals are appropriate, they often lead to fragmentation of care and reinforce the somatic focus of the diagnostic search. Furthermore, unless a single physician takes responsibility for coordinating the referrals and keeping track of the different opinions and diagnostic studies, patients get shuttled from one doctor to another, receiving conflicting advice, multiple medications (often including opiates), and even surgery. This fragmentation of care deprives the patient of the benefit of a coordinated multidisciplinary approach. Although many patients are helped despite this fragmented approach, others continue to suffer and a few are made worse.

There is little question that a significant number of patients with chronic pain can be spared this unhappy experience by adequate evaluation of somatic, psychological, and behavioral factors. In Chapter 8 I outlined a systematic approach to the evaluation of patients with chronic pain. The evaluation should be carried out in all cases in which the cause of pain is uncertain, or persists beyond 3 months, or if the quality and temporal features of the pain are not typical for the presumptive cause. In such patients the emphasis should be on the assessment of exacerbating and perpetuating factors, the most common of which are: psychiatric disturbances, environmental reinforcers of learned pain behaviors, drug abuse, myofascial pain syndromes, nerve injury, and reflex sympathetic dystrophy. The results of the evaluation serve as a guide to treatment.

Although the complete evaluation and treatment of these problems requires specialized training, most physicians should be able to recognize them and make an appropriate referral. In some cases the needed referral is obvious, for example, a patient with reflex sympathetic dystrophy needs an anesthesiologist to perform a sympathetic block. In other cases, the appropriate referral is not clear, either because the cause of the pain is not obvious or because the patient has several problems and it is not clear which is the most important.

VALUE OF A MULTIDISCIPLINARY APPROACH

Patients with chronic pain commonly have multiple problems. For example, a patient who has a deafferentation syndrome like brachial plexus avulsion might also have a major depression. Such a patient would be frustrating to manage if only the deafferentation problem were appreciated and treated. If the depression were unrecognized and persisted, the patient might not report much benefit from a therapy that ought to provide significant relief from the deafferentation pain (e.g., TENS or a dorsal root entry zone lesion; see Chapter 11).

If there is a reason to believe that a patient has more than one type of problem and that no single specialist has the background required for complete evaluation and optimal treatment, referral to a multidisciplinary pain clinic may be the best course of action. Ideally, such pain clinics will have experienced personnel who work together to systematically evaluate all potential factors and then develop a treatment plan that addresses both the medical and psychological problems.

Most urban areas have one or more pain clinics; however, there is little uniformity in the mix of skills available or in the emphasis placed on different aspects of patient care. Pain clinics typically have clinical psychologists, anesthesiologists, and physical therapists. Other personnel may include a neurologist or neurosurgeon, a psychiatrist, a nurse specialist, and a social worker. Some clinics emphasize sympathetic or sensory nerve blocks and myofascial trigger point injections, others are primarily cognitive-behavioral in their orientation.

The efficacy of a pain clinic is critically dependent on its being multidisciplinary. This is because one of the major benefits of a pain clinic is the opportunity to evaluate and treat concurrent somatic and psychological problems in an integrated way. Furthermore, patients are less resistant to psychiatric evaluation and treatment when it is part of a package that includes adequate attention to their somatic complaints. In addition to the benefit of the evaluation and treatment of both medical and psychiatric problems, most pain clinics have personnel that are experienced in the assessment and treatment of environmental factors that sustain pain complaints (e.g., drug abuse, reinforcement by family members, and pathological relationships such as an abusive spouse).

Once the major problems are identified, a treatment plan is developed. In addition to somatic treatments (nerve block, trigger point injection, physical therapy, or antidepressant drugs), which reduce pain, increase mobility, and improve sleep, much of the effort in the pain clinic is directed at increasing the patients' ability to control their own pain. The task is primarily one of education. The first step is to encourage patients to assume increased responsibility for their own care. Specific goals are set that may include increased activity (return to work), travel, social interaction, and decreased analgesic intake. Once goals are set, patients are taught the skills that will enable them to have increased control of the pain. Transcutaneous electrical nerve stimulation, biofeedback, relaxation tapes, guided imagery, and hypnosis are some of the techniques that have been used to accomplish this goal.

In addition to learning skills for pain control, many patients have to "unlearn" maladaptive pain behaviors. Inpatient behavior modification programs are most suited to deal with such problems (see Chapter 7). The patient needs an environment that restricts access to psychoactive drugs, prevents reinforcement for pain behaviors and provides reinforcement for "well" behaviors such as walking. In order for any gains achieved in such behavioral programs to be sustained after the patient is discharged, the educational process must include family members. This is of particular importance if they are contributing in some way to the patient's disability. They have to be shown how their behavior contributes to the patient's problem.

WHICH PATIENTS SHOULD BE REFERRED TO A MULTIDISCIPLINARY PAIN CLINIC?

There are no established guidelines for determining which patients will benefit from referral to a multidisciplinary pain clinic. This is unfortunate because pain clinic evaluation and treatment is usually expensive and time consuming and many patients are not helped. Part of the problem is that we simply do not understand all the somatic and psychological factors that contribute to chronic pain. The patients are complicated and often resistant to approaches that deemphasize drugs and surgery. Another problem is the lack of uniformity of staff skills and therapeutic modalities between different clinics. Despite these limitations, it is appropriate to refer chronic pain patients to a multidisciplinary pain clinic if both somatic and psychological factors appear to be contributing significantly to their problem. Behaviorally oriented pain clinics using operant principles are particularly well suited for patients in whom drug abuse or other environmental reinforcers are suspected of perpetuating pain complaints. Such programs may also be effective for preventing or reversing chronic disability in pain patients (1, 3).

Summary

In summary, I have briefly outlined a practical method for comprehensive management of pain patients. I have stressed the importance of a comprehensive evaluation, especially for patients with persistent pain. This approach will provide some relief for most patients. Others who experience little relief of their pain may nonetheless have an improvement in their level of function. However, lest the reader harbor any illusions that adherence to the evaluation and treatment scheme outlined above will lead to significant benefit for all chronic pain patients, I must say that despite apparently appropriate treatment, many patients do not improve.

In some cases the patient simply does not respond to a treatment that seems appropriate. In other cases, the patient resists certain therapeutic avenues. For example, patients frequently resist psychiatric approaches even when they have severe emotional problems. Often there is a major interpersonal problem, usually with a spouse. In such patients the question is whether to ignore the interpersonal and psychiatric problems and proceed to higher doses of opiates or more invasive steps such as neurolytic procedures or deep brain stimulation. The best rule in such cases is to avoid treating patients as if the psychological problems were separate from the pain problem. Patients should be told that it is unlikely that any treatment will help them if they have major emotional or interpersonal problems. At the present time, the major effect of the comprehensive approach for such patients is to protect them from iatrogenic harm.

Another problem is a fundamental lack of knowledge about the mechanisms of chronic pain. Most chronic pains are perceived as arising from the musculoskeletal system. Although our knowledge of the mechanisms of pain from muscle, joint, and connective tissue has advanced greatly in the past decade, it is still far from complete.

Even when our knowledge of the physiology and chemistry of pain transduction, transmission, and modulation is much more advanced, we will still be far from our goal of adequate treatment for all chronic pain patients because, for many, psychological problems play a major role in exacerbating, perpetuating, and possibly generating their pain and we do not know how this comes about. We do not know what bodily and mental processes are involved in somatization. Furthermore, it seems unlikely that much progress will be made in understanding the psychology of chronic pain until we know more about psychiatric disease. Unfortunately, the definition of the various psychiatric syndromes is still in a state of evolution. The lack of objective markers for psychiatric diseases calls into question their very identity as distinct biological entities and adds a certain arbitrary and metaphysical flavor to discussions about them.

Given the current lack of knowledge, any classification scheme for pain patients is bound to have problems. Nonetheless the International Association for the Study of Pain has recently published such a scheme for chronic pain patients (2). Although primarily descriptive, it is an important advance. At a minimum it represents an attempt to provide a comprehensive common language that can serve as a point of departure to systematize future observations. It is hoped that this document will provide a basic terminology that will stimulate the evolution of knowledge about the basic clinical phenomena. It is certainly an important step toward improving patient care by defining study populations in therapeutic trials.

At the present time pain management is in a promising transition phase. The past two decades have seen unparalleled advances in our understanding of the fundamental mechanisms of pain transmission and modulation. These advances are just beginning to pay dividends in terms of patient management. The use of periventricular gray matter stimulation and the spinal application of opiates are examples. The appreciation of reinforcement of pain behaviors as a factor in maintaining disability is another conceptual advance that has led directly to improved patient care. There is reason to be optimistic about further improvements in patient care as current knowledge becomes more widely appreciated and the results of ongoing basic and clinical research continue to accumulate.

References

1 Fordyce, W. E., Brockway, J., Bergman, J. A., and Spengler, D.: Acute back pain: A control group comparison of behavioral vs. traditional management methods. *J. Behav. Med.* **9:**127–140, 1986.

2 Merskey, H. (ed.): *Classification of Chronic Pain Descriptions of Chronic Pain Syndromes and Definitions of Pain Terms.* Elsevier, Amsterdam, 1986.

3 Turner, J. A., and Chapman, C. R.: Psychological interventions for chronic pain: A critical review. II. Operant conditioning, hypnosis and cognitive-behavioral therapy. *Pain* **12:**23–46, 1982.

Index